THE WORLD MARATHON BOOK

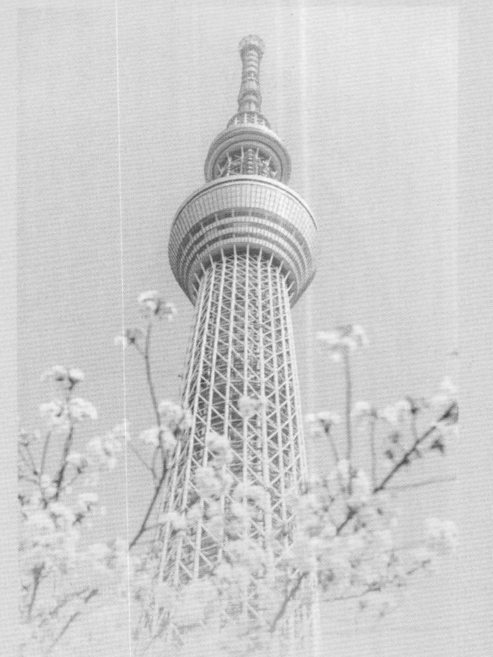
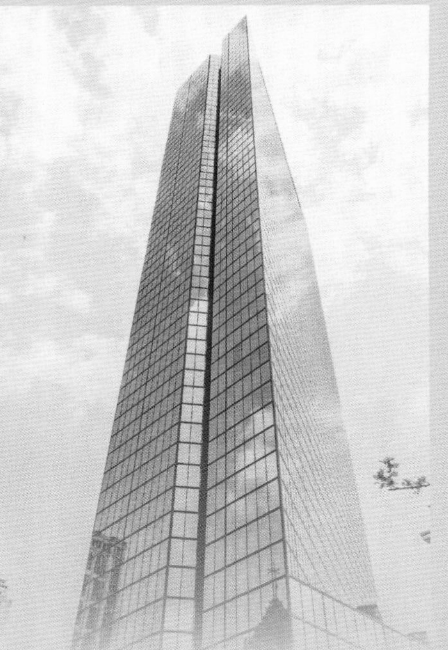
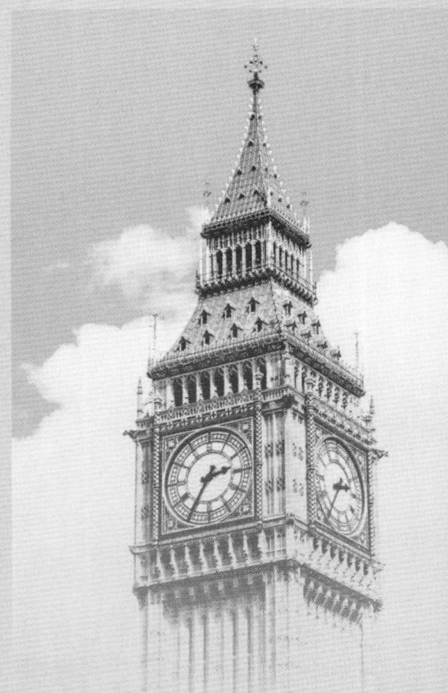

THIS IS A CARLTON BOOK

Published by Carlton Books Ltd
20 Mortimer Street
London W1T 3JW

ISBN 978-1-78739-059-1

Editorial Manager: Chris Mitchell
Project Editor: Ross Hamilton
Design Manager: Luke Griffin
Design: Rockjaw Creative
Production: Ena Matagic
Picture Research: Paul Langan
Contributors: Claire Chamberlain, Ronnie Haydon, Lisa Jackson
Special thanks: Susie Chan, Anne-Marie Lategan, Matthew D Stears, Charlie Watson

A CIP catalogue for this book is available from the British Library

Printed in Dubai

10 9 8 7 6 5 4 3 2 1

IN ASSOCIATION WITH:

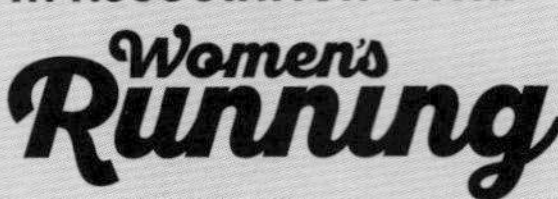

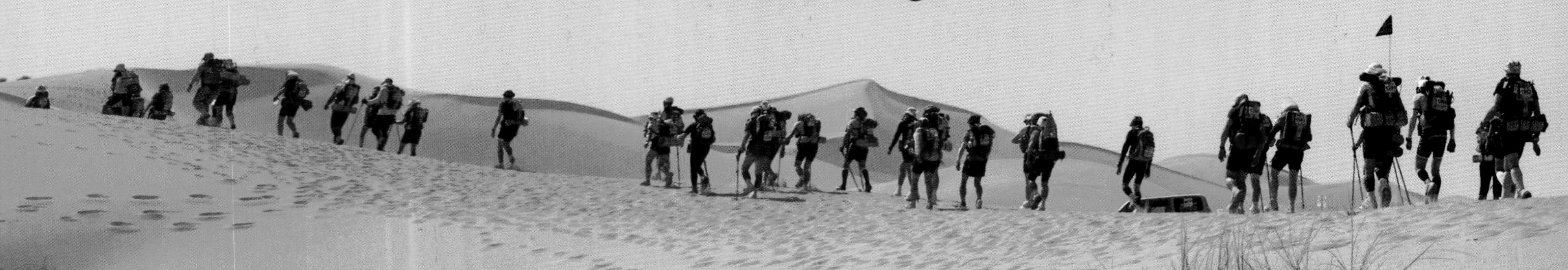

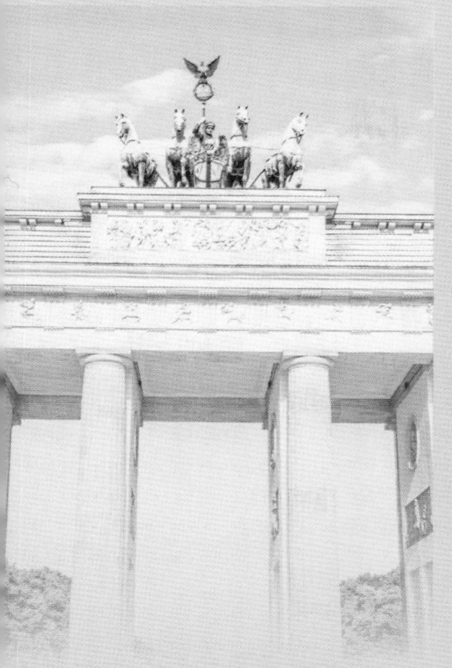
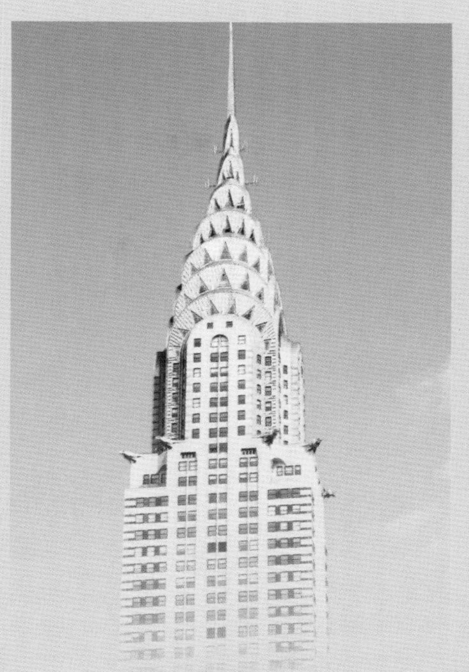
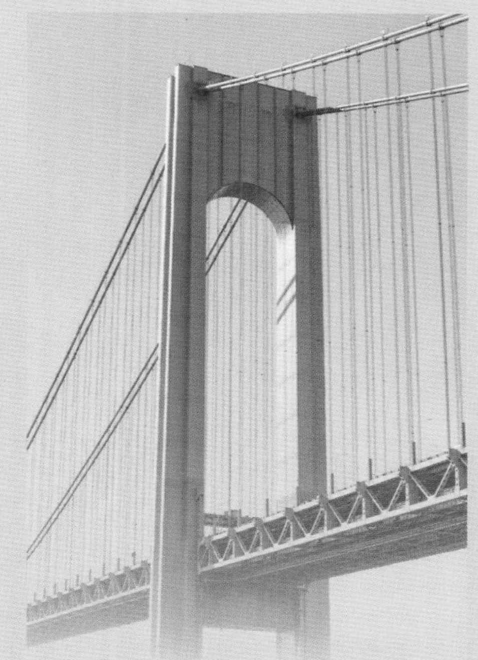

THE WORLD MARATHON BOOK

A CELEBRATION OF THE WORLD'S MOST INSPIRING RACES

CHRISTINA NEAL

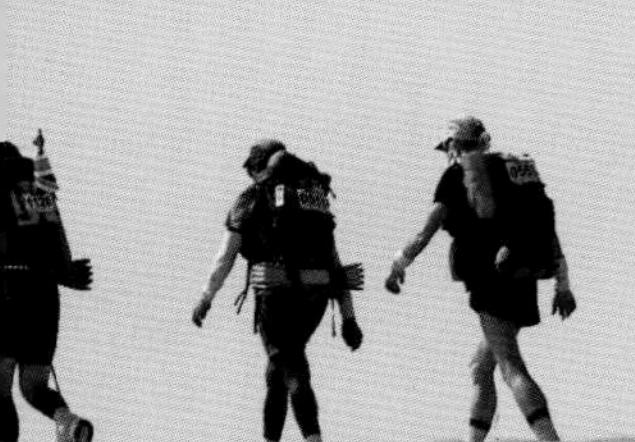
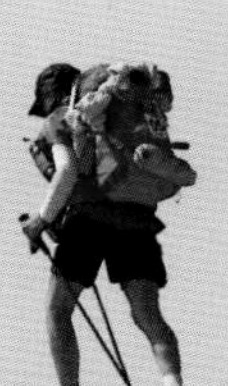
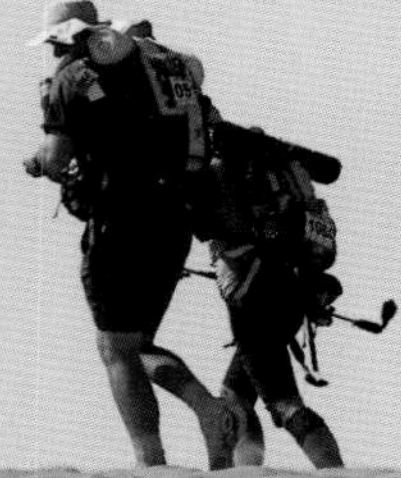
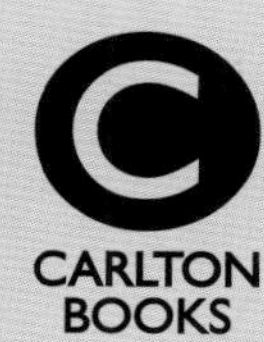

CARLTON BOOKS

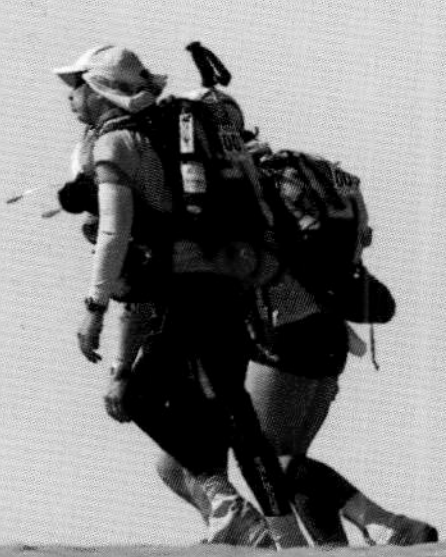
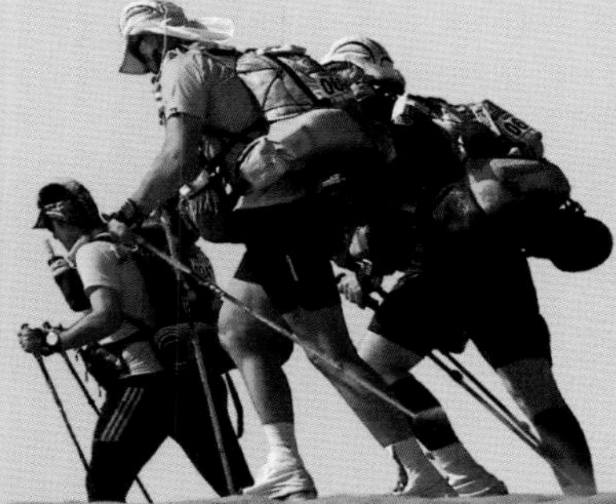

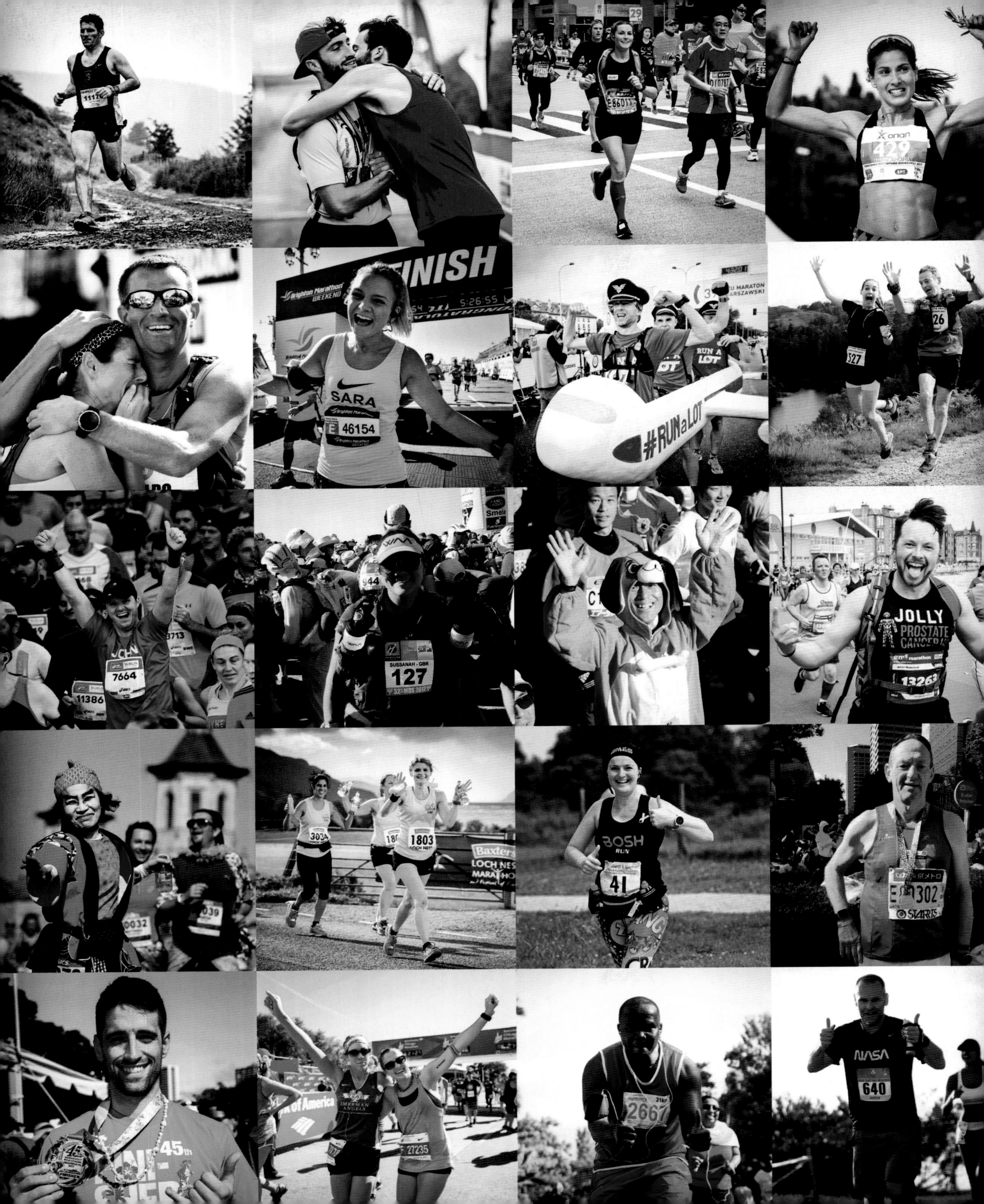

429
FINISH
Brighton Marathon
WEEKEND
SARA
46154
RUN A LOT
#RUNaLOT
7664
11386
3713
SUSSANAH - GBR
127
JOLLY
PROSTATE
13263
3034
1803
LOCH NESS
Baxters
BOSH
RUN
41
45th
IMERMAN
ANGELS
27235
2667
NASA
640

CONTENTS

THE EXPERIENCE OF A LIFETIME

Running a marathon is an incredible experience and one that runners will cherish for a lifetime.

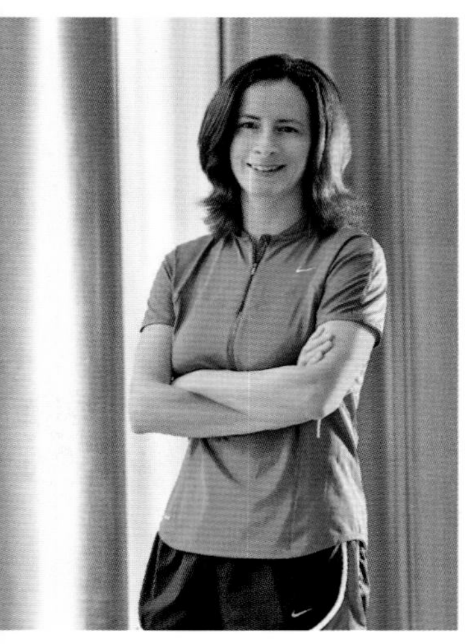

▲ Author, Christina Neal

For many, it can seem like an impossible dream, especially when you first start running and you're building up to completing your first 5K. But, once you've been bitten by the running bug and you've worked your way up to running a 10K and a few half-marathons, your ambitions will grow with your confidence and the urge to go the full 26.2 miles can be all-consuming.

I completed my first marathon in Brighton in 2011. I always said I'd never put myself under pressure to run a marathon, but, in the end, I couldn't resist the challenge. I'm so glad I did it. The Brighton Marathon was the best day of my life. The crowd support was incredible and I felt a huge sense of accomplishment when I crossed the finish line. After I'd been given my medal, I queued up on the pier for a 99 ice-cream. Other people queuing pushed me to the front as they felt I deserved to be served first after running all that way! It's one of my fondest memories of the day. The camaraderie at Brighton was incredible and most marathons are no exception to that, offering fantastic support from fellow runners and the spectators. In short, it's not just about the race: it's about the experience and the memories you make.

In my view, anyone who enjoys running should aim to complete at least one marathon in their lifetime. It's an experience that will stay with you for the rest of your life and a feat that many other people can only dream of achieving.

For many would-be marathon runners in the UK, the London Marathon may seem like the most obvious choice, but there are many other options around the country and overseas. Brighton, Dublin, Edinburgh and Liverpool all host great marathons and, for those who want to travel further afield, there are many overseas options. There are marathons in Malta, Istanbul, California, Tokyo, Boston, New York, Osaka, Paris – a wide variety of locations for you to choose from. Many runners who get the marathon bug and decide to do more than one will usually sign up for races abroad to combine a fantastic cultural experience and a holiday with the achievement of completing another 26.2 miles.

You don't have to stop there, either. You might fancy challenging yourself to an ultramarathon, the definition of which is any distance over 26.2 miles. You could start with a shorter distance of 31 miles, for example, or challenge yourself to a variety of distances ranging from 50 to 100 miles upwards.

The World Marathon Book features 55 of the most popular marathons across the globe and 30 of the world's most famous ultramarathons. For each race, we've included details of where and when they take place, what to expect from the course and why we have chosen to include them in this book. And, for good measure, we've also included some training plans to get you race-fit.

By the time you've finished reading this book, I hope you'll be eager to pin on a race number and go the distance!

"It's an experience that will stay with you for the rest of your life..."

Christina Neal, Editor-at-Large,
Women's Running

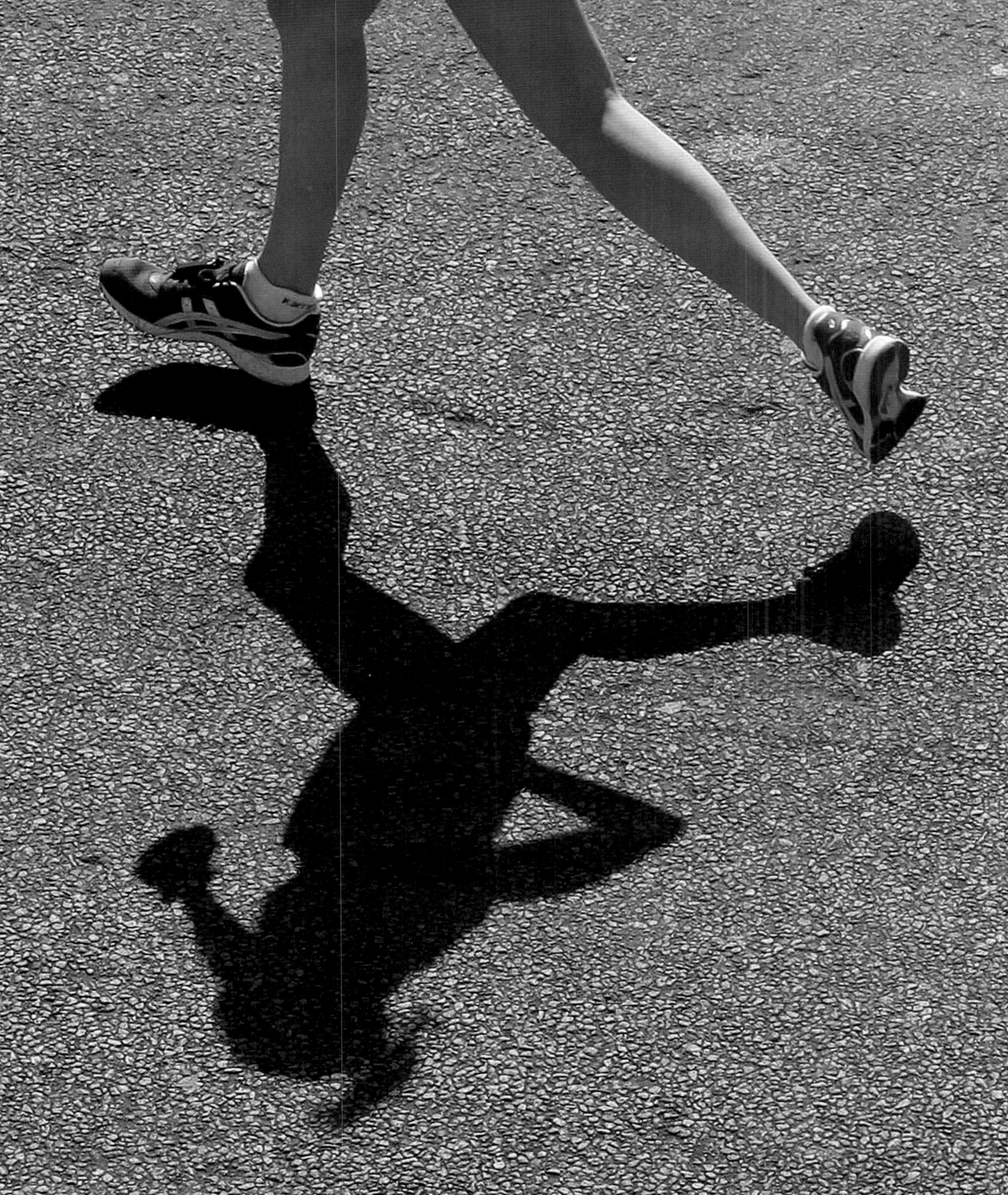

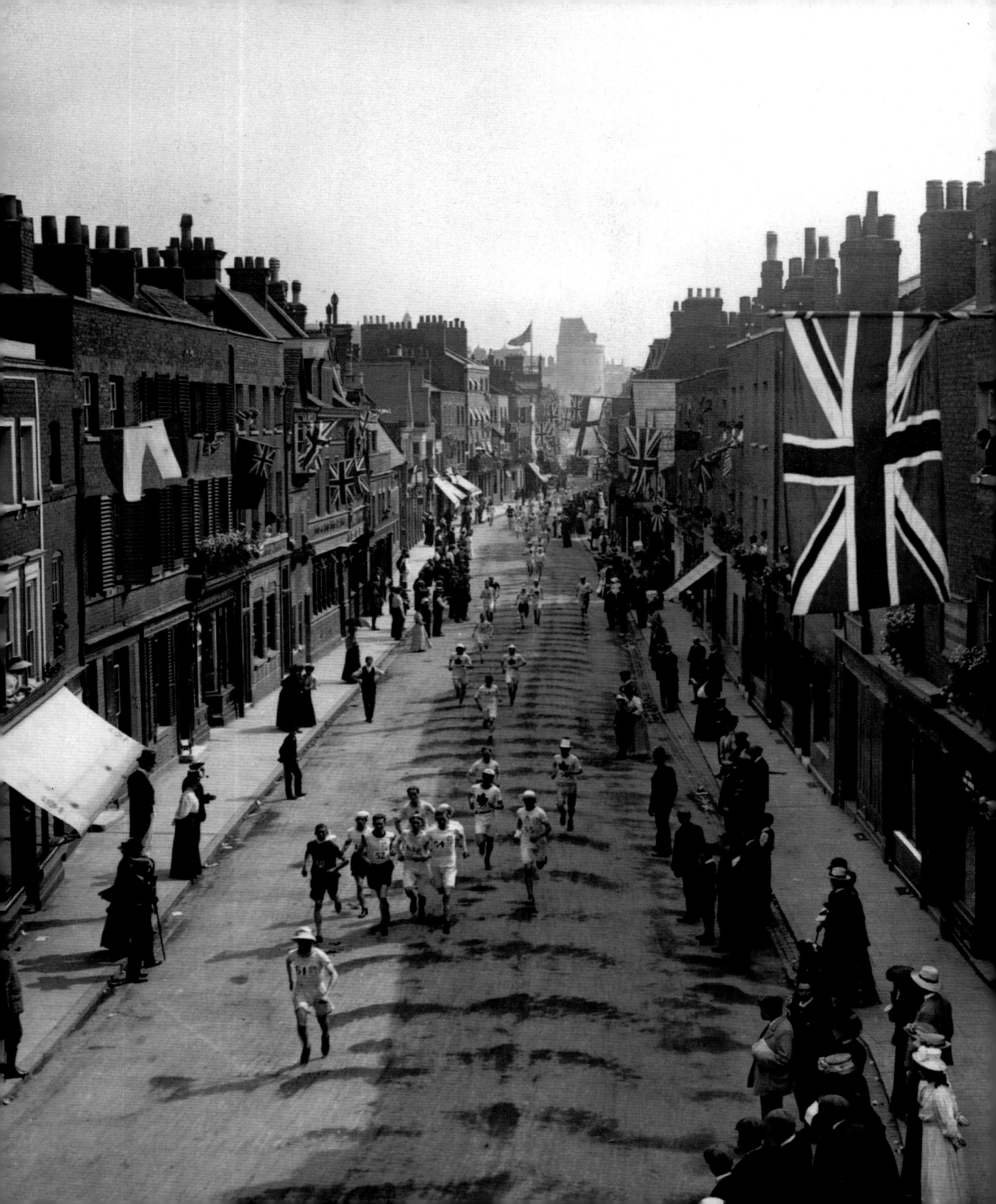

ORIGINS OF THE MARATHON

LEGENDARY BEGINNINGS

The origins of the marathon go all the way back to 490 BC, and have their roots in the superhuman feat of Pheidippides, a Greek messenger. But marathons are far more than just the stuff of myth and legend – they've endured to become a thoroughly modern phenomenon.

It all began in Greece, in the year 490 BC. Legend has it that a massive army from Persia crossed the Aegean Sea and landed at Marathon, a city in Greece about 25 miles from Athens. The Persians had come to capture and enslave Marathon, before moving on to do the same to Athens. They had 50,000 highly trained warriors; whereas the defending army at Marathon had only 9,000, so the Greeks were outnumbered five to one.

Long before Steve Jobs, communication involved either sending a messenger on horseback, or else using a professional runner. The Greeks needed help, and due to the rocky and mountainous terrain that would have severely hampered a horse, a runner was sent to get reinforcements. That runner's name was Pheidippides (or, by some accounts, Phillippides).

Pheidippides set off and ran from Marathon to Sparta (a city in southern Greece) to ask the Spartans for help. Unfortunately, the army at Marathon clearly needed help right now, and the Spartans – for religious reasons – would only come when the moon was full. So Pheidippides ran all the way back to Marathon with this disappointing news: a 150-mile round trip!

Learning that the odds were significantly in their favour, the Persian commander sent half of his army across to Athens to conquer it, leaving the other half to attack Marathon. However, the Greeks at Marathon had some clever commanders and, to make a long battle short, the Persians were defeated, losing a hefty 6,400 warriors to the Greeks' mere 192.

Pheidippides, not one to take a break, was one of the men who fought the Persians at Marathon. When the battle was won, he was then chosen to run the 25 miles from Marathon to Athens to relay the news of the victory. He made it, but was so exhausted that, after shouting, "Rejoice, we conquer!", he collapsed and died. Perhaps it wasn't the most propitious start to marathon running, but the sport has since had much better fortune.

Still, if the distance from Marathon to Athens was about 25 miles, why is the marathon always an exact 26.2 miles? Having been revived in 1896 in the modern Olympics, it was at the 1908 Olympic Games, held in London, that the final distance was permanently established. The royal family wanted the marathon's finish line to lie directly in front of the their "viewing box", and the course was consequently lengthened to 26.2 miles. Later, after 16 years of extremely heated discussion, this 26.2 mile distance was enshrined at the 1924 Olympics in Paris, France, as the official marathon distance. And millions of runners have not looked back since!

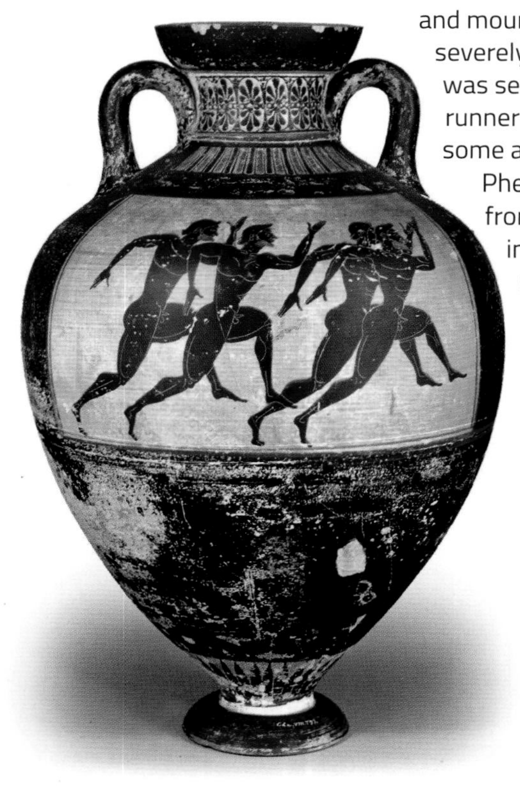

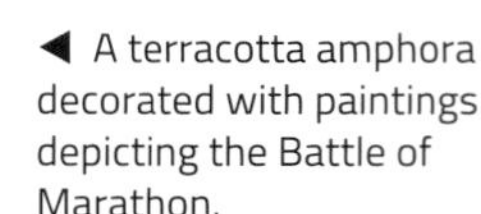

◀ A terracotta amphora decorated with paintings depicting the Battle of Marathon.

▶ Greek shepherd Spyridon Louis was the inaugural victor of the modern Olympic marathon at the 1896 Athens Olympics.

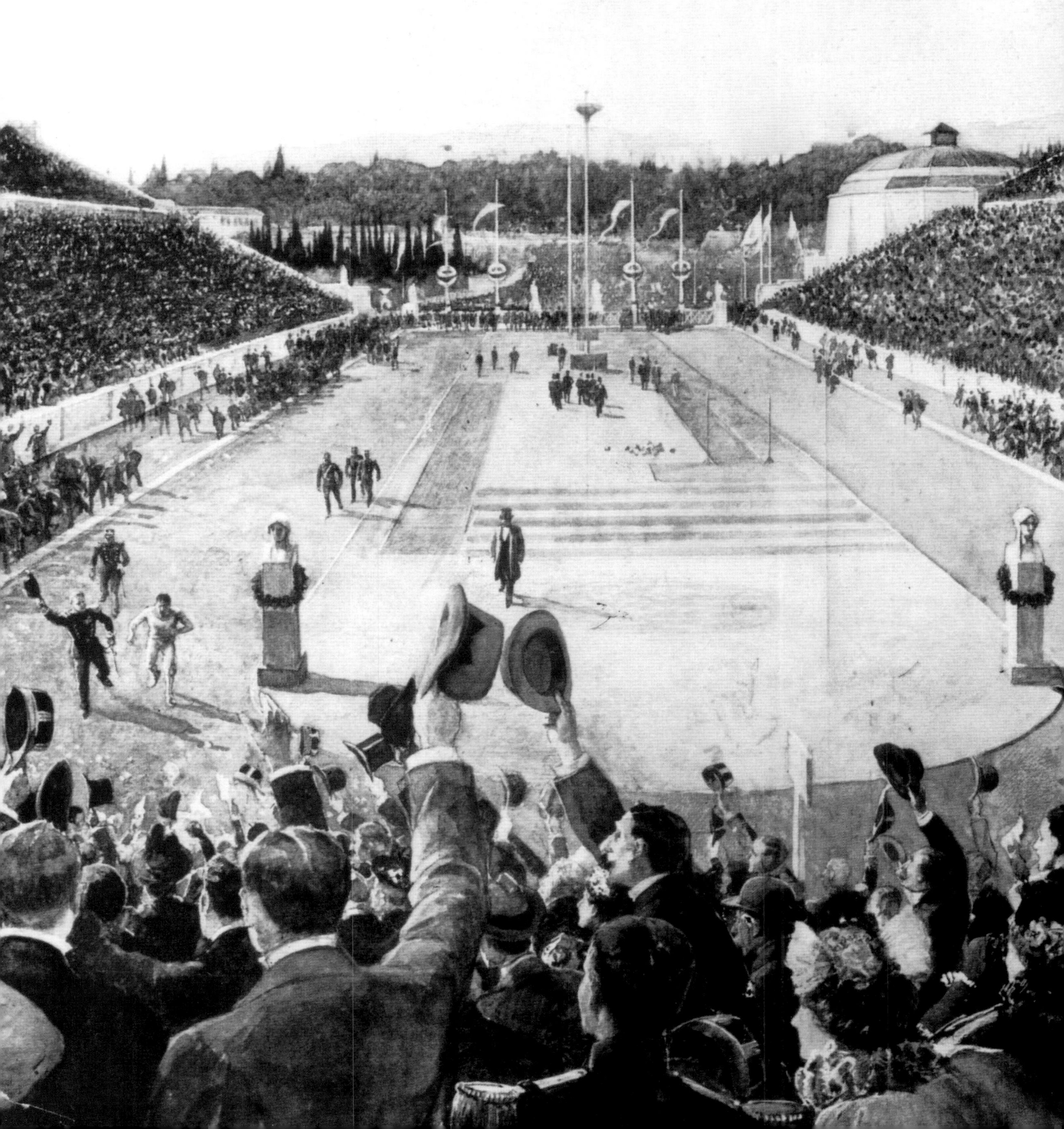

THE BIRTH OF THE MODERN MARATHON

Since its revival at the 1896 Olympics in Athens, the modern incarnation of the marathon has flourished over more than a century – though its surge in popularity around the world hasn't been without controversy...

Mention the word "marathon" nowadays and most of us tend to think of puffed-out runners pounding the streets of London with the common goal of completing 26.2 miles in search of that sense of personal achievement. You may think that anyone who runs a marathon is crazy, dedicated, brave or amazing. It doesn't matter. Everyone knows what a marathon is and, whatever you think of anyone who completes one, it's an incredible achievement and one of the most amazing feats anyone can accomplish in their lifetime.

But have you ever wondered where the idea of a marathon came from? What was the deciding factor behind the 26.2-mile distance? Why not just 26 miles or even 20 miles, which are still highly respectable distances in their own right? The marathon distance is very specific. It is officially 42.195 kilometres or 26.219 miles, or you could say it's 26 miles and 385 yards.

First, let's look at the word "marathon". The name comes from the legend of Pheidippides, a Greek messenger who was apparently sent from the battlefield of Marathon in Athens to announce the Greeks' victory over the Persians in 490 BC. Pheidippides ran the entire distance without stopping – apparently 25 miles – and then, after announcing the victory, promptly collapsed and died from exhaustion.

However, the Greek historian Herodotus claims that Pheidippides actually ran from Athens to Sparta to seek help during the war, and then ran back, which would have been a distance of 150 miles each way. So there is some debate about the accuracy of the story.

The first modern marathon took place at the 1896 Olympics in Athens, although the distance didn't become standardised until 1921. For the next few Olympics, the distance was almost 25 miles, but the 1908 Olympic Games in London had the course extended. One of the reasons for this was to accommodate the British royal family. Queen Alexandra had apparently requested that the race could start on the lawn of Windsor Castle, so that the smallest royals could watch from their window, and finish in front of the Royal Box at the Olympic Stadium. This distance just happened to be 26.2 miles.

MAINSTREAM APPEAL

The organizers of the Olympics had the idea of having a special event to feature in the first modern Olympic Games. They wanted an event that would make the Olympics popular and generate lots of appeal. The idea came from French linguist Michel Breal, and was supported by Pierre de Coubertin, a French historian and founder of the modern Olympics. The Greeks were also on board with the idea of a marathon and staged a selection race for the Olympic Marathon, on 22 March 1896, which was won by Greek athlete Charilaos Vasilakos in 3 hours and 18 minutes. The future winner of that first marathon, Spyridon Louis, came in fifth at a second selection race two weeks later.

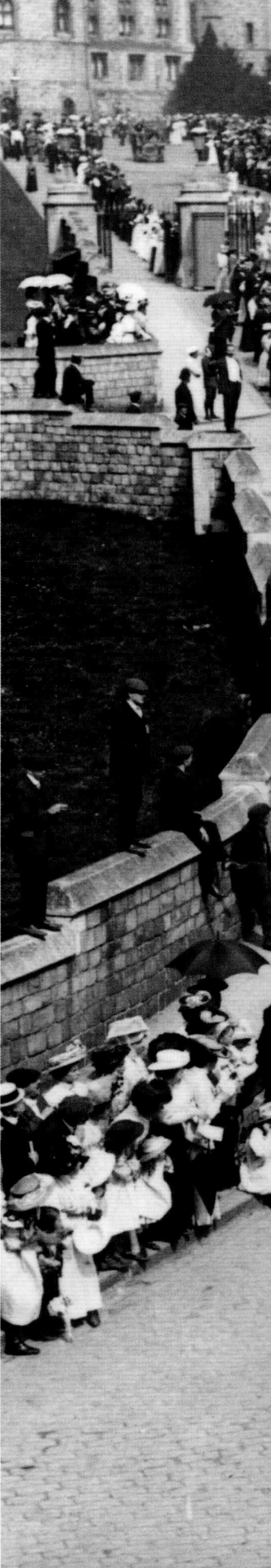

▶ With Windsor Castle in the background, runners make their way down Eton Hight Street during the 1908 London Olympics, the first time the 26.2 miles was officially completed.

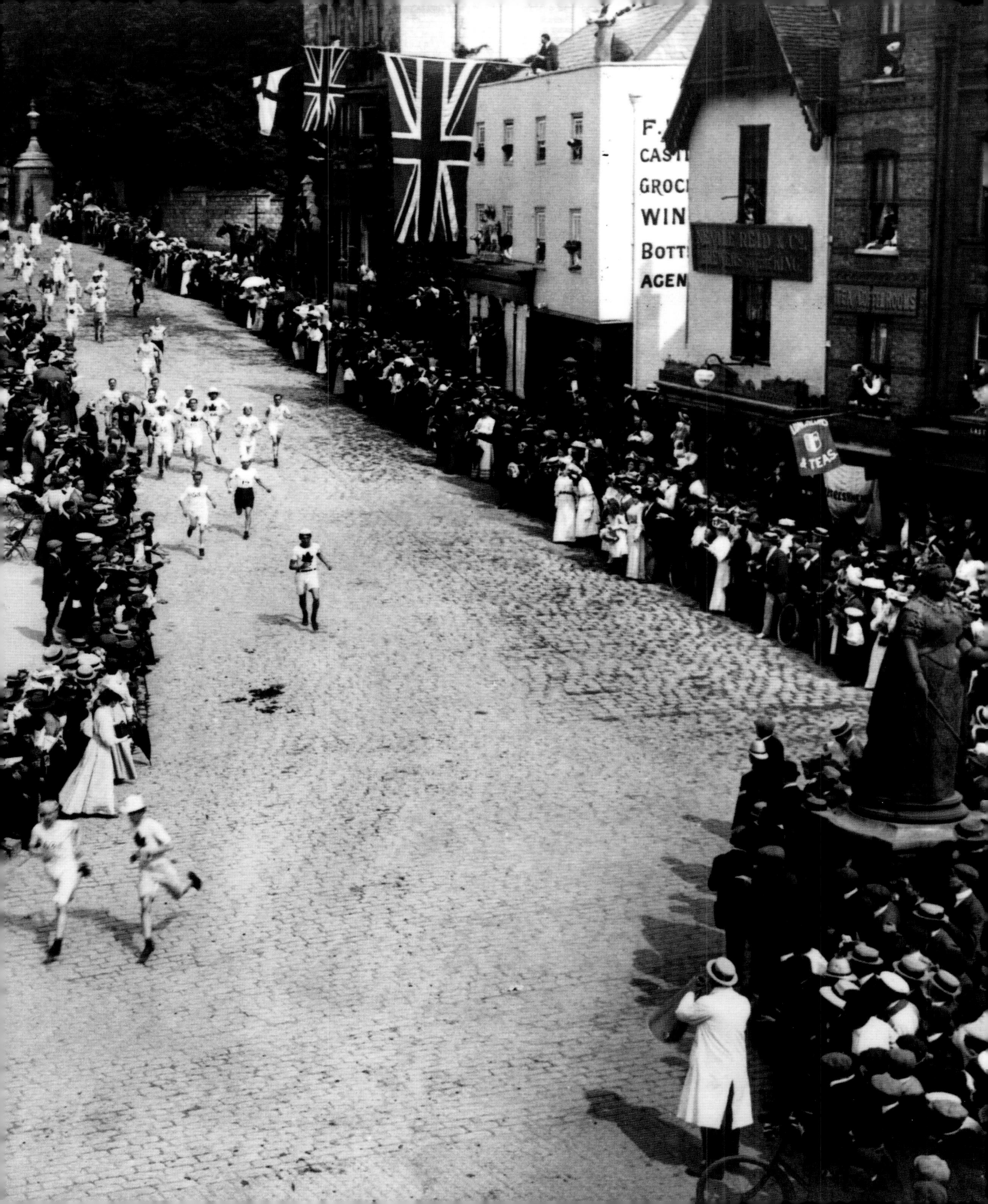
F.
CASTL
GROC
WIN
BOTT
AGEN
& TEAS

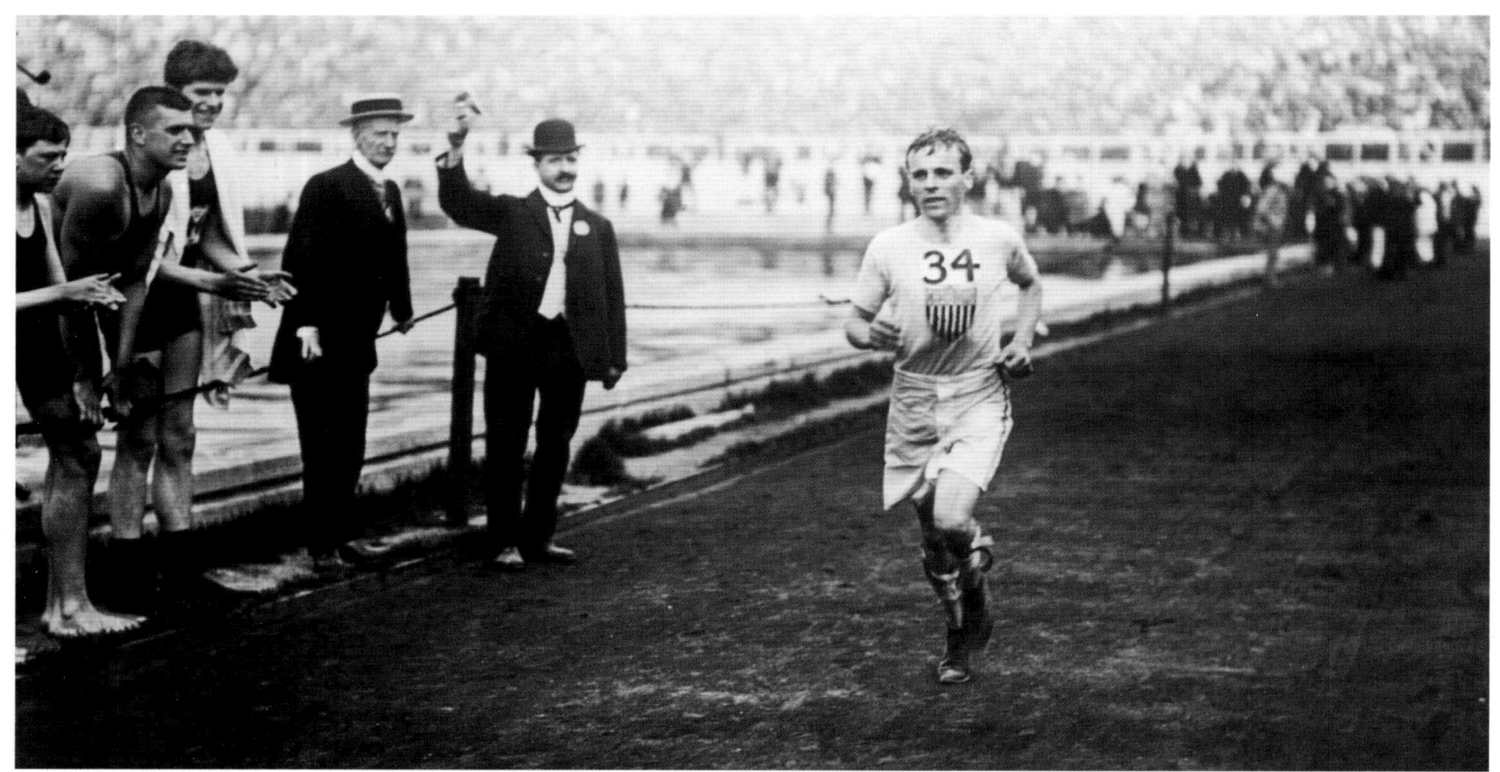
34

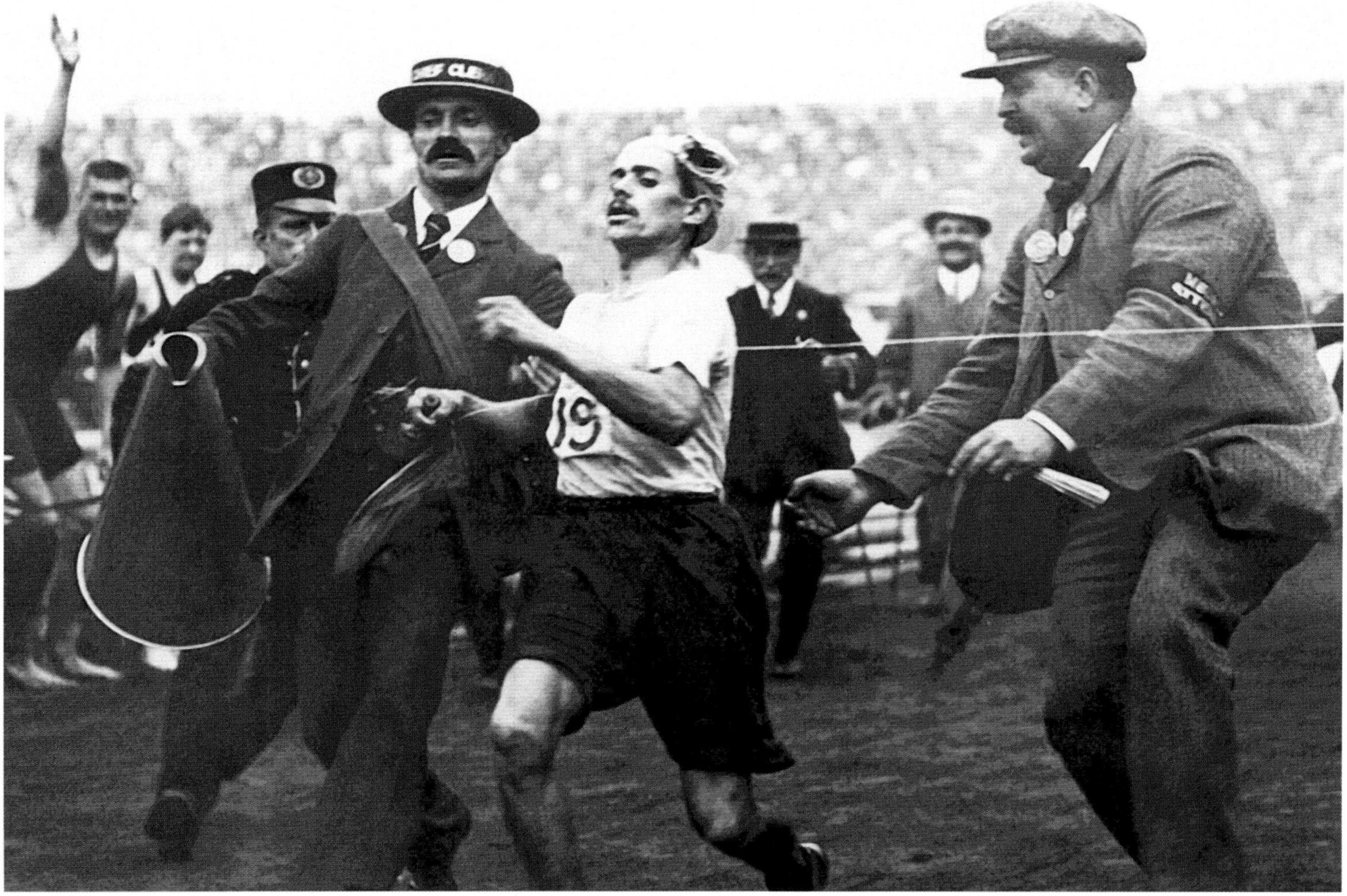

Louis, who won that first marathon on 10 April 1896, was a Greek water carrier, who ran it in a time of 2 hours, 58 minutes and 50 seconds. It was a male-only race. These days, it's traditional for the men's Olympic Marathon to be the last event of the athletics calendar.

The British Olympic Association and the International Olympic Committee held a meeting at The Hague in May 1907 and agreed that the 1908 Olympics in London would include a marathon. Jack Andrew, honorary secretary of the Polytechnic Harriers, offered to take over the task of organizing the marathon. Interestingly, the media had already jumped the gun and announced that the route would entail the runners starting at Windsor Castle and finishing at the Olympic Stadium in Shepherds Bush, London. It had been agreed that the marathon distance would be fixed to around 26 miles to a given stadium, plus a lap of the track. The full Olympic route ran from Windsor via Eton, Slough, Langley, Uxbridge, Ruislip, Harrow, Sudbury, Wembley and Willesden to White City Stadium. It was reported in the book *Marathon Makers* by John Bryant that the first mile of the 1908 Olympic Marathon course was 174 yards short.

At the 1908 Summer Olympics, American athlete Johnny Hayes won the marathon in 2:26:04, which boosted the popularity of marathons in the US. He won the race after Italian competitor Dorando Pietri was disqualified for getting help before the finish line.

For many years, women were considered incapable of being able to run a marathon. It was believed that their bodies lacked the ability to cope with the level of endurance required, and many people truly thought that it might cause a woman's uterus to fall out. The Amateur Athletics Union actually prohibited women from running further than 1.5 miles.

There were no distance races for women and, although a few women had run the marathon distance, their achievements weren't included in any official race results. French athlete Marie-Louise Ledru was credited as the first woman to run a marathon, in September 1918, and was reported to have completed the Tour de Paris Marathon in 5 hours and 40 minutes, finishing in 38th place. Violet Piercy was credited and timed as running a marathon in October 1926 and is recognized by the International Association of Athletics Federations as setting the first women's world best in a time of 3:40:22 on a course between Windsor and London.

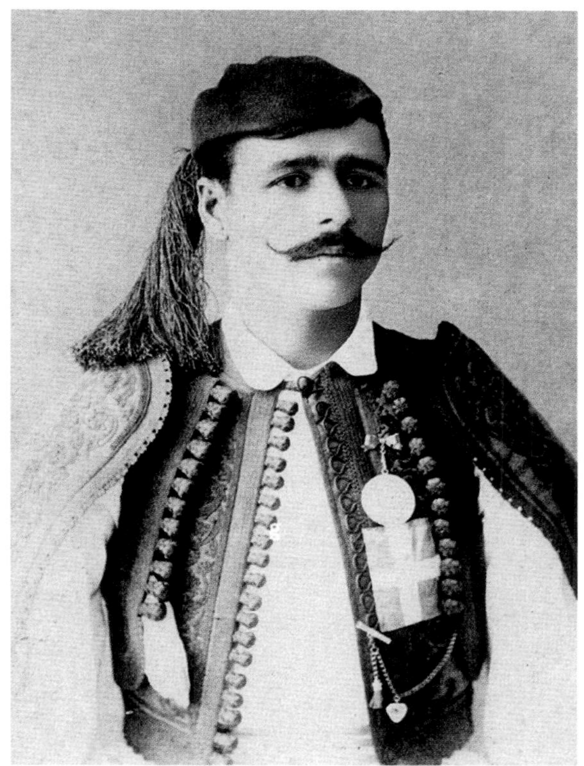

But, many years later, women were still struggling to be taken seriously as endurance runners. Arlene Pieper became the first woman to finish a marathon in the US when she ran the Pikes Peak Marathon in Colorado in 1959. She ran with her daughter, Kathy. This challenging event began at the base of Pikes Peak and climbed over 7,000 feet, so it was a real test of strength as well as endurance.

The Boston Marathon was a male-only event that didn't officially allow women to compete until 1972. Roberta "Bobbi" Gibb was the first woman to run the entire Boston Marathon in 1966 (without a race number). Bobbi turned up at the Boston Marathon on 19 April 1966 at the age of 23, and knew she wasn't supposed to be taking part, as the race directors had previously rejected her written request to run. When the gun went off, she jumped in among the 500 male runners taking part and finished the race in an impressive time of 3:21:40, coming 124th out of the 500 runners. She was mobbed by reporters at the finish line and simply told them she loved running, and didn't care about beating men. It was clear that she just enjoyed the experience of running and said, "I didn't see any reason why men and women couldn't run together."

More controversy was on the way a year later. Kathrine Switzer ran the Boston Marathon in 1967 as a numbered runner after entering the

▲ Spyridon Louis lived a quiet life following his victory in Athens, becoming a farmer and later a police officer.

◤ Eventual winner Johnny Hayes heads towards the marathon finish line at the 1908 Olympics.

◀ Dorando Pietri of Italy, on the verge of collapse, is helped across the finish line of the marathon at the 1908 Olympic Games. He was subsequently disqualified.

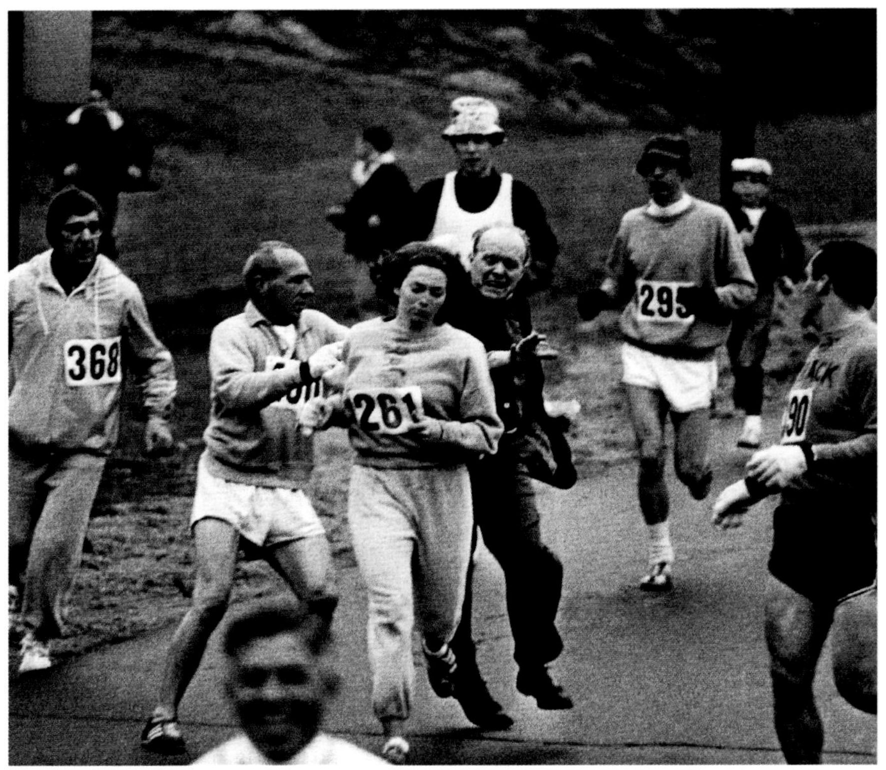

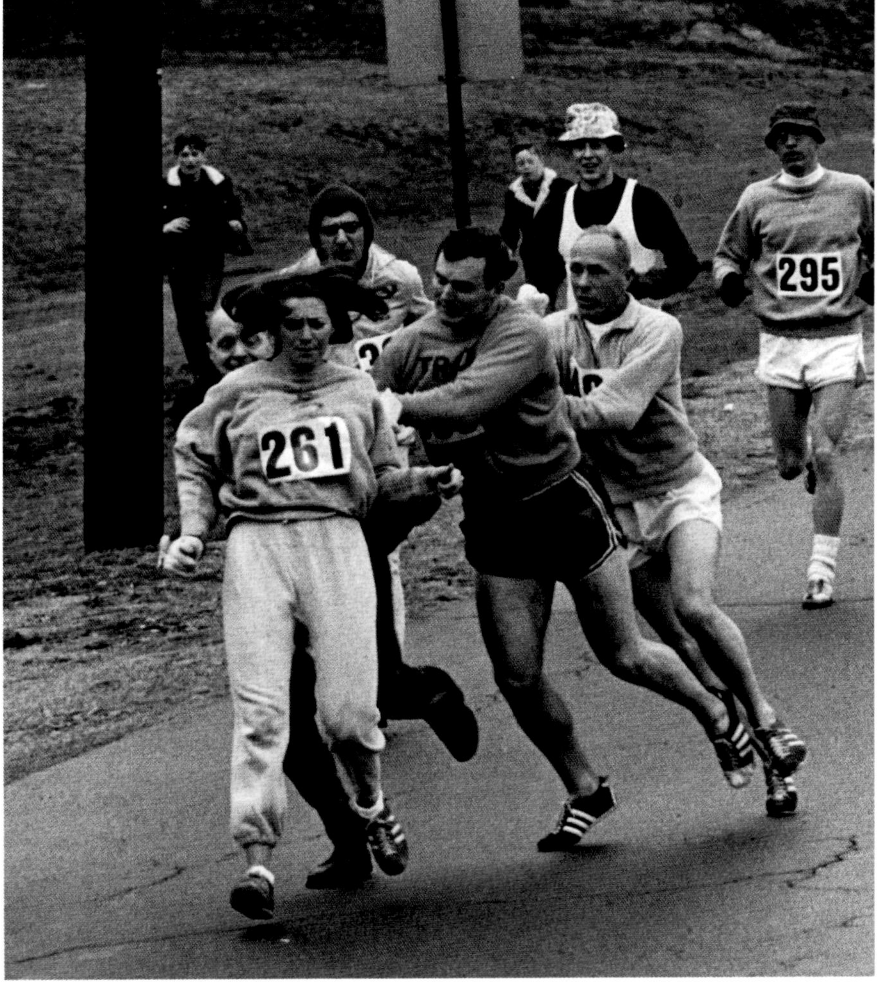

"I didn't see any reason why men and women couldn't run together"

race under the name of "K V Switzer". Kathrine achieved overnight fame because of the attempts of race organizer Jock Semple to rip off her number and eject her from the course during the race. Fortunately, Switzer was running with her coach, Arnie Briggs, and her boyfriend, Tom Miller, and Tom pushed Semple away, enabling her to continue running and finish the race. Switzer went on to run 35 marathons (coming second in the Boston Marathon in 1975 with a time of 2:51:37) and won the 1974 New York City Marathon with a time of 3:07:29. She also campaigned for a women's marathon to be included in the Olympic Games.

In 2017, Switzer ran the Boston Marathon again, 50 years after completing it for the first time, and completed the race in a time of 4:44:31.

But not everyone is prepared to put in the hard work to run a marathon. In 1980, Rosie Ruiz came first in the Boston Marathon after crossing the finish line in a time of 2:31:56. She hadn't been seen on the course during the earlier stages of the race and it was later confirmed by witnesses that the 23-year-old had hidden in a crowd of spectators, then joined the course about half a mile from the finish line. She had sprinted to the end. Kathrine Switzer later wrote in her book *Marathon Woman* that Ruiz didn't have the same exhausted look of a marathon runner as she crossed the finish line. Strangely enough, six months beforehand, Ruiz had done the same thing in New York, having ridden the subway for several miles in the middle of the race.

FIRST OLYMPIC WOMEN'S MARATHON

The very first women's Olympic marathon wasn't introduced until 1984 at the Summer Olympics in Los Angeles. The event was won by Joan Benoit Samuelson, from Cape Elizabeth in Maine. Samuelson won the marathon in a speedy time of 2:24:52, finishing several hundred metres ahead

▲▼ Kathrine Switzer (#261) is mobbed by race organizer Jock Semple in an attempt to prevent her from running the Boston Marathon in 1967.

MARATHON FACTS

- One of the world's most popular marathons, the New York Marathon, was first held in 1970. It involved a few laps around the Park Drive of New York's famous Central Park. Only 127 runners took part. Now it attracts around 50,000 every year.
- The average finishing time for marathon runners is around 2 hours or so for world-class elite runners to 4:20 for recreational male runners and around 4:45 for female runners.
- At the time of writing, the fastest marathon time in history was run by 32-year-old Kenyan Eliud Kipchoge in 2017, who recorded a time of 2:00:24 at the Monza Formula 1 track in Italy. Before that, the official marathon record was 2:02:57, set by Dennis Kimetto in Berlin in 2014.
- In the US, almost half a million Americans ran a marathon in 2012 according to Running USA. Ninety-three marathons took place in the USA that year.
- There has been a surge in popularity for marathons among women over the decades. In the eighties, women made up around 10.5 per cent of marathon runners. Today, the figure is around 41 per cent.
- Japanese runner Shizo Kanakuri has the world record for the slowest marathon time of 54 years, 8 months, 6 days, 5 hours and 32 minutes. He dropped out of the 1912 Olympics in Stockholm and didn't report that he had done so. He was invited back to finish the race 50 years later.
- The youngest marathon runner is Jennifer Amyx, who was only five when she ran the Johnston YMCA Marathon in Pennsylvania in 1975.

of Grete Waitz (who, in 1979, had become the first woman in history to run the marathon in under two and a half hours), Rosa Mota (a Portuguese marathon runner) and Ingrid Kristiansen (a former Norwegian long-distance runner). This victory was even more impressive as Samuelson had suffered a knee injury months before during a 20-mile training run and had undergone arthroscopic (keyhole) knee surgery just 17 days before trials for the Olympic Marathon took place. At the trials, she beat runner-up Julie Brown by 30 seconds, winning in 2:31:04. No one could deny her fitness and running ability.

WORLDWIDE MARATHONS

These days, there are around 800 marathons worldwide each year, with most competitors being recreational runners with busy, full lives, rather than elite athletes who devote themselves to their training. Running a marathon is not a pursuit reserved for the elite. If you have a busy life, but you have the desire to train and get yourself fit for the race, then you can do it. Anyone with a clean bill of health can run a marathon if they are prepared to put in the hard work, and you don't need to be super-fit or super-fast to do it. You just need to have the urge.

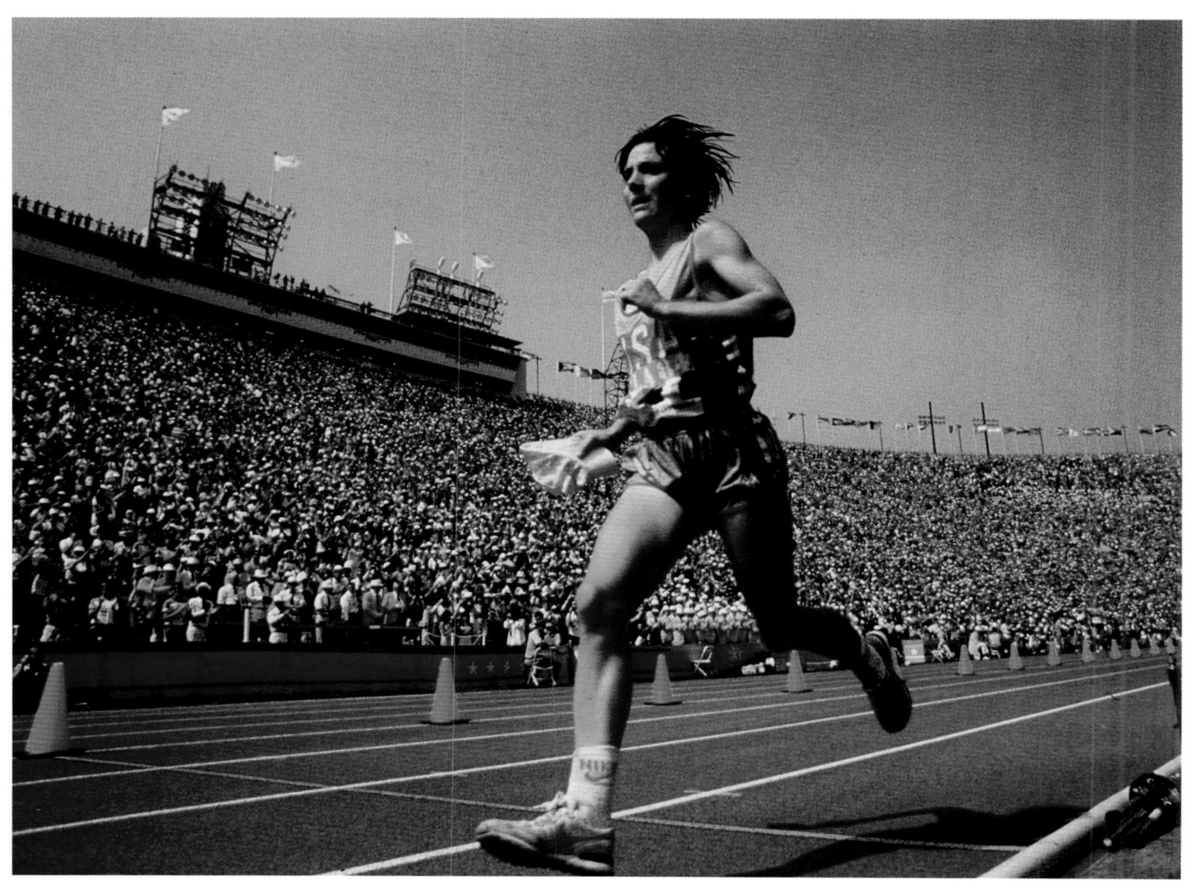

◀ Joan Benoit comes into the Coliseum to run the last portion of the Women's marathon at the Olympic Games in Los Angeles. She won the gold medal.

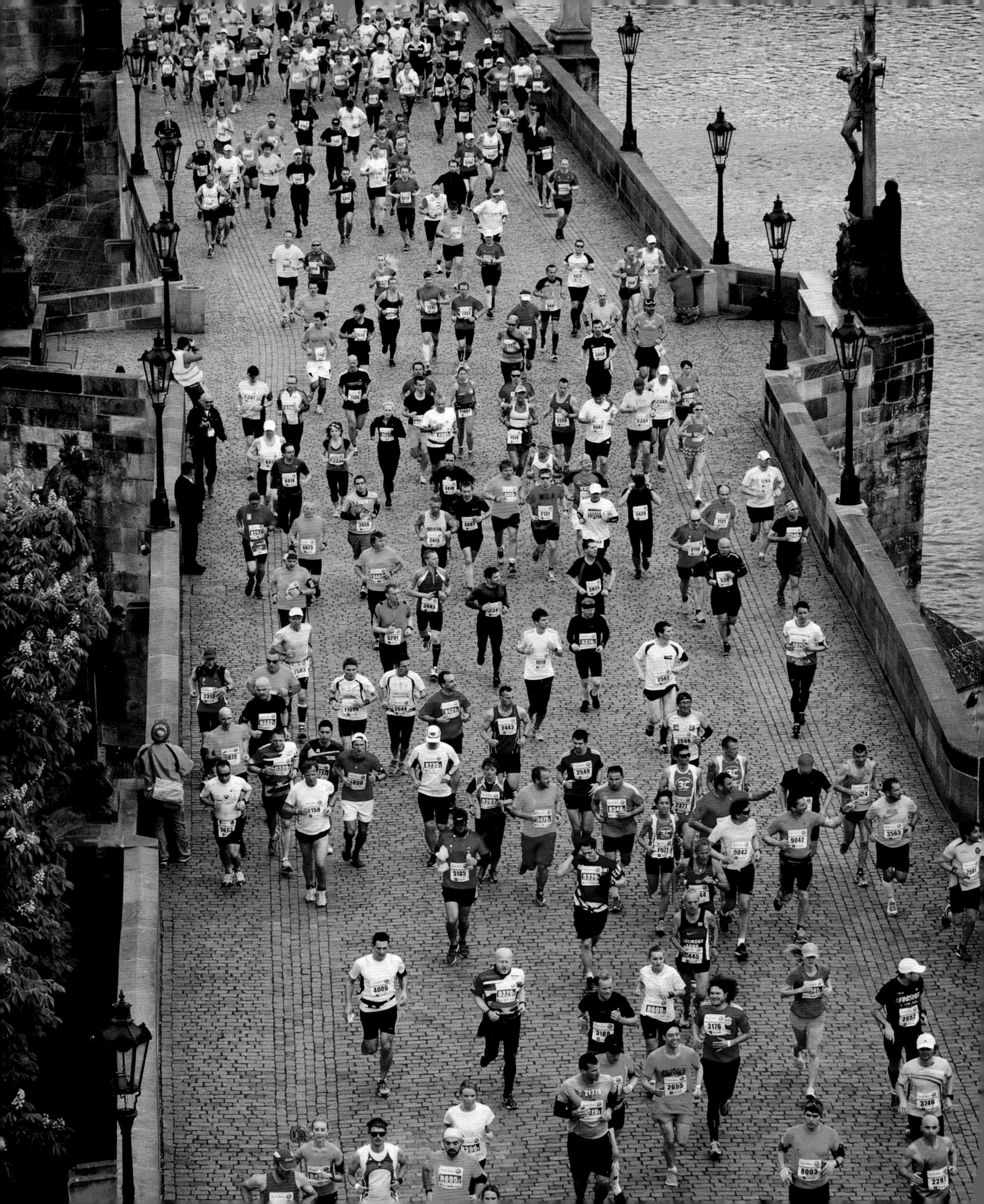

MODERN MARATHONS

MODERN MARATHONS

Thanks to their popularity, there's now more choice than ever when it comes to choosing where to run a marathon. Interest shows no signs of decreasing either – more than half a million people completed a marathon in 2014 in the US alone.

Marathons are now known as mass-participation events, which means anyone in good health can train for one and get marathon-fit. The question is, though: which one do you want to choose? Some, such as the London Marathon, operate a ballot system and are difficult to get into, as demand is, unsurprisingly, high. With that in mind, you might want to consider a marathon abroad. There are plenty of options, and you'll find a selection of some of the best modern marathons in this chapter.

ATHENS, GREECE
Established:
1972
When: Early November

ATHENS CLASSIC MARATHON

This is a marathon steeped in history. The race, dubbed "the Authentic Marathon", was inspired following a battle 2,500 years ago: the Battle of Marathon in 490 BC. Greek forces fought a Persian army and, after the battle, which the Greeks won, the legend has it that Greek messenger Pheidippides ran straight from the battlefield to Athens to relay news of the victory, covering approximately 25 miles. After announcing the victory, he collapsed and died from exhaustion. Despite his unfortunate fate, this inspired the marathon that launched at the 1896 Olympics.

The first 32K of this race between the village of Marathon and Athens are a challenging uphill slog. This is the marathon that defeated Paula Radcliffe in the 2004 Athens Olympics (she pulled out due to exhaustion and cramps from extreme heat). However, cruising downhill to the finish in Athens's beautiful marble-clad Panathenaic Stadium, where the first modern Olympic Games were staged, is likely to be an unforgettable experience.

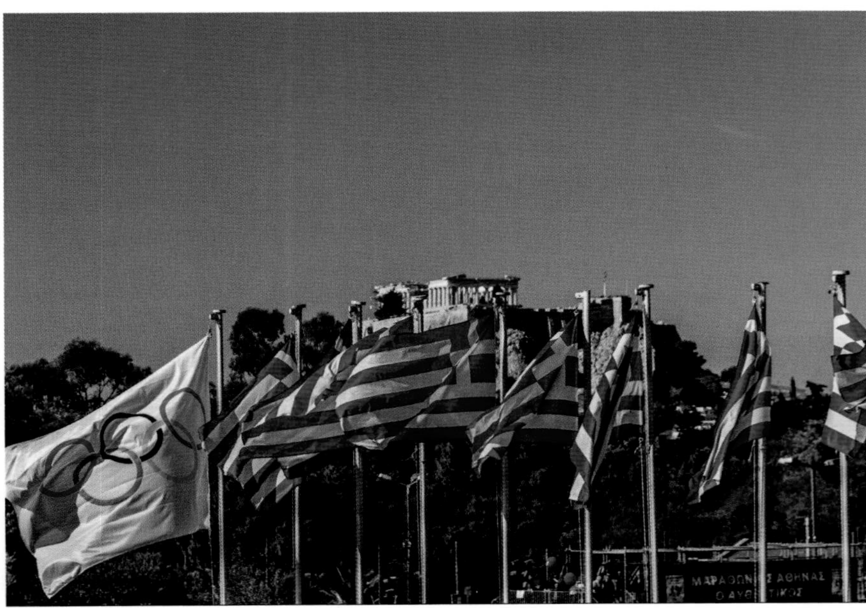

◣ Where better to run your race than the birthplace of the modern marathon?

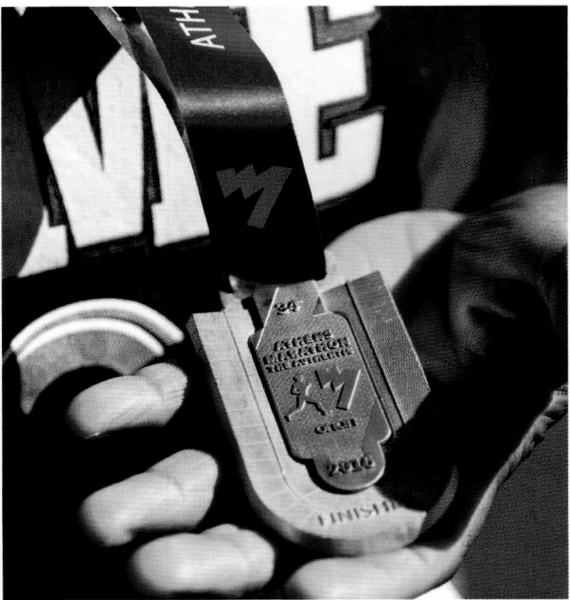

▼ Finisher medals hark back to the arena from the 1896 Olympic Games.

CALIFORNIA, USA
Established:
1986
When: April

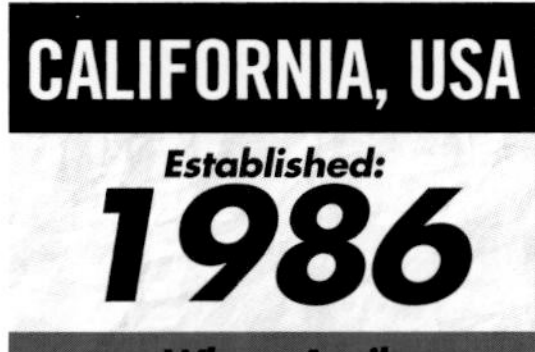

▶ Bridges and coastal views aplenty await runners in the Big Sur Marathon.

BIG SUR MARATHON

This scenic race has a start time of 6.45 a.m., so you'll need to be an early riser and be able to cope with the six-hour cutoff time. The race has various rolling hills and claims to be the largest rural marathon in the world. The course goes along the California Scenic Highway 1, the country's first nationally designated Scenic Highway, from Big Sur to Carmel. The scenery is fantastic, with great coastal views, as well as mountains, trees and the Bixby Bridge (one of the most photographed bridges in California due to its aesthetic design), located at the halfway point of the race, where you'll be greeted by a musician playing a baby grand piano.

There's a 520 foot ascent from Miles 10 and 12 known as "Hurricane Point", which offers amazing views of the Pacific, but be prepared for the hills, though the strawberries you'll get at Mile 23 could well make up for it! A challenging but scenic, friendly race.

The event also includes a marathon relay, 21-mile, 11-mile, 5K and 3K race distances. This makes it an excellent choice if you want a race experience in sunny California while enjoying a break with family and friends, as there's distances to suit all abilities.

BRIGHTON, ENGLAND
Established:
2010
When: April

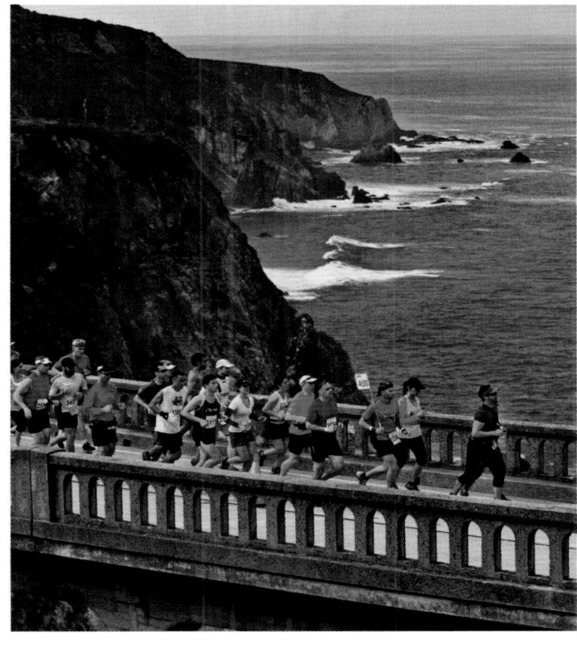

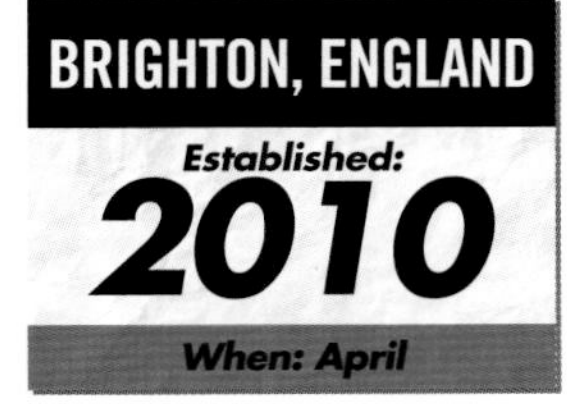

▼ The marathon route takes in the seaside resort's most famous attractions.

BRIGHTON MARATHON

This event has become hugely popular and has grown considerably since its launch in 2010 in the city often referred to as "London by the Sea". The very first race attracted 7,589 competitors, and the number of entrants had grown to 18,000 by 2012. The route has been changed several times, with some of the narrow parts replaced to make it a more comfortable experience.

The race starts in Preston Park, then heads through the town and past the station and out towards the small village of Ovingdean, then back towards the power station at Hove. There's deafening crowd support and some interesting views, including the Royal Pavilion, and the race finishes on the seafront by Madeira Drive, just past Brighton Pier, where you can treat yourself to a well-deserved ice cream afterwards.

For other family members or friends who don't want to run a marathon, there's a 10K on the same day and Kids and Teens Mini Miles the day before. Brighton offers a great sense of community support, the locals are relaxed yet encouraging, and it's a well-organized event.

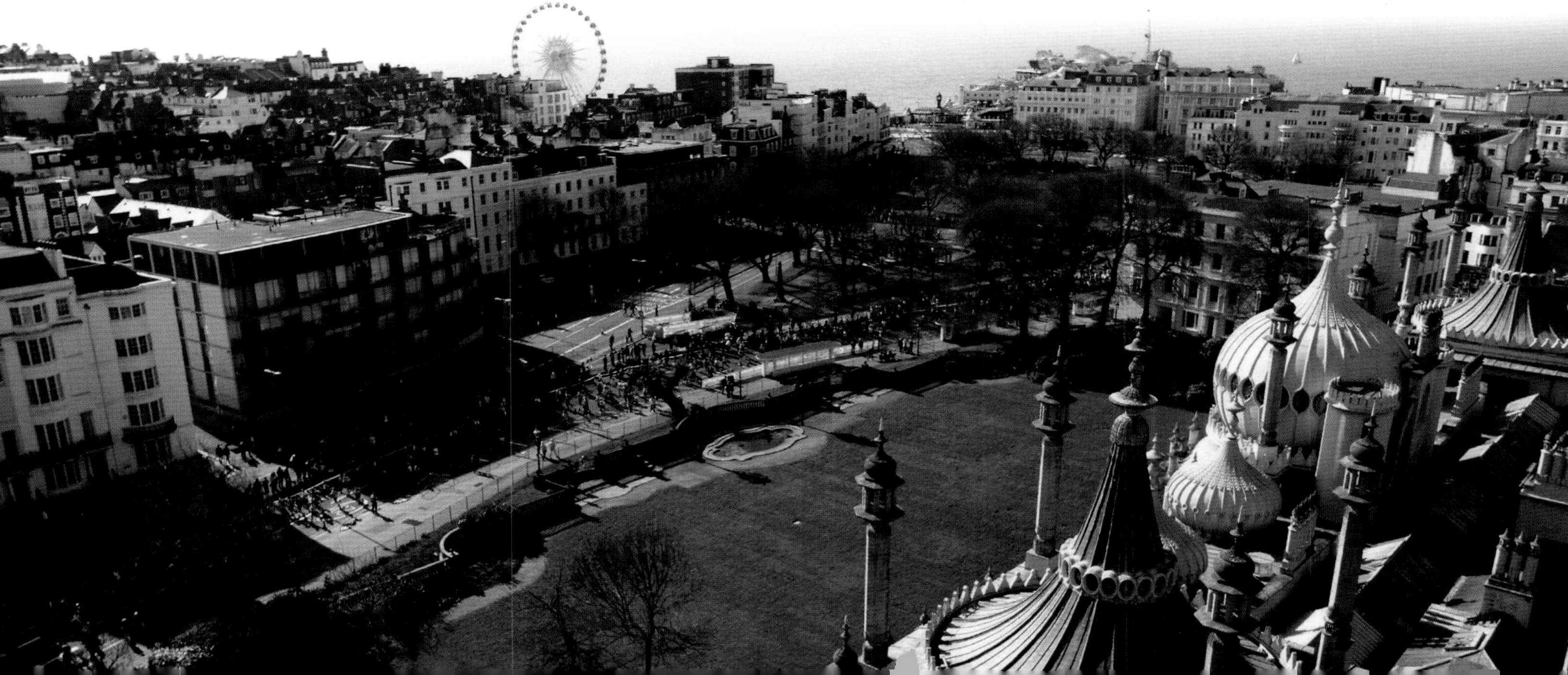

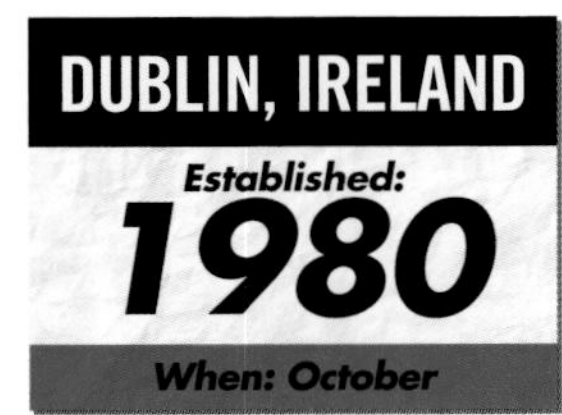

DUBLIN MARATHON

This is a single-lap course that starts and finishes in the city centre and is now claimed to be the fifth-largest marathon in Europe. With an average of around 19,500 participants, the event starts in Merrion Square (a Georgian garden square) and takes you past the River Liffey and through Phoenix Park (the largest enclosed park in any capital in Europe), which offers some gorgeous views. You'll also pass the University College, Dublin. Temperatures during this race are usually around a comfortable 50 degrees Fahrenheit. The race is mostly flat with just a few slight inclines, and the people of Dublin are very friendly, offering great support around the course, though some runners have reported that the race is very crowded at the start. However, it's a fast course, and the Irish are known for their sense of humour – one runner reports a spectator shouting to her, "If you hurry, you can still win." The post-race reward can be second to none – enjoy a wonderful evening sinking several Guinnesses and swapping post-marathon war stories with the friendly locals in McDaid's, a super-cosy, bookshelf-lined pub.

EDINBURGH, SCOTLAND
Established:
2003
When: May

EDINBURGH MARATHON

The capital city of Scotland has one of the fastest marathon courses in the UK with a flat route offering good personal-best potential. But remember that the temperatures in Scotland can be unpredictable – expect anything from snow to searing heat. That said, it's worth the risk – Edinburgh is Scotland's most popular marathon and offers a scenic course. Edinburgh Castle is the backdrop for the marathon and pipers will see you off at the start line. The race goes through Holyrood Park and then towards the coast, with a downhill stretch in this section and a nice view of the sea at around Mile 5. The route has changed over the years – with the course adapted to make it flatter. Around 16,000 runners take part. If you don't fancy the idea of doing the whole 26.2 miles, you can enter the marathon distance in a relay team of four. There are also a half-marathon, 10K, 5K and junior races.

QUEENSLAND, AUS
Established:
1978
When: June/July

GOLD COAST MARATHON

In 2018, this marathon celebrated its 40th anniversary and it's easy to see why. It's a race that typically attracts around 25,000 runners of all abilities from countries worldwide. The event also offers a wheelchair marathon, a half-marathon, a wheelchair 15km, a Southern Cross University 10k run, a Gold Coast Airport fun run and 4k and 2k junior dashes. There's no shortage of choice. It has an unusual start time of 10.20 p.m., which means you'll be running way past midnight and into the early hours.

The marathon is an IAAF (International Association of Athletics Federations) Gold Label Road Race, and is known as one of the most prestigious marathons in the world. The fast, flat and scenic course goes alongside Queensland's gorgeous surf beaches, and is ideal if you're hoping to achieve a marathon personal best.

Before the start, there's usually a speech from the former Australian marathon runner, Rob de Castella, who says in no uncertain terms what the race has in store. But he also reminds runners that the reward of completing the race will more than make up for some of the tough moments to come.

The route takes you south and past Southport Bridge, before going along the Main Beach, Surfers Paradise, Mermaid Beach and Miami, before you turn at Burleigh Heights. The first 6k of the race is flat, then you'll encounter a small incline, before taking a few turns at the 17k mark, then heading back onto the Gold Coast Highway.

Queensland is a popular holiday destination, so you'll have a chance to relax while you're there, but do allow plenty of time to cope with the time difference and overcome jetlag if you're travelling from abroad. Surprisingly, you won't find race conditions too hot – humidity is low with minimal wind and mild temperatures. It is claimed that around 60 per cent of participants achieve a personal best time each year, and the race can also be used as a qualifier for the Boston Marathon.

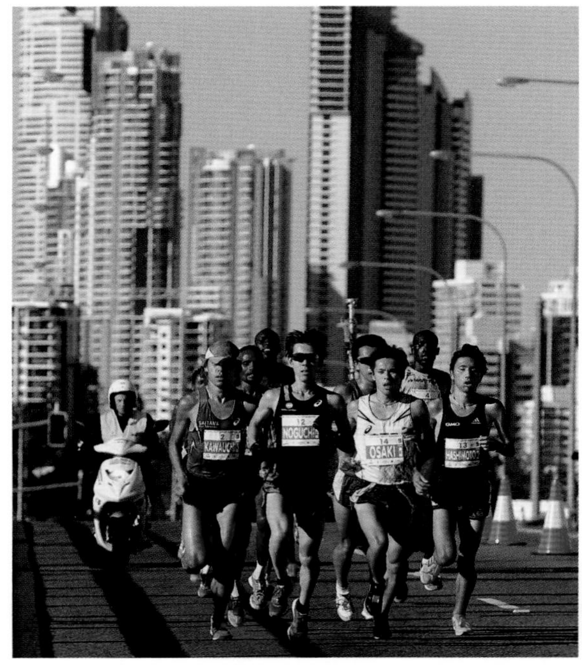

▶ Surfers Paradise is one of the more idyllic marathon locations you could hope for.

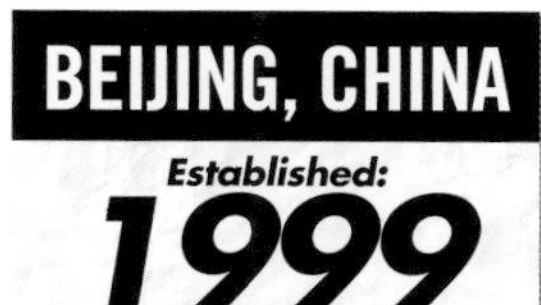

▶ There aren't many marathons that take place on a wonder of the world.

GREAT WALL MARATHON

Launched in 1999, this race must be one of the world's most challenging marathons but offers some amazing views. It attracts an average of 2,500 runners from more than 60 countries, and the iconic Great Wall of China offers some breathtaking surroundings. The race starts and finishes in the Yin and Yang Square in the old Huangyaguan Fortress. There are 5,164 steps to climb and the next stage of the course is completed on the Great Wall of China itself, some of which is around the fortress walls. Weather can be unpredictable, with previous temperatures ranging from 61 to 95 degrees Fahrenheit, and the race has an eight-hour cut-off time. Sounds generous, but not when you take all those steps into account!

There's a 700m ascent before you conquer the Great Wall from West to East. In case you're not sure whether you can manage the world's most challenging marathon – but the location sounds appealing – there's a half-marathon option, as well as an 8.5k race and a fun run.

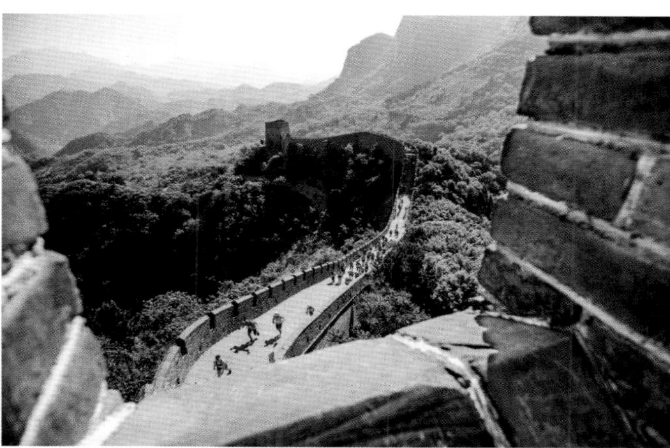

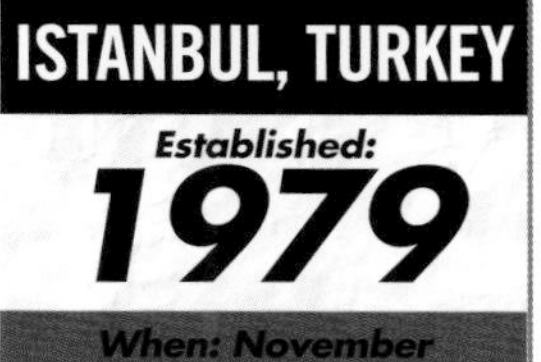

◥ Globetrotting runners can tick both Europe and Asia off their lists in Istanbul.

ISTANBUL MARATHON

The course is mostly flat and traffic-free, and, interestingly, covers two continents, Asia and Europe. Formerly known as the Istanbul Eurasia Marathon, it was launched in 1979 and completed by many Turkish athletes, who used the race for training and often went on to compete on an international level.

The race starts on the Asian side of the city and crosses the First Bosphorus Bridge (one of three suspension bridges), passing historic sites, including the Blue Mosque, a historic mosque so named because of blue tiles surrounding the interior walls. The Hippodrome, which was the meeting point of the Romans and the Ottoman Empire, is where the race finishes. The race attracts runners from many countries. Scenic, historical and friendly, the event also has a 15k, 10k and a fun run.

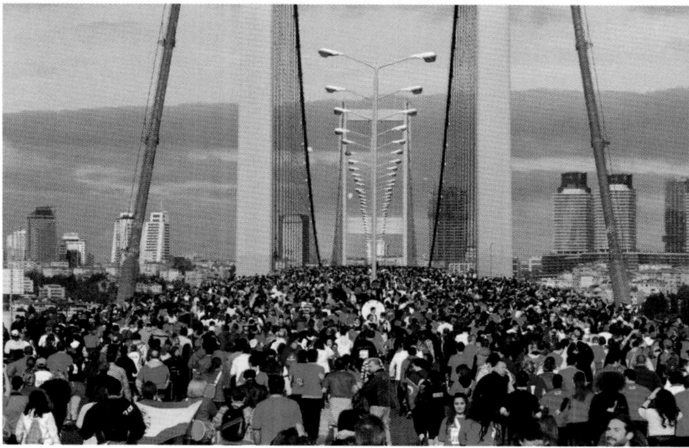

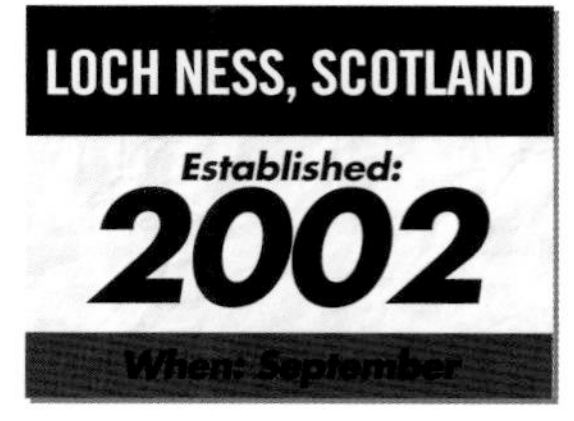

◥ Winding trails, beautiful scenery, and not a monster in sight.

LOCH NESS MARATHON

This race was the winner of the Best Marathon at the 2017 Running Awards in the UK. Runners are transported by bus to the start line in a remote woodland at 5.30 a.m., so you'll need to be comfortable getting up very early. But it's worth the early start. The race follows a breathtaking route that starts in a moorland setting in a wood that Macbeth's witches would have whooped over. The course heads downhill before hitting the scenic shores of Loch Ness.

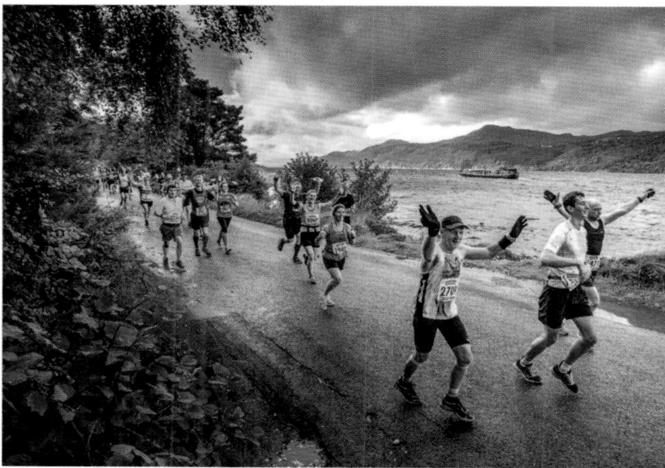

Keeping an eye out for Nessie is a wonderful way to distract yourself from the route's rollercoaster hills. You'll run along the shores of Loch Ness, across the River Ness and finish in Inverness in the Highlands. There's a fun and friendly atmosphere and the event includes a 10K and a 5K fun run. Some of the more remote parts of the course have few spectators but the Highland views are stunning and more than make up for it. Around 8,000 runners take part and you can be sure of good crowd support at the finish line.

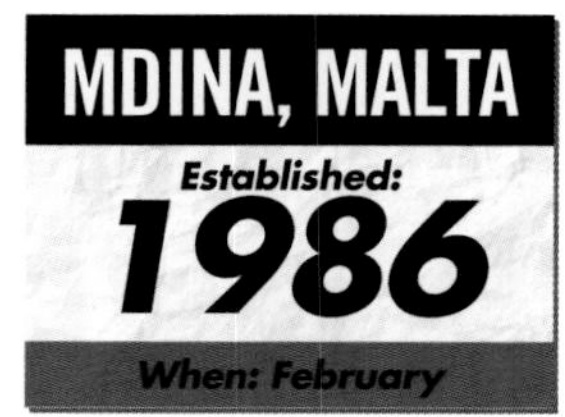

MALTA MARATHON

Devising a course on a small island of 122 square miles is quite an achievement and may explain why the route has changed frequently over the years. The race typically attracts more than 4,500 participants and offers beautiful historical sites. It starts at 7.30 a.m. from the bastions of Malta's old capital, Mdina, through the main road of Rabat and goes through the countryside down to Attard (a quiet town best known for its San Anton Gardens), through the towns of Attard and Mosta, and then back to Attard. You'll pass the American Embassy, and the finish line is in Sliema, the main coastal resort in Malta. The event also includes a half-marathon and both distances are mostly downhill.

ARLINGTON, USA
Established:
1976
When: October

MARINE CORPS MARATHON

One of the largest marathons worldwide, the Marine Corps Marathon chooses to celebrate the courage and discipline of all of its finishers. This event is intended to showcase physical fitness and promote the standards of the Marine Corps, and is organized by the men and women of the Marine Corps. It has been voted the "Best Marathon in the Mid Atlantic", "Best Marathon for Charities" and "Best Spectator Event" and attracts runners from all 50 US states and also from 60 countries.

The race played host to 23,519 finishers in 2012, despite the forthcoming Hurricane Sandy. The course varies from year to year, but more recently has started in Virginia and moved into the George Washington Memorial Parkway. There's a climb on the first few miles but the race offers plenty of distractions, including the Jefferson Memorial (a memorial dedicated to the third US president, Thomas Jefferson) and the National World War II Memorial. It also passes the Pentagon before finishing at the Marine Corps War Memorial.

▲ Charles Bridge is just one of the historic sights on the route through Prague.

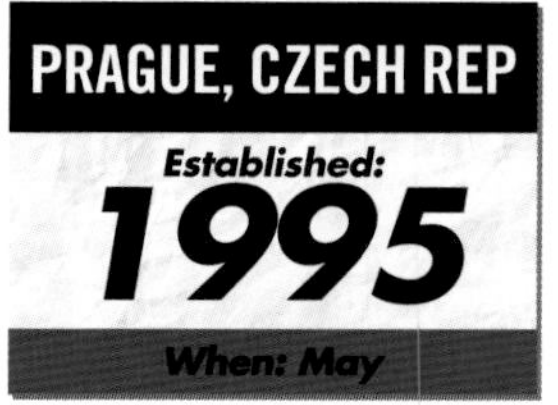

PRAGUE MARATHON

A scenic marathon that starts and finishes in the historic Old Town Square in the heart of the city, where you get a good view of the town hall's famous astronomical clock built in the early fifteenth century. This race has a lot to offer the sight-seeing enthusiast as they make their way around the course, crossing the Vltava River over the Charles Bridge, before winding their way through the city.

Founded in 1995, the route is mostly flat with narrow, cobbled streets from around Mile 8, which look great but may be hard on those with bad knees. It's generally a spacious course, with lots of crowd support at the end, and offers beautiful scenery. Runners have been known to describe it as a "magical" experience. With a castle and Gothic buildings that look uncannily like Hogwarts, it's an utterly charming race.

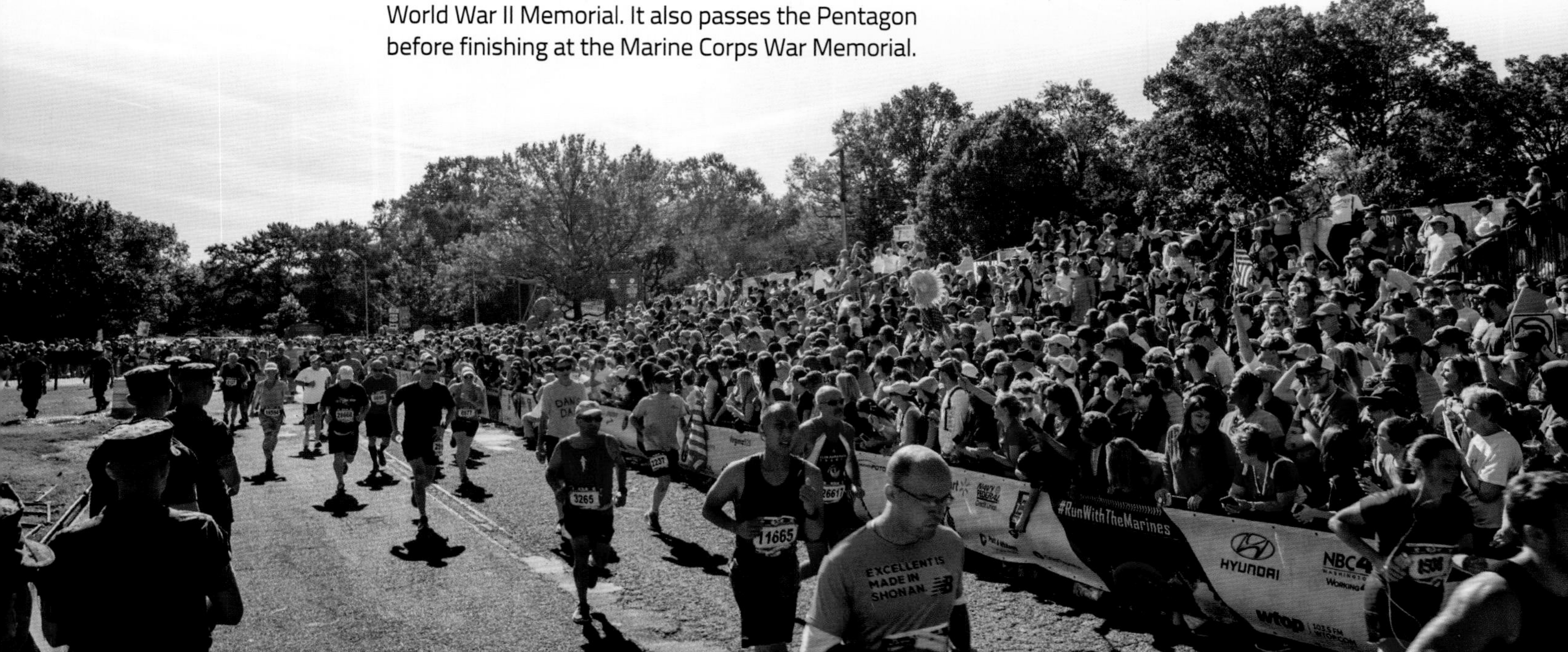

▼ Excellent organization has led to the Marine Corps Marathon winning various prizes and accolades.

REYKJAVÍK, ICELAND
Established:
1984
When: August

REYKJAVÍK MARATHON

The Viking name of Reykjavík translates to "smoky bay", but the name actually refers to the steam that rises from Iceland's geothermal springs. This race was first launched in 1984 and had just 56 participants. Since then, it's clearly grown in popularity and it's easy to see why, though it's still a small event with around 1,000 runners (a half-marathon on the same day attracts around 2,000 runners). Despite this, there is a lot of crowd support, with large crowds gathering to cheer on the runners.

The race offers a great chance to enjoy the most beautiful parts of the capital. The course starts in the east of the city, away from the traffic at the bank of the Ellioaa River – one of the country's best salmon-fishing rivers. The route goes along the sea south of the city and past Nautholl, which has a sand beach heated up by geothermal water during the summer. After the first 10.5K, runners turn around and head back, eventually running the route twice. It's a mostly flat race, with only small elevations at 3K and 4.5K. The event also includes a 10K, a 3K fun run and children's run distances.

RIO DE JANEIRO, BRAZIL
Established:
1979
When: June

THE RIO DE JANEIRO MARATHON

Home of the 2016 Olympics, Rio de Janeiro hosts a marathon every June and also offers a half-marathon distance for those who don't want to commit to the full 26.2 miles. The crowd support during these events is incredible: around 100,000 local people turn out to cheer on the runners.

The race starts at the Tim Maia Pontal Square and finishes at the Aterro do Flamengo, a large park and public recreation area. It's a flat race and takes you past sights offering gorgeous ocean views and mountains. You'll also get to see some of Rio de Janeiro's most famous areas, including Copacabana, one of Rio's liveliest neighbourhoods; Ipanema, a popular surfing area; and, of course, Flamengo.

Despite the flat course and amazing support from the crowds, you may struggle to get a personal best as the warm and humid weather conditions can make it difficult. Temperatures on race day can exceed 86°F, which means you'll need to make sure you stay hydrated and be prepared to slow down if necessary.

However, the friendly atmosphere and the fantastic sights and sounds of Rio de Janeiro will more than make up for the heat.

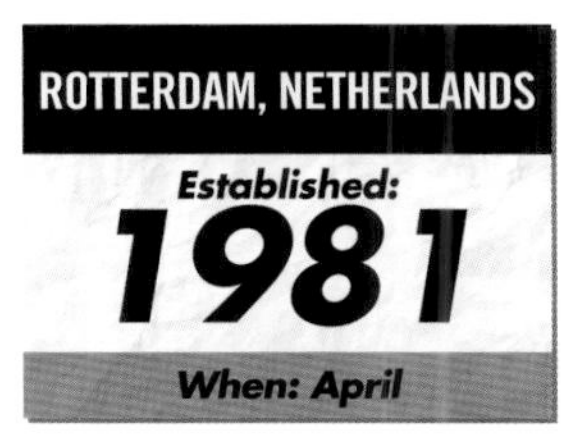

ROTTERDAM MARATHON

One of the fastest marathon courses in the world, this race was launched in 1980 and starts at the foot of Erasmusbrug (an 800-metre-long bridge in the centre of Rotterdam). It is a huge sporting event, with more than 35,000 runners taking part and around 925,000 spectators coming out to cheer on the participants. The Dutch are some of the world's most enthusiastic party people, so you're sure to enjoy the experience, and the route is as flat as a Dutch pancake. You'll enjoy great views of Rotterdam and some unique, ultra-modern architecture. Think Rubik's Cubes on pedestals. The atmosphere is friendly and relaxed, so this race is a good choice for your marathon bucket list.

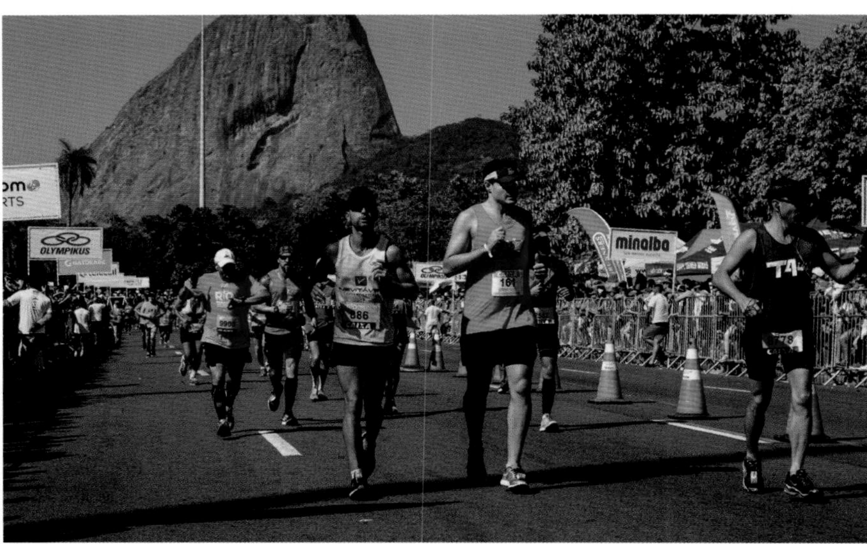

▼ Heat and humidity are a big factor in Rio, but the views can't be beaten.

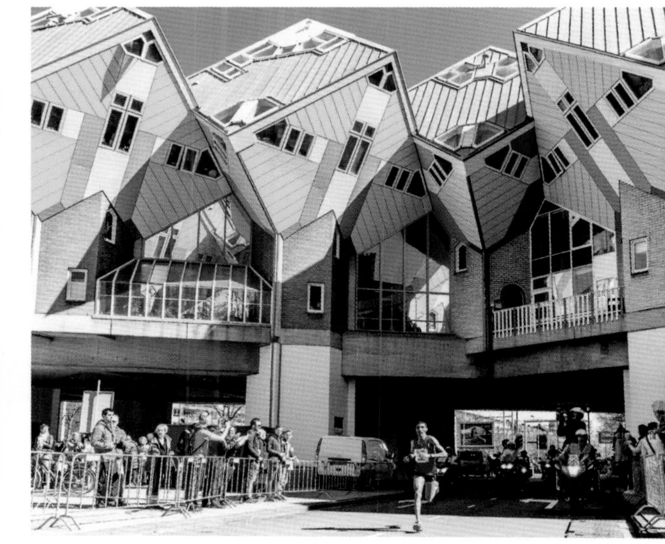

▼ Rotterdam's distinctive architecture is on display throughout the marathon.

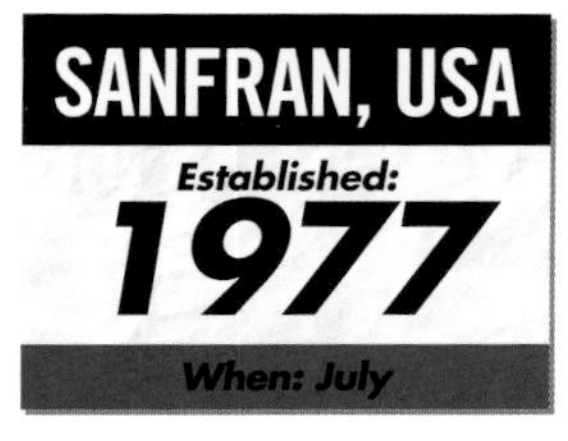

▶ The bright side to the San Francisco marathon's early start is that runners can be finished by lunchtime.

SAN FRANCISCO MARATHON

You'll need to be an early riser to tackle the San Francisco Marathon, as this popular race has a 5.30 a.m. start. A loop course around the city, it attracts around 27,500 runners and begins at Mission Street and The Embarcadero before passing through Fisherman's Wharf (home to many hotels and restaurants) and through the Marina. It finishes in Folsom Street, the location of Folsom Prison, which opened in 1880 and is one of the state's oldest prisons, made famous by Johnny Cash. The marathon route consists of many scenic parks and heads up towards AT&T Park – home of the San Francisco Giants. The home stretch of the race takes you under the Bay Bridge and back to the Ferry Building. The course is described as "rolling" and can be used as a qualifying race for the Boston Marathon.

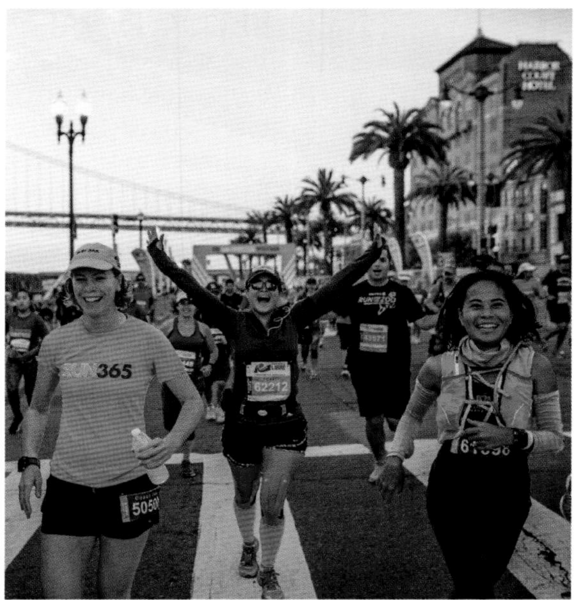

SNOWDONIA, WALES
Established:
1982
When: October

SNOWDONIA MARATHON

Voted the "Best British Marathon" twice, this scenic marathon has been in existence for over 30 years and is a popular choice for many runners. The route circles Mount Snowdon, the highest peak in Wales. It has a very civilized 10.30 a.m. start and climbs to the top of the Pen Y Cwyryd junction, then goes along an old road to a campsite. Some of the course is farm track, and there's a downhill section, too.

The later stages of the race involve a steep 1,200-foot climb at Bwlch y Groes, but there is a downhill finish. Crowd support is good, with locals coming out to support runners in all weathers, even heavy rain (and for that reason you're advised to bring waterproofs with you, just in case). Good organization, great views and descents, but make sure you're used to trail running before you sign up.

▼ Be prepared for a significant climb when running in Snowdonia.

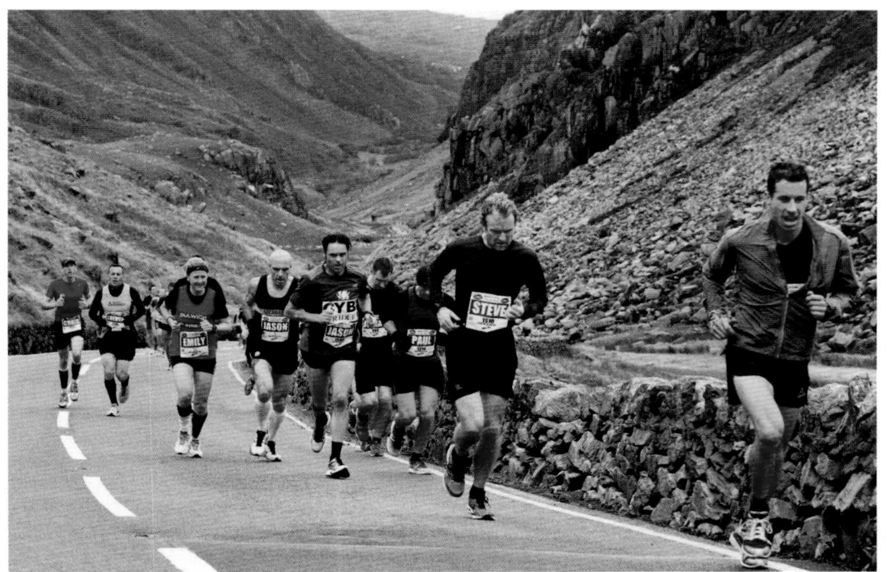

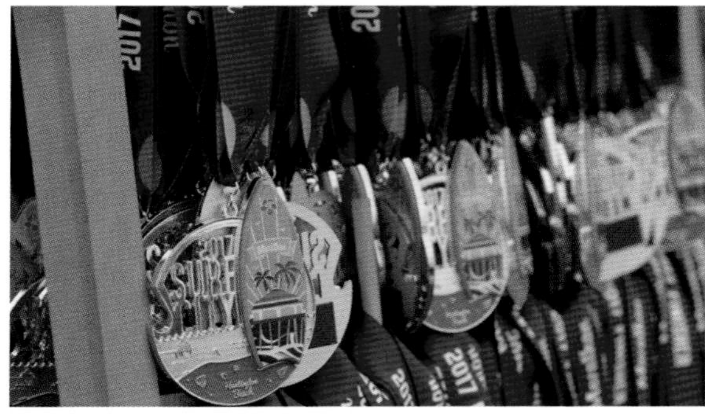

▲ Surf City's marathon medals are typically distinctive.

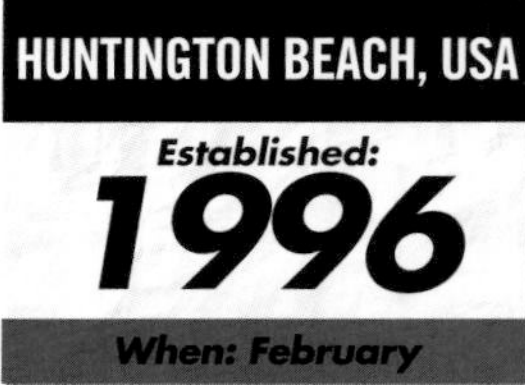

SURF CITY MARATHON

With average race-day temperatures normally around 68 degrees Fahrenheit, this race takes place on the morning of Superbowl Sunday, with the route offering oceanfront views. The race covers the best bits of Huntington Beach, taking you from the Pacific Coast Highway to Central Park. There are plenty of water stations around the course and the event is well organized, with a huge medal to look forward to at the end, along with a free shuttle service to the start line from most car parks. There are also two free beers for runners and live musical entertainment, so there's a real party atmosphere waiting for you when you've completed the course. The event also includes a half-marathon.

ARIZONA, USA
Established:
1995
When: December

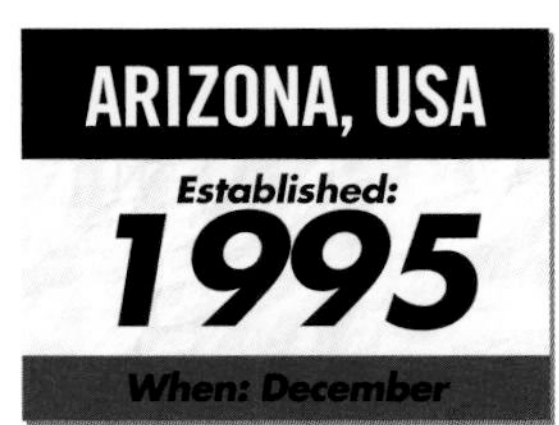

TUCSON MARATHON

Ultra-runner Pam Reed is the race director for this popular downhill marathon, which takes place in the Arizona desert. Reed is the former two-time overall winner (she beat men as well as women!) of the Badwater 135-mile ultramarathon in 2002 and 2003. So Pam knows a thing or two about what makes a good long-distance event, and this race is well known for its mainly downhill course, which descends 2,200 feet along the Santa Catalina Mountain range.

Many runners use it to qualify for the Boston Marathon. The race starts in the Old West historical town of Oracle at 7 a.m. and takes you past the Santa Catalina mountains, which blush pink with the dawn as you cruise downhill. The course goes through the desert on paved roads and finishes at Golder Ranch fire station in Catalina. One of the most scenic marathon courses you'll find anywhere.

VALENCIA, SPAIN
Established:
1981
When: December

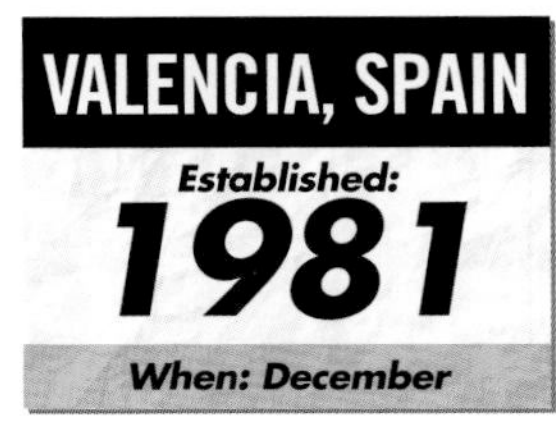

VALENCIA MARATHON

Described as "flat, warm and fast", this is a well-organized marathon in the heart of Valencia. The course covers mostly suburban areas, with part of the route taking you along the scenic coast. There are some sights to see, including the Jardín del Turia (one of the largest urban parks in Spain) and Mercado de Colón (a market in the city centre). The route finishes at the Museo de las Ciencias Principe Felipe (a modern science museum). There's plenty of live music on the course to keep you motivated while you run. Typically, around 17,000 runners take part. As there's much to see and do in Valencia, it's a great opportunity for anyone wanting to combine a marathon with a cultural experience.

VERMONT, USA
Established:
1989
When: May

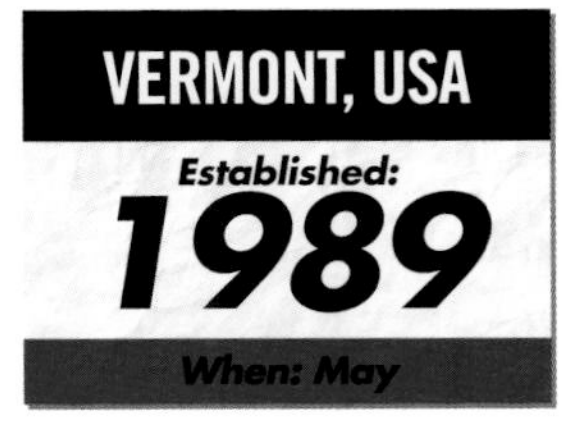

VERMONT CITY MARATHON

Vermont is located in the northeast of the US and offers incredible scenery, lakes and greenery. This course starts at Battery Park and takes you through tree-lined residential streets and Burlington's marketplace, before you head to an out-and-back section on the course at about three and a half miles in. You'll then go along the Northern Connector, a divided highway closed to traffic, where you'll get to enjoy views of the Green Mountains, before heading back through the city streets.

The race offers musicians to keep you entertained and good crowd support throughout. You'll also enjoy a steep downhill section at Mile 21.5, which leads you into the Burlington bike path, taking you over beautiful lake views for the remaining miles of the course.

WARSAW, POLAND
Established:
1979
When: September

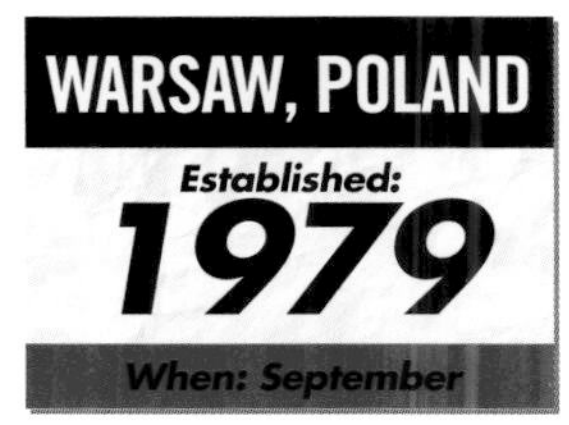

WARSAW MARATHON

This race starts on the Poniatwoski Bridge, a historic bridge built in the early 1900s, next to a spectacular National Stadium built for the 2012 European Football Championships. You'll cross the Vistula River (the longest and largest river in Poland) and the Tomb of the Unknown Soldier – a national tomb dedicated to soldiers who have given their lives in war – in the famous Pilsudski Square (the largest square in the capital), where a military band will be performing.

On a more practical level, this race is famed for having more toilets than many runners have ever seen at the start line of a race. Another plus is the flat and fast route, offering the best major sights in the first third of the race, so you won't be too tired at that stage to appreciate them. "A super-impressive marathon," according to one runner who has completed more than 100 marathons.

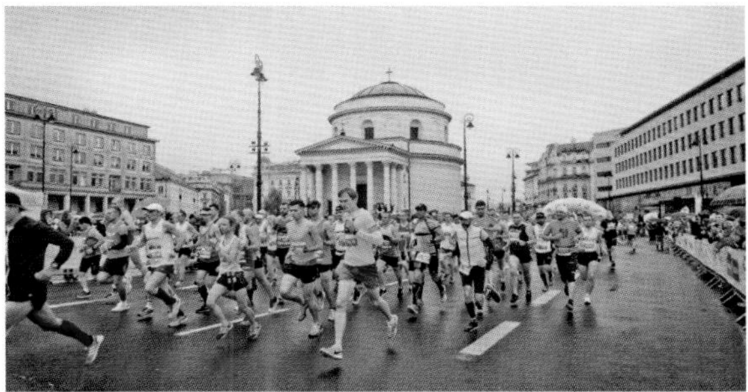

▼ Warsaw is a great marathon destination for historical sights and potential PB times.

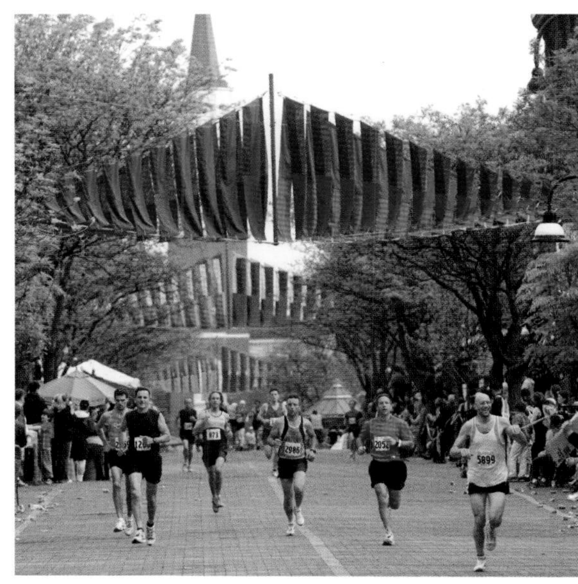

► A springtime date makes Vermont an especially green place to race.

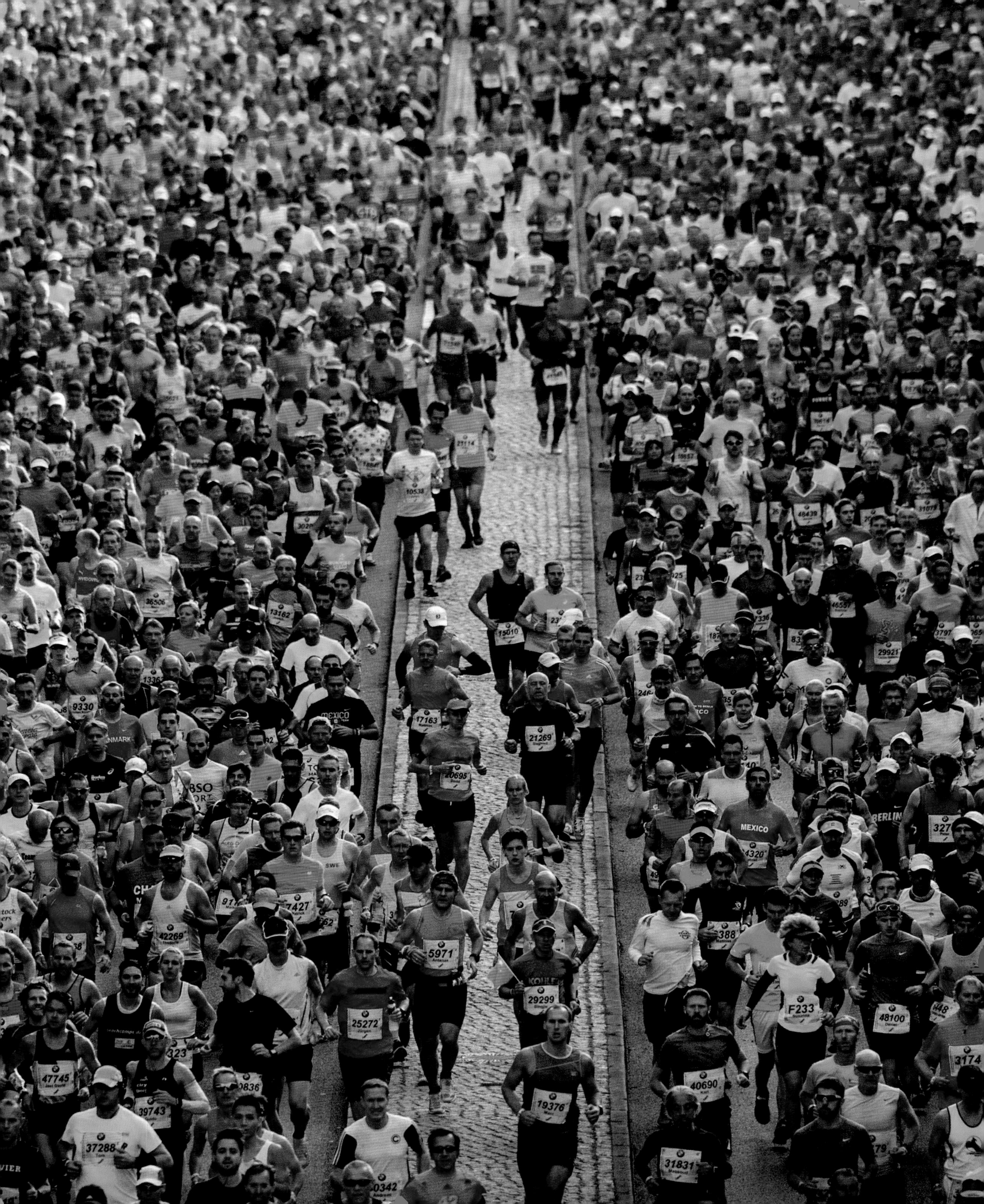
10538
36506
13162
15010
29921
9330
MEXICO
17163
21269
20695
MEXICO
BERLIN
SWE
42269
5971
29299
25272
F233
48100
47745
39743
19376
40690
37288
31831

GREAT MARATHONS

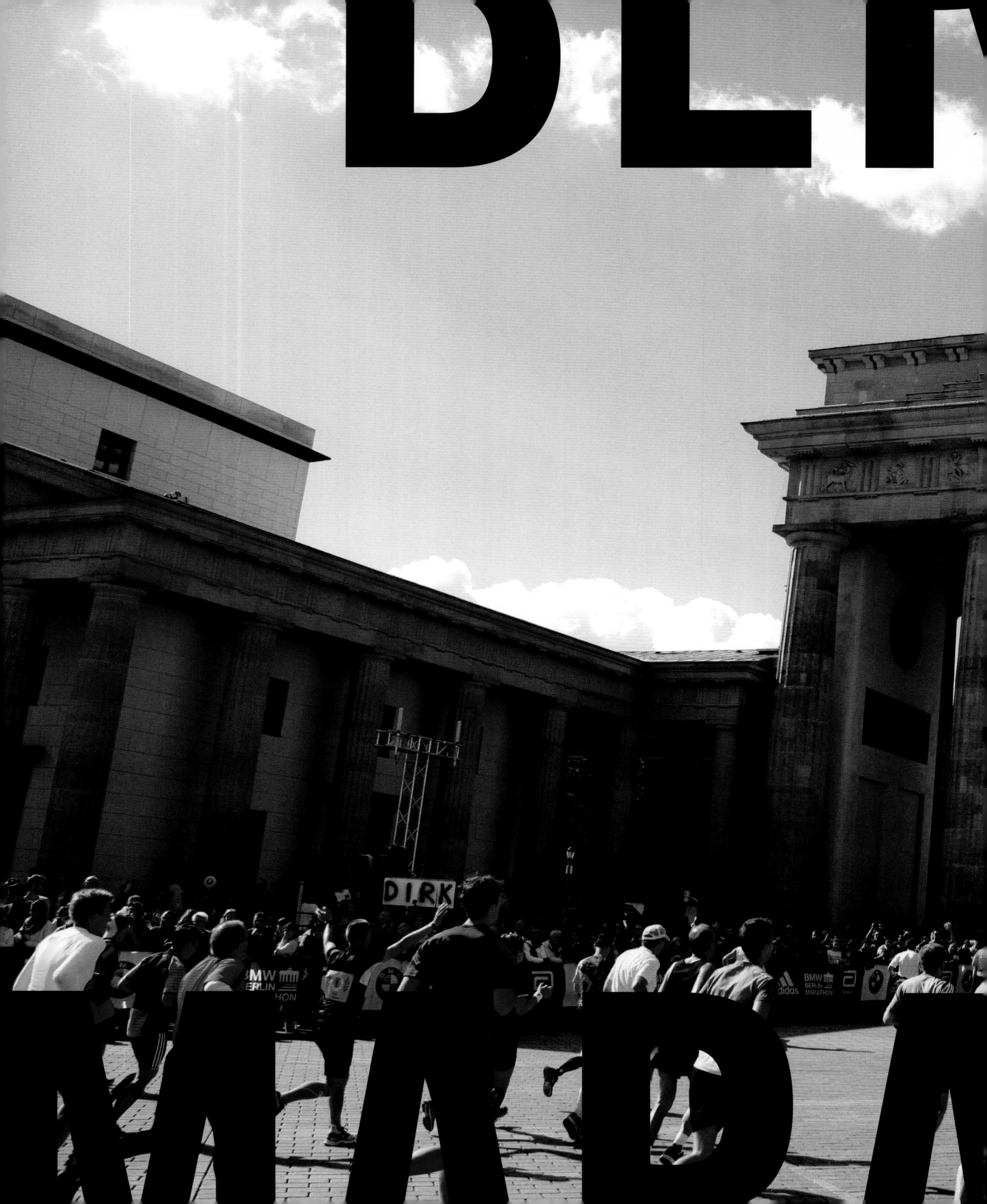
DIRK
BMW BERLIN MARATHON
adidas

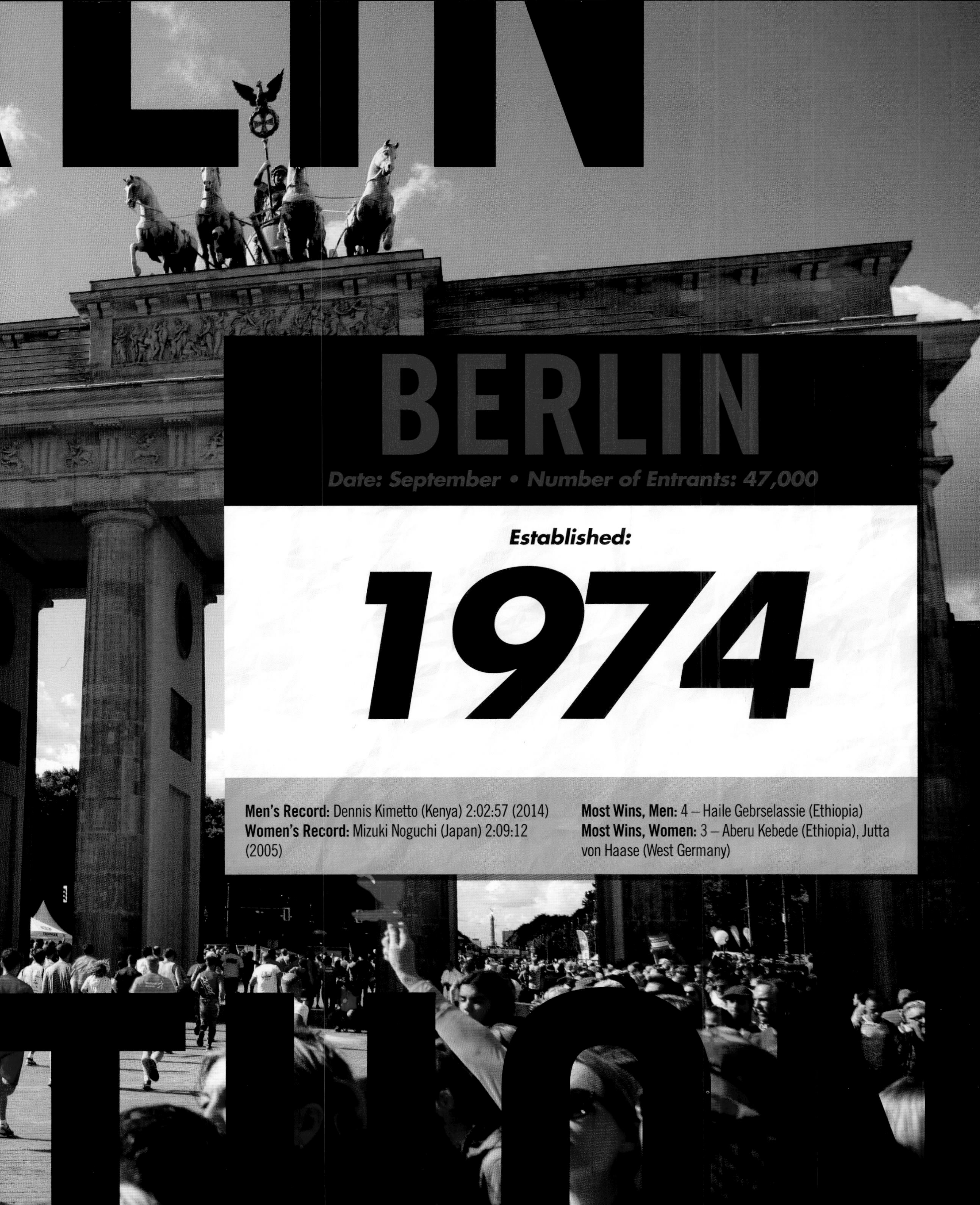

BERLIN
Date: September • Number of Entrants: 47,000
Established:
1974
Men's Record: Dennis Kimetto (Kenya) 2:02:57 (2014)
Women's Record: Mizuki Noguchi (Japan) 2:09:12 (2005)
Most Wins, Men: 4 – Haile Gebrselassie (Ethiopia)
Most Wins, Women: 3 – Aberu Kebede (Ethiopia), Jutta von Haase (West Germany)

THE BMW BERLIN MARATHON

The BMW Berlin Marathon is one of the largest and best-known road races in the world. With a fascinating backstory and a reputation as a world-record-breaking event, it's easy to see why this particular 26.2-mile course is famous across the globe as one of the six World Marathon Majors.

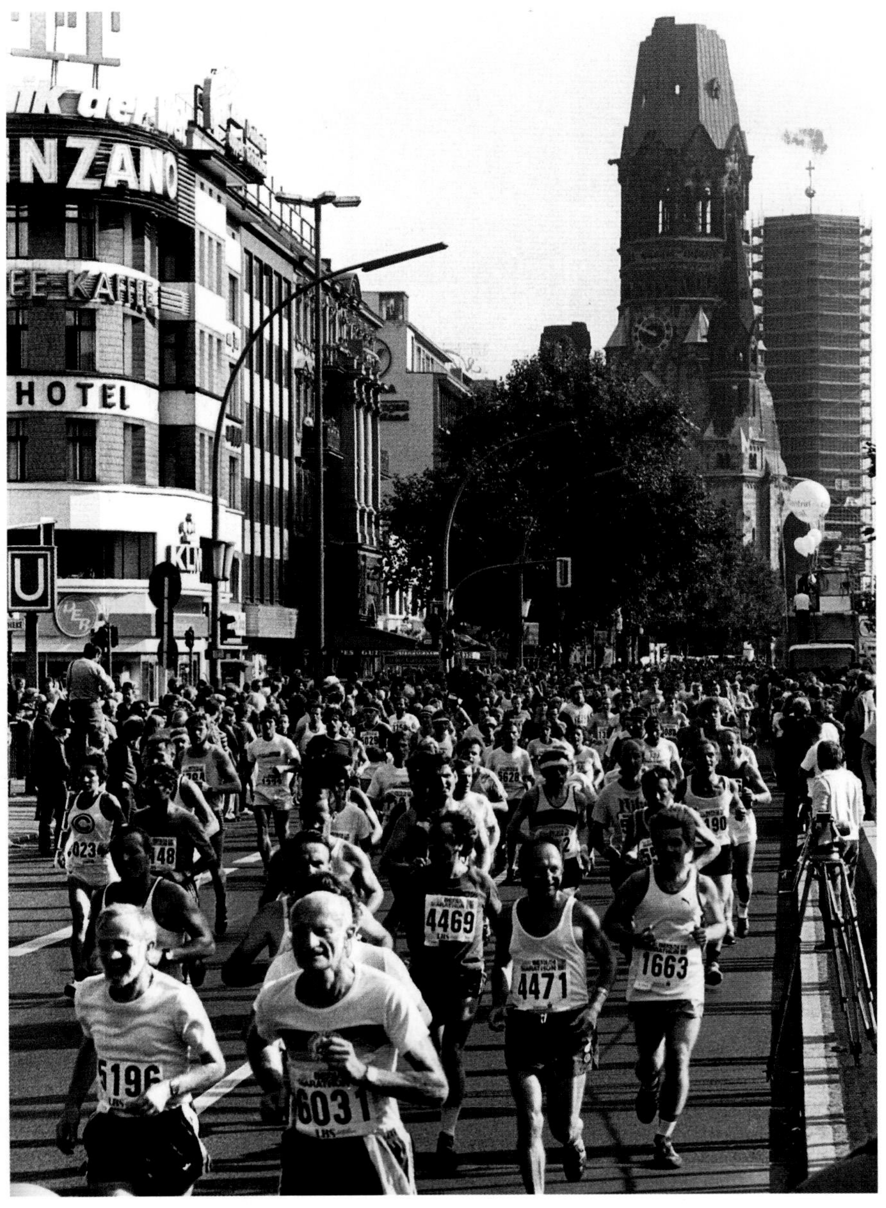

◀ In 1981, the marathon was allowed to be run through the streets of Berlin for the first time.

▶ The 1990 Berlin Marathon marked the first time the course included both East and West parts of the city.

THE HISTORY

The inaugural Berlin Marathon took place on 13 October 1974, organized by a group of runners from the prestigious German athletics club SC Charlottenburg. Its route was a far cry from the modern-day event, however: it started on a minor road next to the organizers' stadium and then led runners along the Grunewald, a forest in West Berlin. A modest 286 athletes entered the first Berlin Marathon and the winners were local runners Günter Hallas, who crossed the finish line in 2:44:53, and Jutte von Hasse, who finished in 3:22:01.

The Berlin Marathon continued to follow the same route along the Grunewald each year until, on 27 September 1981, after much negotiation with the local government and police, the race was finally allowed to be held on the city streets through West Berlin, starting in front of the Reichstag and finishing along the wide and picturesque boulevard of Kurfürstendamm.

However, it was after the collapse of the Berlin Wall, in November 1989, that the marathon route underwent its most historic change: on 30 September 1990 – three days before German reunification – 25,000 marathon runners followed the course through the Brandenburg Gate and into both parts of Berlin. The event was momentous – symbolic of a new era for the German capital – and it was reported that many of the participants had tears in their eyes.

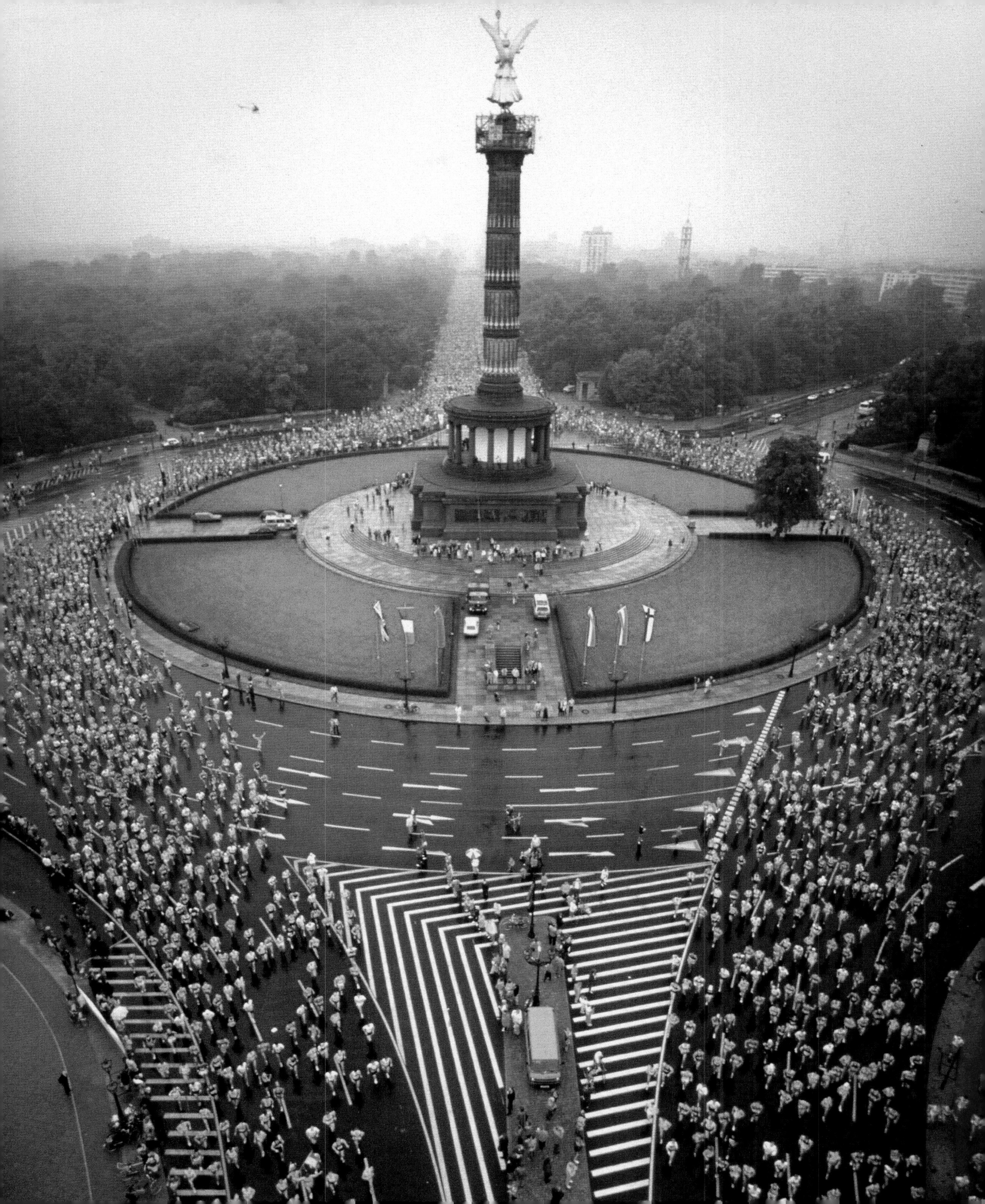

RECORD BREAKERS

Its rich history is not the only reason behind the Berlin Marathon's fame and notoriety: this World Marathon Major has also been the setting for many a world record. Even if you're not an elite athlete, the race is also hugely popular with club and fun runners alike, thanks to its exceptional personal-best (PB) potential.

As far back as the seventies, the Berlin Marathon made a name for itself as a fast course. The first world record was set there in 1977, when the National Marathon Championships were held at the race for the first time. The German long-distance runner Christa Vahlensieck clocked a super-speedy time of 2:34:48.

This was not the last time the race sped into the history books. In fact, to date, no fewer than 10 world records have been set at the BMW Berlin Marathon, across both the men's and women's races. It was in 1998 – on the 25th anniversary of the race – that Berlin really established itself as one of the fastest marathons in the world. Brazilian athlete Ronaldo da Costa crossed the finish line in a time of 2:06:05 and, in doing so, became the first runner to complete a marathon in an average speed of more than 20km/hr. In the following year, 1999, it was the women's race that saw the world record broken, when Tegla Loroupe from Kenya crossed the finish line in 2:20:43.

From that point on, the records just kept coming: in 2001, Japanese athlete Naoko Takahashi became the first female runner to break the 2:20 mark, winning in an impressive 2:19:46; while, in 2003, Kenyan elite Paul Tergat became the first runner to go below 2:05, finishing in a remarkable 2:04:55.

Then, in 2006 – with a field that had grown to 39,636 runners – up stepped Haile Gebrselassie. The Ethiopian superstar won the race for three years running, completing it in 2:05:56 in 2006, in warm weather conditions, before setting new world records in both 2007 and 2008, in times of 2:04:26 and 2:03:59 respectively.

At the 40th Berlin Marathon, in 2013, Kenyan athlete Wilson Kipsang knocked an impressive 36 seconds off Gebrselassie's record, winning in 2:03:23. But it was Kipsang's fellow countryman, Dennis Kimetto, who raced into marathon history the following year, 2014, setting the 10th world record on the Berlin course and smashing through the mythical 2:03 barrier, in an unprecedented time of 2:02:57.

It's not just the elites who enjoy posting super-speedy times in Berlin, either. There have been many fun runners in fancy dress who have entered the record books, too. In 2017, the UK's Jennifer McBain entered *The Guinness Book of World Records* as the fastest marathon runner dressed as a fast-food item (she was sporting a hot-dog outfit), in a time of 3:19:53. In the same year, foursome Michael Wong, Sarah Mattison, Chain Lee and Nam Gip, all from the US, also claimed a Guinness World Record, for the fastest marathon in a four-person costume, completing the course in 4:53:33 while joined together dressed as a colourful caterpillar.

No other marathon has seen so many global records, and many runners head here to bag a personal best. But just what exactly is Berlin's magic formula when it comes to runners achieving fast times?

One of the driving factors is the race profile: the BMW Berlin Marathon is an exceptionally flat course, starting at 38m above sea level, and never getting higher than 53m or lower than 37m. But there are several additional factors that can be taken into account, too. The first is that there are very few twists and turns along the course, meaning athletes can maintain a steady speed. The second is the climate. Late September in Berlin sees practically ideal running conditions, with very little wind and a temperature that falls between 12°C and 18°C.

The final consideration is the terrain: the BMW Berlin Marathon is run on asphalt, rather than concrete, which some say could contribute to a faster race and is almost certainly a lot kinder to runners' joints.

Taking all the above into account, it's no wonder athletes love Berlin so much, and – even if you're not racing at the elite level – it's worth bearing the BMW Berlin Marathon in mind if you're chasing that elusive PB!

▶ Dennis Kimetto won the Berlin Marathon in 2014, setting a new world record time in the process.

▼ Mizuki Noguchi celebrates her win in the 2005 Berlin Marathon. Her record time has yet to be broken.

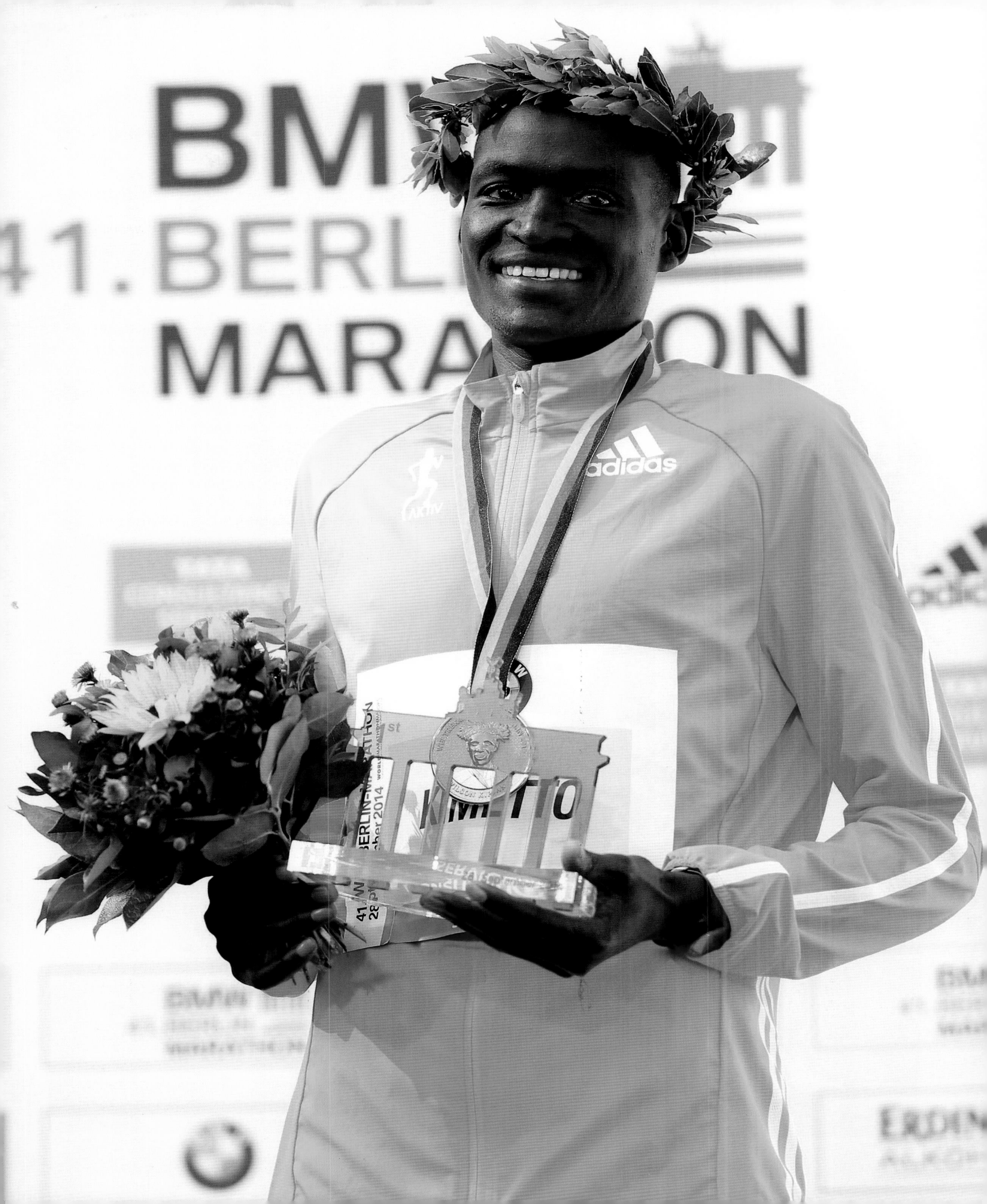
adidas

THE COURSE

The Berlin Marathon's appeal is not just that it's fast and flat: it's also vibrant and well supported. The modern-day marathon course is a far cry from its origins along the Grunewald in 1974, and, these days, participants experience a fabulous historic sightseeing tour of the city while they pound along Berlin's streets.

The course comprises a 26.2-mile loop, which starts and finishes at one of Berlin's most outstanding monuments, the Brandenburg Gate. From here, runners pass the Reichstag, before being able to take in a series of other famous landmarks and monuments, including the Fernsehturm (Berlin's television tower), Rathaus Schöeneberg (the city hall in front of which American President John F. Kennedy delivered his famous anticommunist speech that included the proclamation, '*Ich bin ein Berliner*') and the Konzerthaus Berlin (the city's impressive classical-music venue).

The course then turns northwest, leading runners along the Kurfürstendamm – the most famous and elegant boulevard in Berlin. At the 34km mark, the Kaiser Wilhelm Memorial Church becomes visible – it's one of Berlin's most important churches and is a memorial of peace and reconciliation.

Almost at the homeward stretch, runners continue on towards Potsdamer Strasse and then Potsdamer Platz, where they cross the line of the Berlin Wall. They then run along the Leipziger Strasse, before reaching the Spreeinsel. Here, runners can see the ruins of the Palast der Republik (Palace of the Republic), before arriving at Unter den Linden, Berlin's picturesque boulevard lined with lime trees, which runs all the way to the finish line at the Brandenburg Gate.

If the fast course and historic sightseeing tour aren't enough to entice you, perhaps the fantastic support will. The Berlin Marathon boasts a phenomenal crowd of more than a million people,

▼ Konzerthaus Berlin is one of several historic buildings to take in on the route through the city.

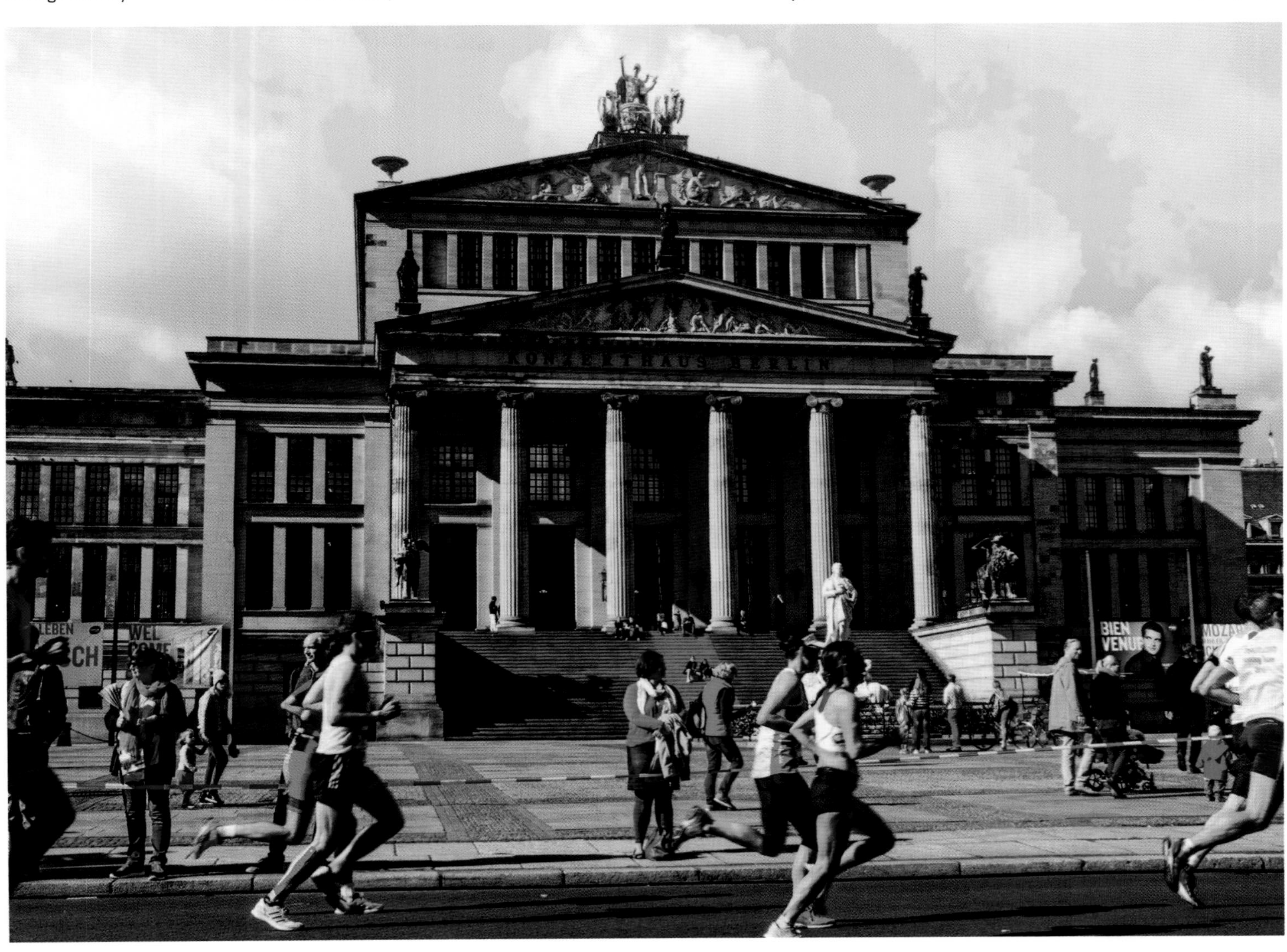

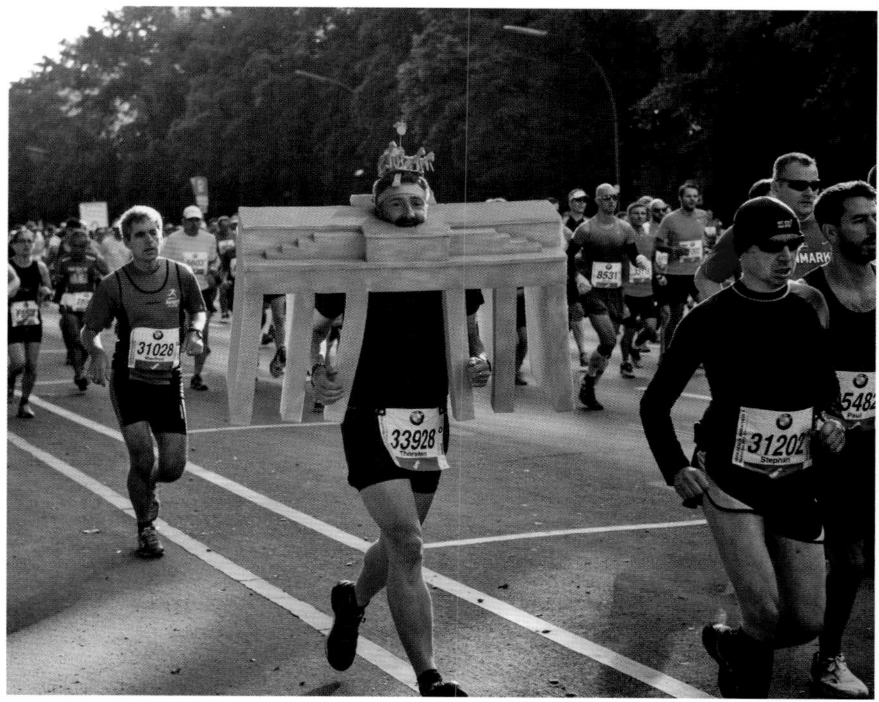

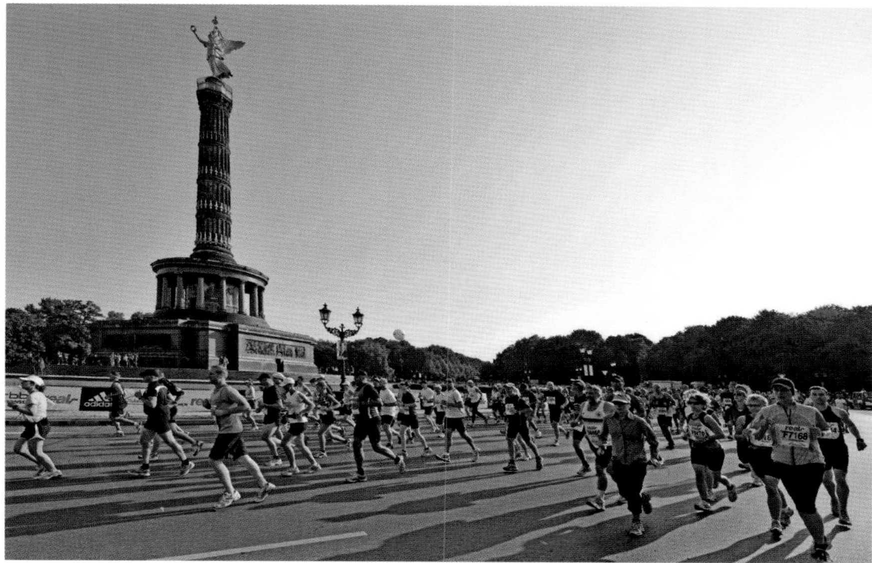

which is surely enough to spur you on to that finish line. What's more, with more than 80 bands and music stations situated approximately every 500m along the route, you could even dance your way round.

The marathon and its sensational atmosphere is enough to bring runners back time and time again – including Günter Hallas, the race's first winner back in 1974, who has gone on to run in the event almost every year since. Having only missed a few marathons in the years since the race began, Hallas takes part simply for the love of it. He is, of course, an inspiration to many fellow runners.

▲ Runners in Berlin pass through the Grosser Stern, complete with its iconic Victory Column.

▲▲ The standard of costumes in Berlin can be very high.

HOW TO ENTER

As with many large-scale marathons, there are several ways to enter if you fancy giving it a go. The first is by registering for the Entry Draw as a single runner. This is open for three weeks, roughly 11 months prior to race day. If your name is drawn (about a month after registration closes), only then will you be charged for your race place. If you'd like to run alongside two or three friends, simply select the "Entry Drawing Teams" option and enter together. If your team is drawn in the ballot, you all get to run together (this is not a relay option).

If you can complete 26.2 miles more quickly than the average marathon runner, you could be eligible to enter via the "fast runners" route. To qualify as a "fast runner", entrants need to have previously completed a marathon in under a certain time, which varies for both men and women depending on your age.

If you can prove you have already completed the BMW Berlin Marathon 10 times, you become part of the Jubilee-Club, and can receive a guaranteed place in the future. For a guaranteed entry without having to hang around to find out whether you've bagged a place via the draw, you can enter via a tour operator or charity partner. Alternatively, you can approach a number of tour operators who enable you to book your place as part of a holiday package.

Finally, if you'd like to complete the BMW Berlin Marathon a little differently, you could try the option to inline-skate the course the day before the main running event! Yes, on the Saturday of the marathon weekend, some 6,000 inline skaters take to the marathon course, to glide 26.2 miles to the finish line, cheered on by some 250,000 supporters. All runners who enter the Skating Marathon with a special code qualify for the "skate to run" initiative, receiving guaranteed entry into the following year's running marathon.

There can hardly be a more novel and fun way to cross-train than by getting your skates on and taking part in one of the world's most spectacular marathons on wheels. For any skaters, it's an opportunity that's not to be missed.

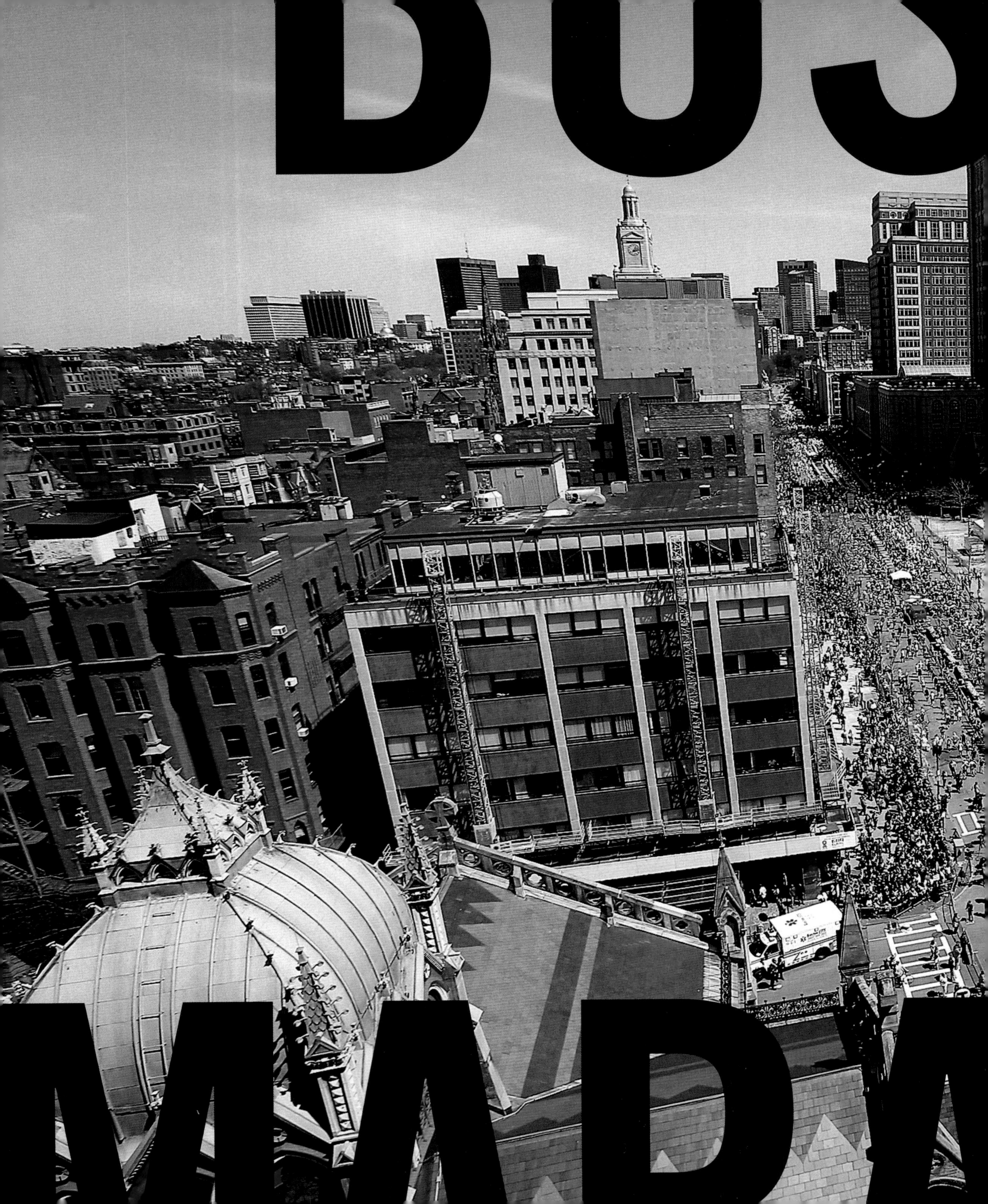

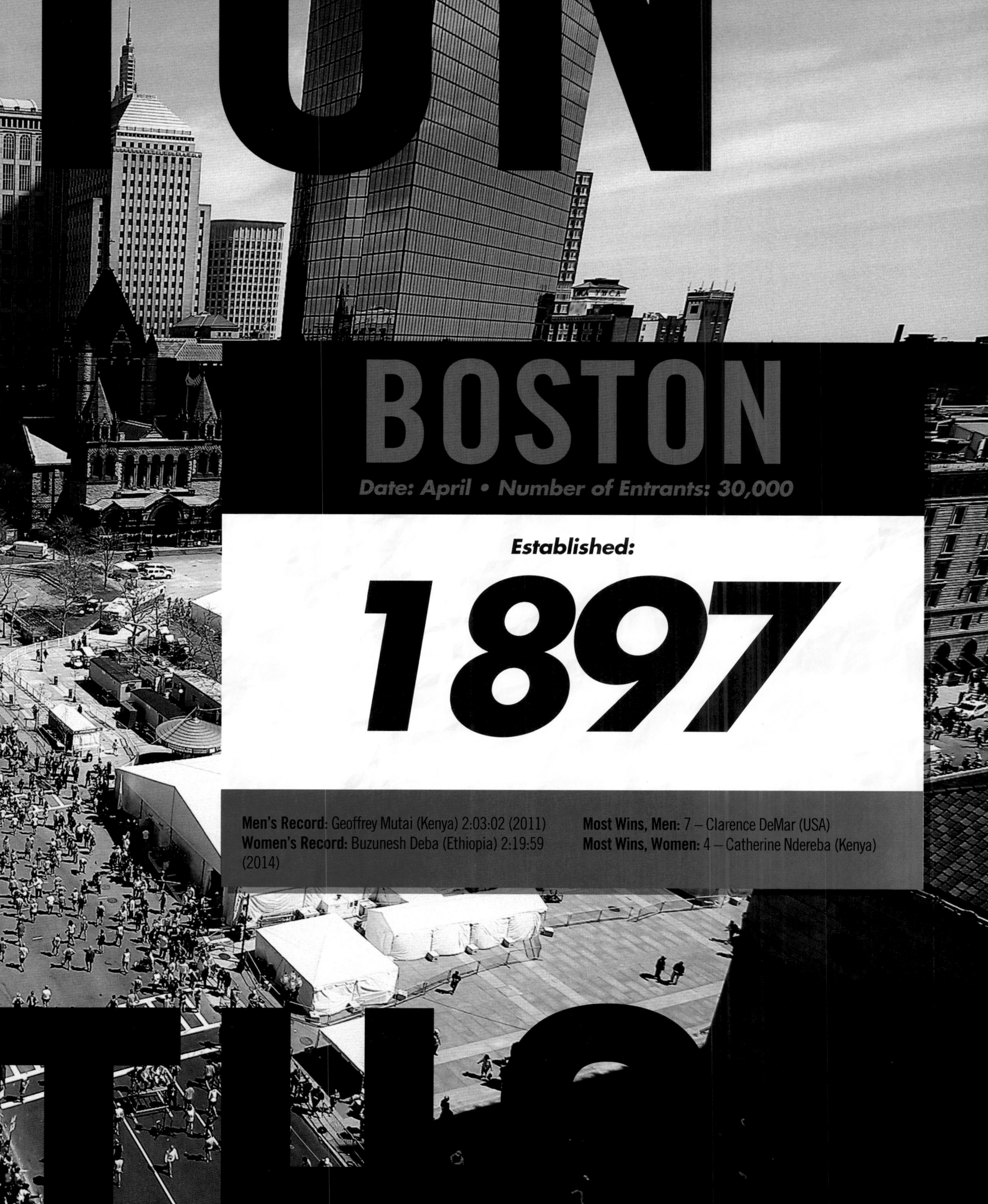

BOSTON
Date: April • Number of Entrants: 30,000
Established:
1897
Men's Record: Geoffrey Mutai (Kenya) 2:03:02 (2011)
Women's Record: Buzunesh Deba (Ethiopia) 2:19:59 (2014)
Most Wins, Men: 7 – Clarence DeMar (USA)
Most Wins, Women: 4 – Catherine Ndereba (Kenya)

THE BOSTON MARATHON

The Boston Marathon is unique for several reasons – not least in that it's the world's oldest annual marathon. Taking inspiration from the marathon event at the first modern Olympic Games, several members of the Boston Athletic Association founded their own event in 1897. The inaugural 24.5-mile race was won by John J. McDermott, who led a field of just 15 runners.

The Boston Marathon has run every year since its inaugural race in 1897, traditionally taking place on Patriot's Day. This is observed on the third Monday of April each year, and is often affectionately referred to by Boston locals as "Marathon Monday".

The second factor that makes the Boston Marathon stand out from the crowd is that not just anybody can run it. In order to enter, you must have previously run a qualifying time in another marathon, and entrants must meet a time standard that corresponds to their age and gender. A full list of age groups and qualifying times can be found by visiting the Boston Athletic Association website, but, as an example, if you are a man aged 40 to 44, you would currently need to have run a recent marathon in a time of 3:15:00 or below (for a woman aged 40 to 44, the qualifying time is currently 3:45:00 or below).

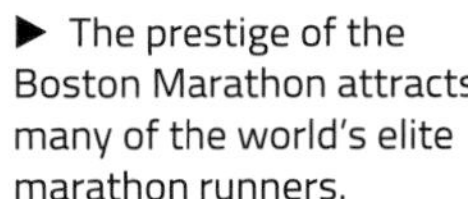

▶ The prestige of the Boston Marathon attracts many of the world's elite marathon runners.

▼ The history of the marathon is deeply intertwined with the modern history of Boston itself.

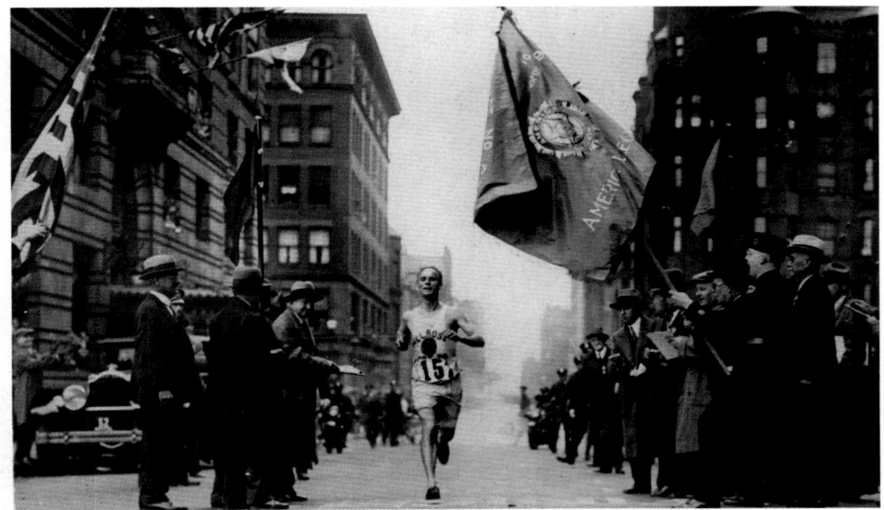

You therefore need to be pretty fast on your feet to gain your place at the start line – and, even then, it may not be enough. In recent years, due to the fact the enormous number of entries has exceeded the field size, the fastest qualifying times in each age and gender category have not been selected until all the places have been filled. In the 2017 event, for example, the cut-off for qualifying times was finalized as those who beat their qualifying standard by two minutes and nine seconds or faster.

If you're not fast enough to meet the qualifying standard but wish to run the Boston Marathon, there is still hope. Even if you don't have a qualifying time, you can enter via the Boston Marathon Official Charity Program.

In years gone by, there was one other way you could have run the Boston Marathon – although it was decidedly unofficial: you could become a "bandit" runner.

"Bandits" have a long tradition in running events – people who have not gained official entry to the race, but who run the course anyway. While other races have always been keen to remove them from the course, the Boston Marathon organizers generally tolerated them, simply asking that they start after all the official, registered runners had crossed the start line. However, since 2014, the bandits have officially been outlawed.

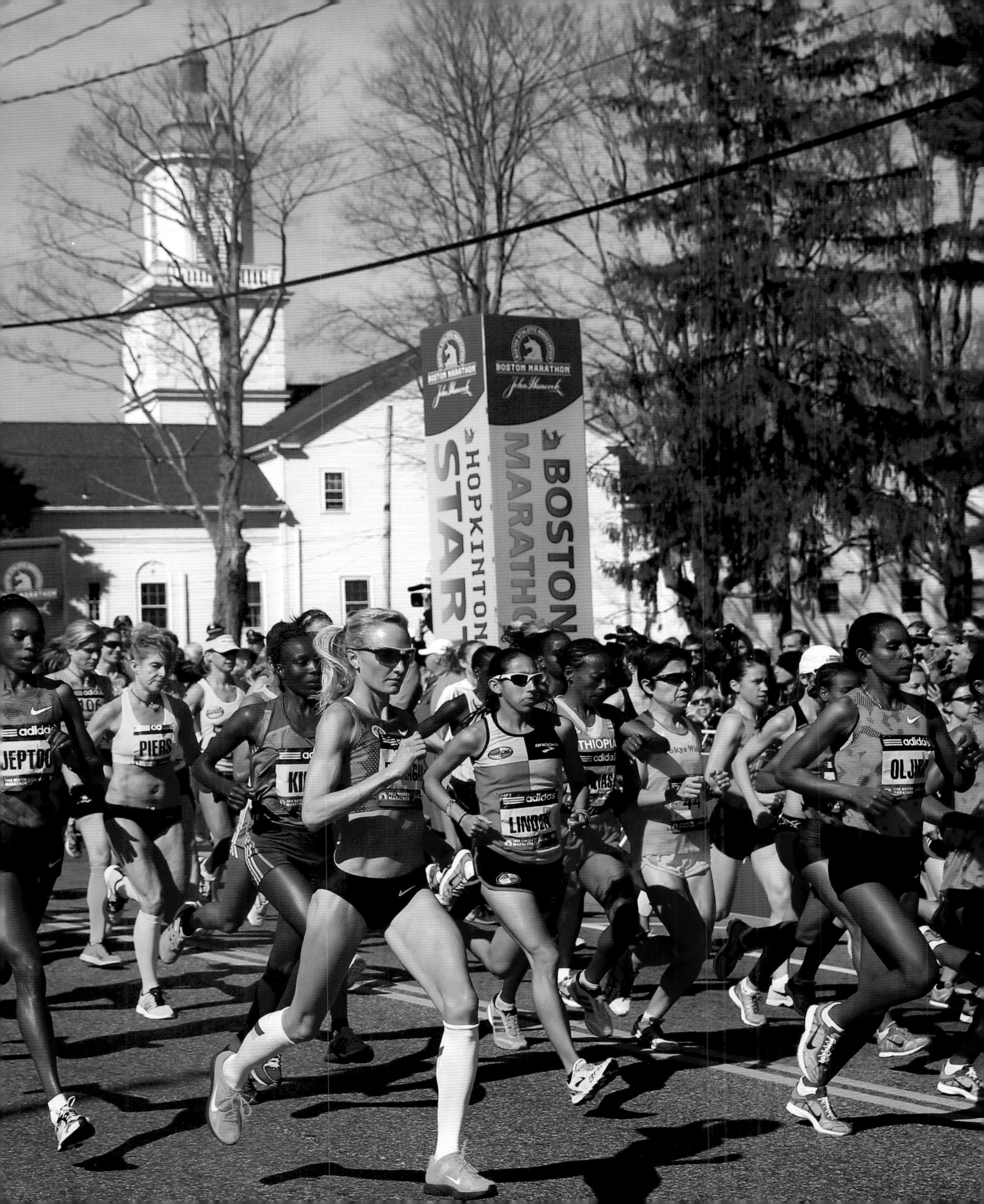
BOSTON MARATHON
John Hancock
HOPKINTON
BOSTON
JEPTOO
PIERS
adidas

THE COURSE

The Boston Marathon's start and finish lines have been moved over the years, but much of the course remains faithful to its original design.

The race follows a point-to-point route, starting in the rural New England town of Hopkinton and then following Route 135 through the towns of Ashland, Framingham, Natick and Wellesley. From there, it continues along Route 16, through Newton, and then finally into Boston, finishing near the John Hancock Tower in Copley Square.

Overall, the course profile has a considerable net elevation drop of 140m. In fact, the drop is so large that it exceeds the standards of the International Association of Athletics Federations, and, therefore, performances here are not eligible as world records – a fact that meant Kenyan athlete Geoffrey Mutai could not claim the world record in 2011, when he ran the fastest marathon time until that point, crossing the line in 2:03:02. However, there are some tricky inclines – most notably the famous "Heartbreak Hill", which subjects runners to a steep uphill section just after the 20-mile mark.

But, even when the course is taking its toll on your energy reserves, there should be enough support to keep you going. With an estimated half a million supporters turning up to cheer each year, the atmosphere is fantastic for even the most weary of runners. Notable spectator hotspots include TJ's Food & Spirits, a lively biker bar at Mile 2, and Wellesley College's infamous "Scream Tunnel" at the 12.5-mile mark. Because of the way the course bends, the cheers and shrieks of the college's students and faculty staff can be heard by runners long before they see them – but, when

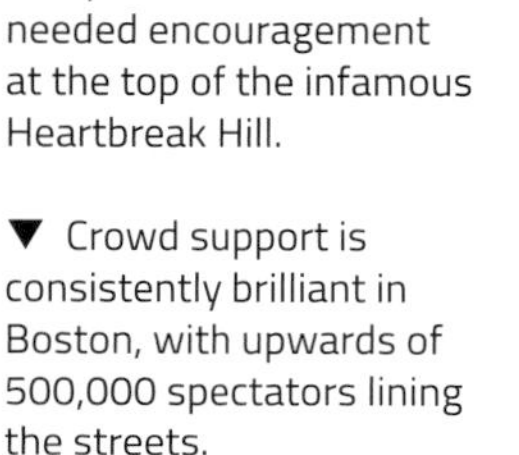

◥ Spectators deliver much-needed encouragement at the top of the infamous Heartbreak Hill.

▼ Crowd support is consistently brilliant in Boston, with upwards of 500,000 spectators lining the streets.

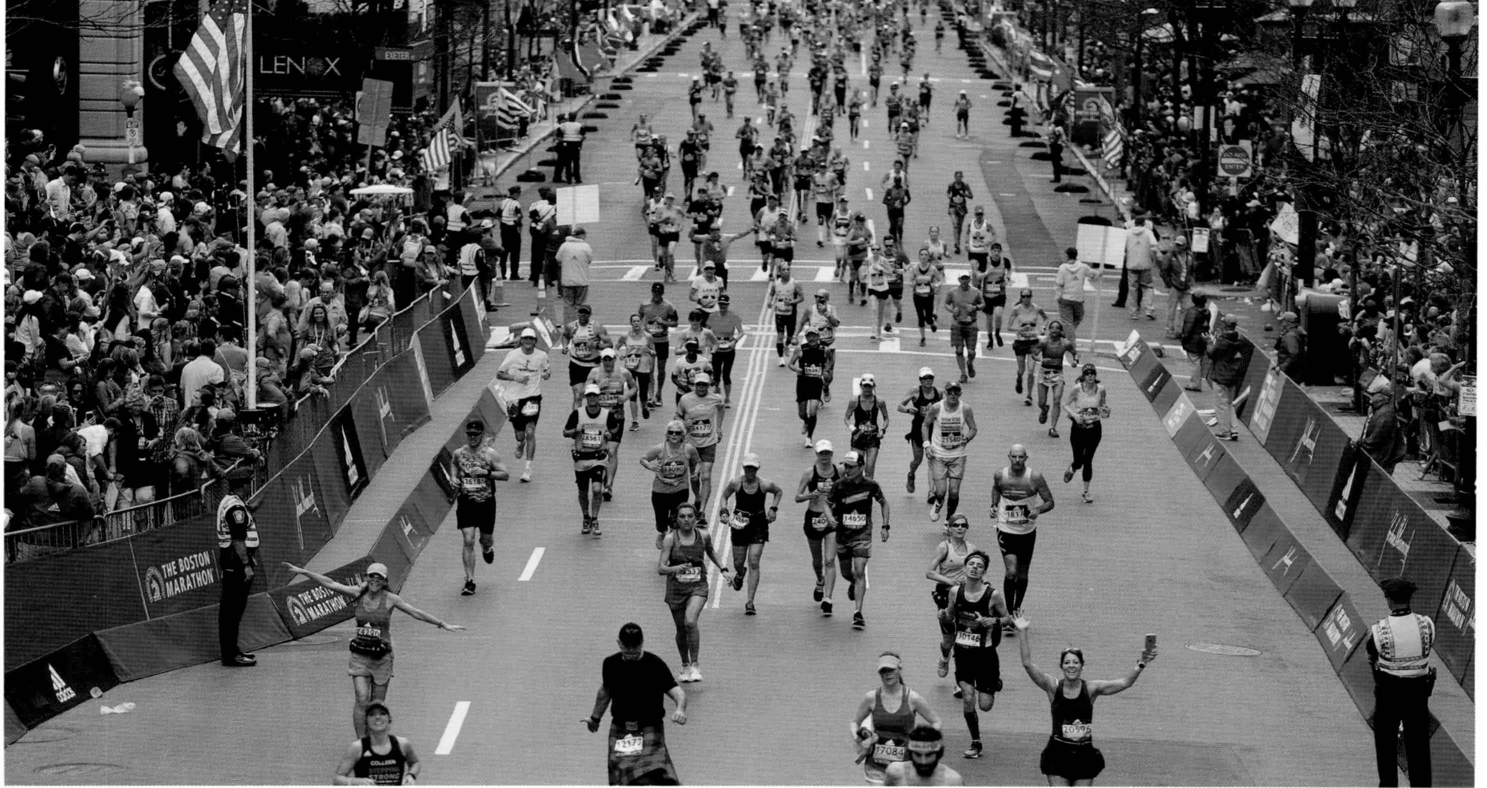

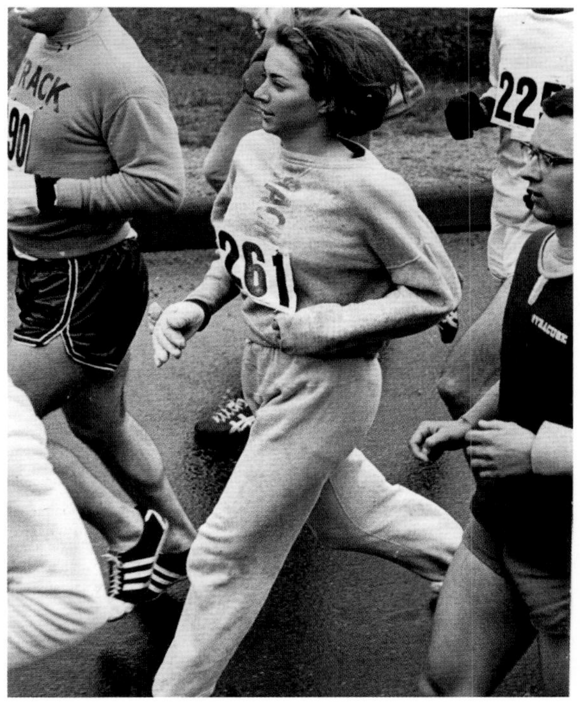

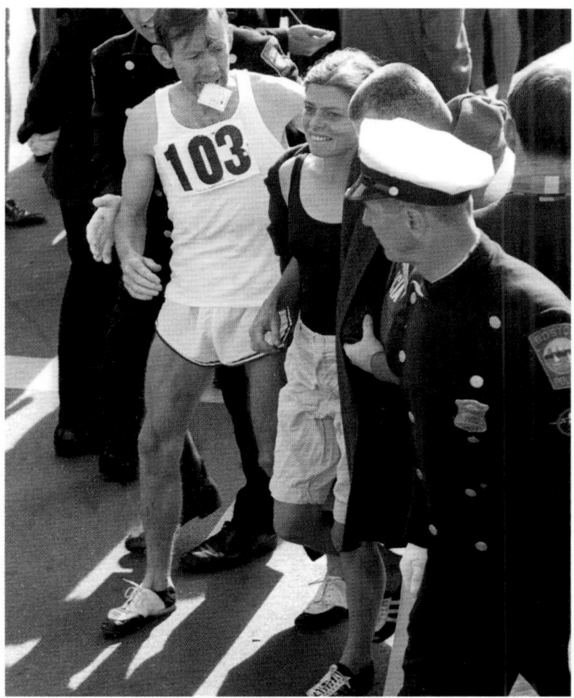

◀ Roberta Gibb became the first woman to run and complete the Boston Marathon in 1966.

◀◀ Kathrine Switzer defied organizers and other athletes alike to run the Boston Marathon in 1967.

they do get a glimpse, they are spurred on not only by the deafening cheers, but also by some great banners and signs, and even the offer of kisses – a tradition that's rumoured to have started at the first race, in 1897, when the college girls reportedly cheered on a particular Harvard favourite.

EQUAL RIGHTS

While, these days, it seems absurd that women were ever banned from running the marathon distance, it was not until 1972 that they were finally allowed to enter and run the Boston Marathon. Which is why a certain "KV Switzer" caused such a stir during the 1967 race.

Kathrine Switzer registered for the all-male Boston Marathon using her initials in place of her first name and, in the mêlée at the start line, where officials were checking off bib numbers, her gender went unnoticed.

It wasn't until approximately four miles into the race that she started to attract attention – a photo press truck was making its way through the throng of runners, but then slowed in front of her so the photographers could snap images of the female runner who was wearing an official race number – 261. Moments later, however, Kathrine heard the pounding of leather-soled shoes behind her and turned instinctively to see who it was. In her own words, here is what happened next:

"A big man, a huge man, with bared teeth was set to pounce, and before I could react, he grabbed my shoulder and flung me back, screaming, 'Get the hell out of my race and give me those numbers!' Then he swiped down my front, trying to rip off my bib number, just as I leapt backward from him."

The man – race official Jock Semple – did not succeed in his attempts to remove Switzer forcibly from the course, and she went on to cross the finish line in a time of 4:20 – becoming the first woman to complete the Boston Marathon officially and an instant hero in the women's-rights movement.

However, unbeknown to many, another woman, Bobbi Gibb, had actually completed the Boston Marathon course the year before, in 1966, as a bandit. She also ran as a bandit the same year as Switzer – finishing in a time of 3:27:17 – and again, in 1968, and is now recognized by the Boston Athletic Association as the pre-sanctioned-era women's winner for those three consecutive years.

During this time, a growing number of women were unofficially running the marathon course, including Sara Mae Berman, who was the pre-sanctioned-era women's winner in 1969, 1970 and 1971.

It was only in 1972 that the Amateur Athletic Union finally saw sense and began to sanction women's-division marathons, and the first officially sanctioned women's-division event at the Boston Marathon was won by Nina Kuscsik, in a time of 3:10:26.

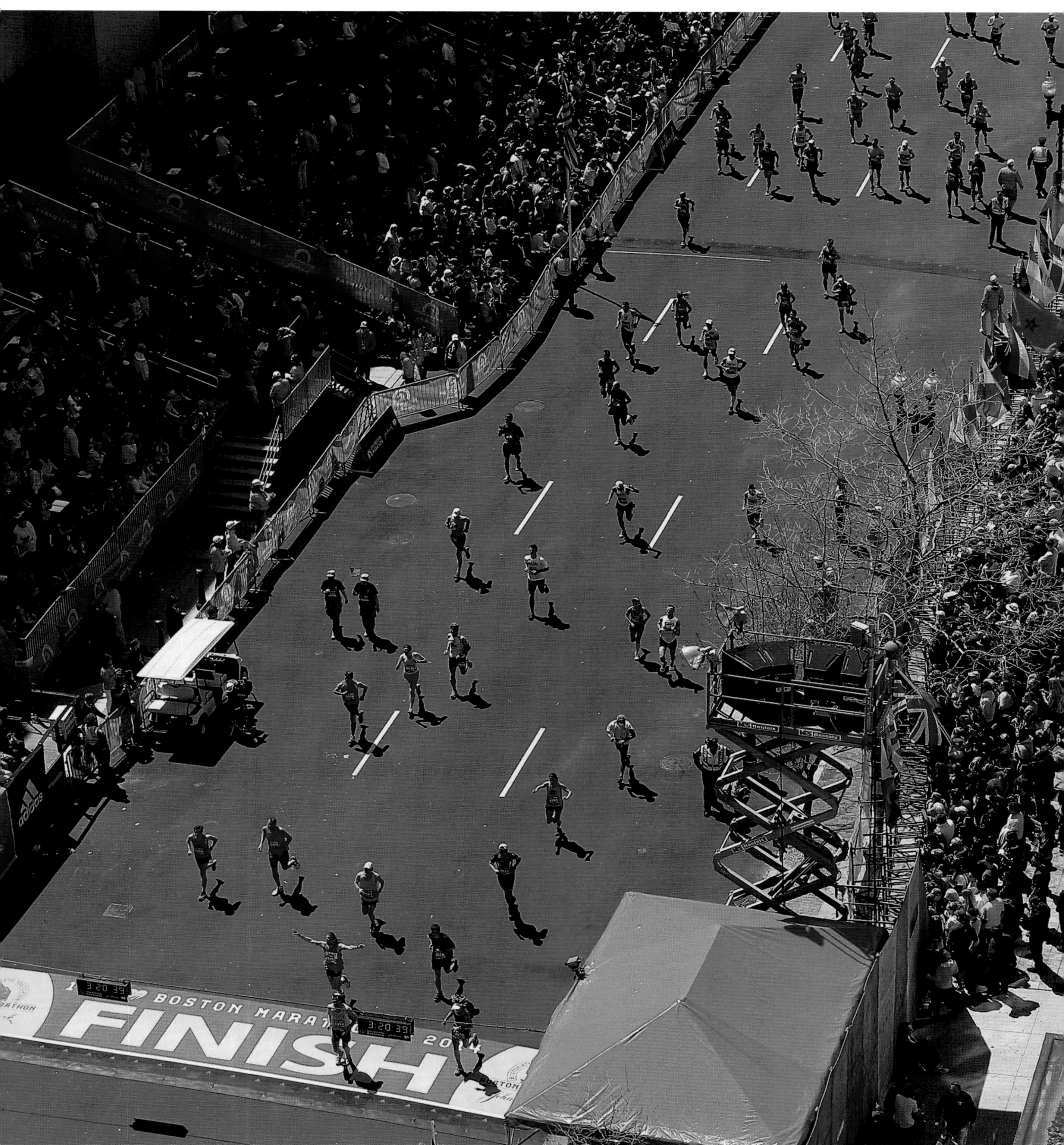
3:20:39
BOSTON MARATHON
FINISH
3:20:39
2014
PATRIOTS' DAY
adidas

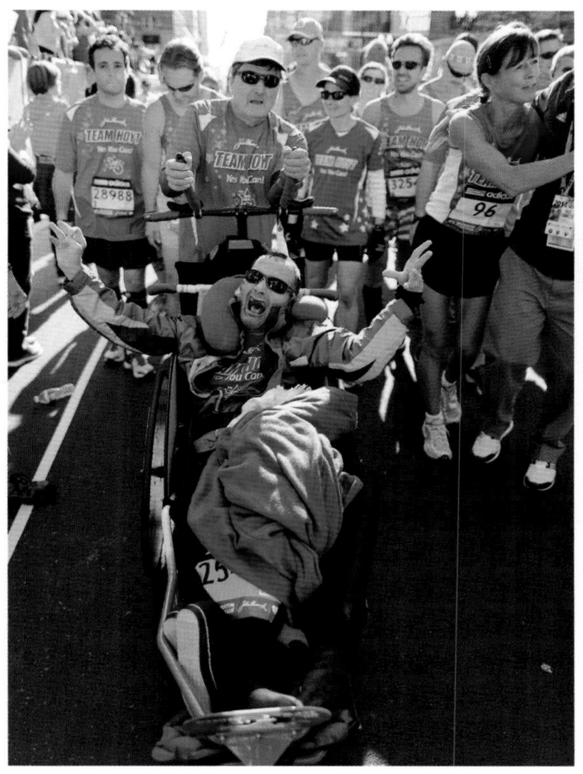

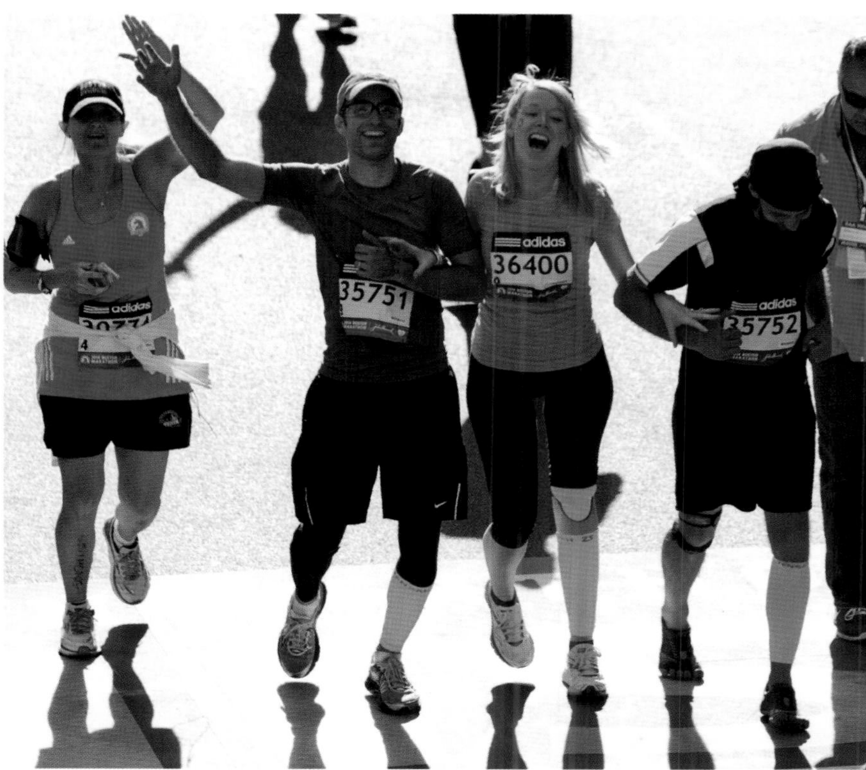

RUNNING HEROES

It's not just the elites crossing the finish line first each year who are the heroes of the Boston Marathon. As with any epic 26.2-mile race, there are a fair share of regular heroes, too. Heroes like Adrianne Haslet-Davis, a professional ballroom dancer who lost her lower left leg in the 2013 bombing while spectating the race. After a long and difficult road to recovery, Haslet-Davis learned to run wearing a prosthetic running blade and completed the Boston Marathon in 2016, three years after her terrifying ordeal.

Then there's Team Hoyt – father-and-son duo, Dick and Rick. Rick has cerebral palsy and, although doctors feared he would never be able to communicate or lead a normal life, Dick and his wife Judy refused to give up hope. When a computer device was invented to allow Rick to communicate with them, they learned of his love of sport and, in 1977, Rick asked his father if they could take part in a race together, to prove that life could go on, no matter your disability.

"Team Hoyt" have gone on to run the Boston Marathon 32 times (including in 2013, when they were forced to stop a mile short of the finish line due to the bombings), with Dick pushing Rick in a wheelchair. They took part in their final Boston Marathon in 2014 – when Dick was 74 and Rick was 52. In 2013, a bronze statue of the pair was erected in the town of Hopkinton, to honour the fact that they have inspired runners and spectators alike for three decades. And, in recognition of his incredible connection to the event, Dick was named Grand Marshal of the 2015 Boston Marathon.

Offering one of the largest marathon-prize purses to the winners (the male and female champions each receive $150,000, plus an additional $25,000 if they beat the course record), the incentive for the elite athletes is clear. But Boston's lure goes far, far deeper than that: take part in this race and you become part of road-racing history, running the streets that marathon runners have pounded for more than a century. But only if you're fast enough!

▲ Adrianne Haslet-Davis showed tremendous courage to complete the marathon, just a year after losing her leg in the 2013 bombings.

◤ Dick and Rick Hoyt show the trademark passion that has made them local legends in Boston.

◀ Turnout has been anything but diminished since the horrendous bombings in 2013.

"After a long and difficult road to recovery, Haslet-Davis learned to run wearing a prosthetic running blade and completed the Boston Marathon in 2016, three years after her terrifying ordeal"

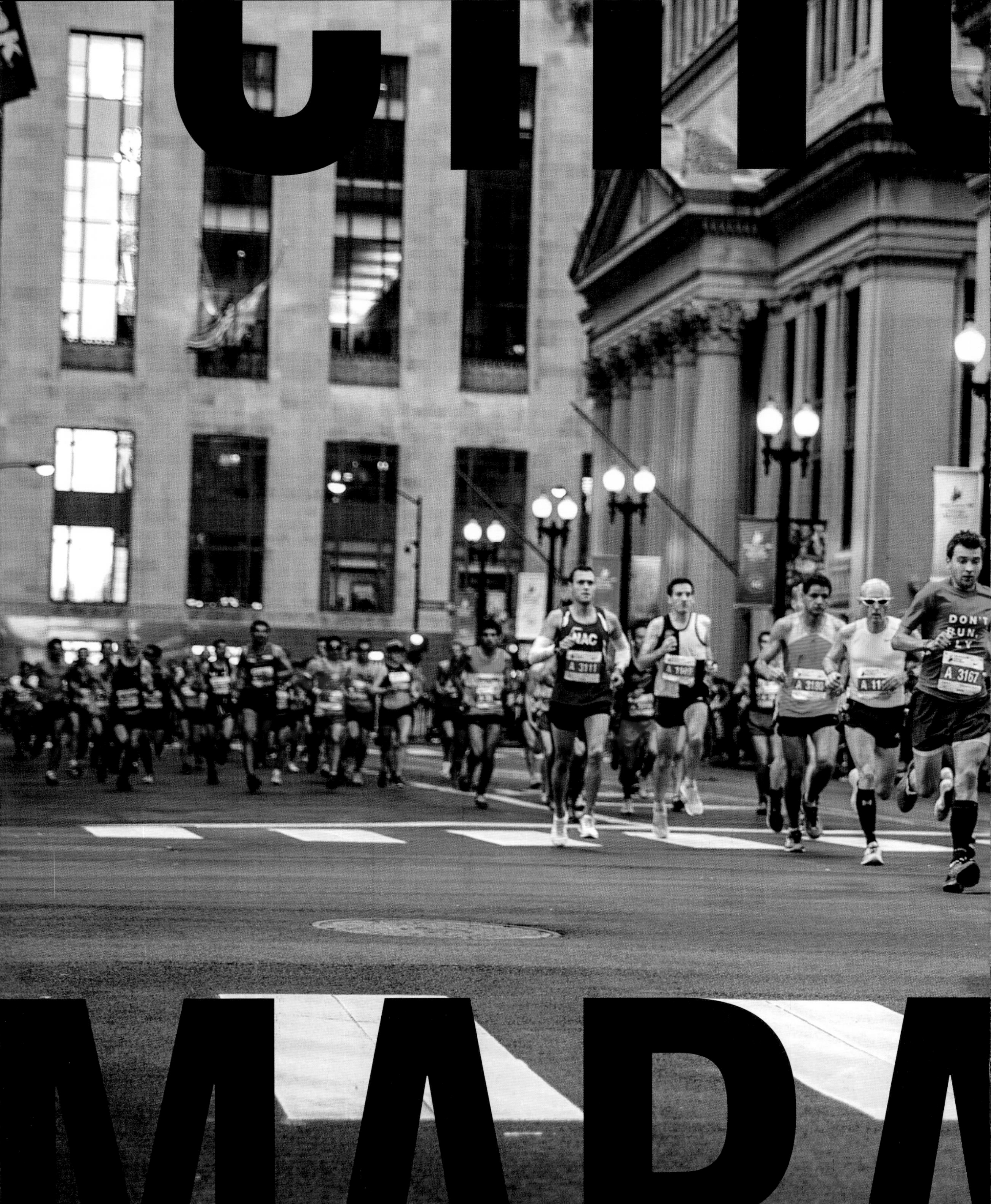
NAC
A 3111
A 3180
A 3167

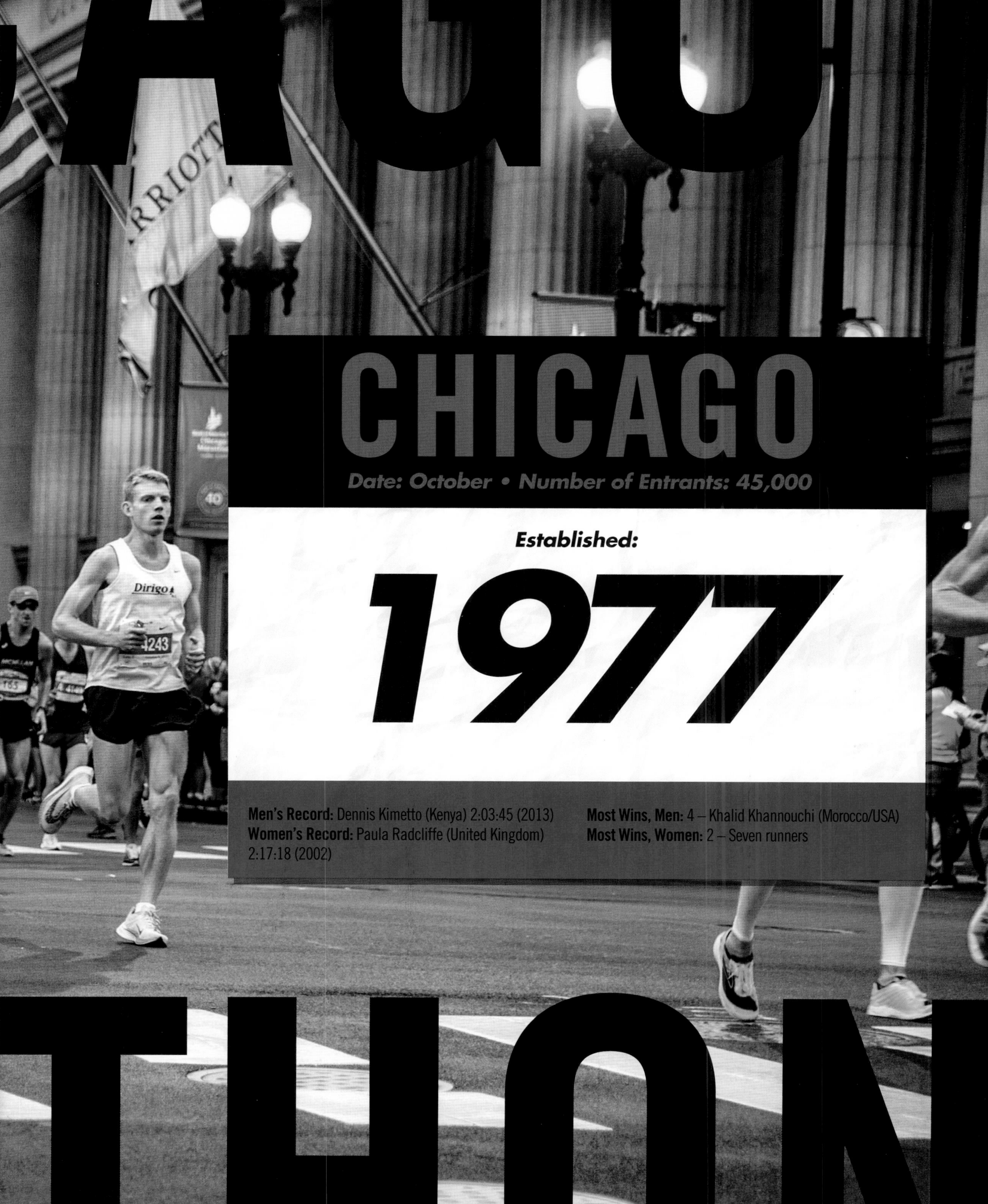

CHICAGO

Date: October • Number of Entrants: 45,000

Established:

1977

Men's Record: Dennis Kimetto (Kenya) 2:03:45 (2013)
Women's Record: Paula Radcliffe (United Kingdom) 2:17:18 (2002)

Most Wins, Men: 4 – Khalid Khannouchi (Morocco/USA)
Most Wins, Women: 2 – Seven runners

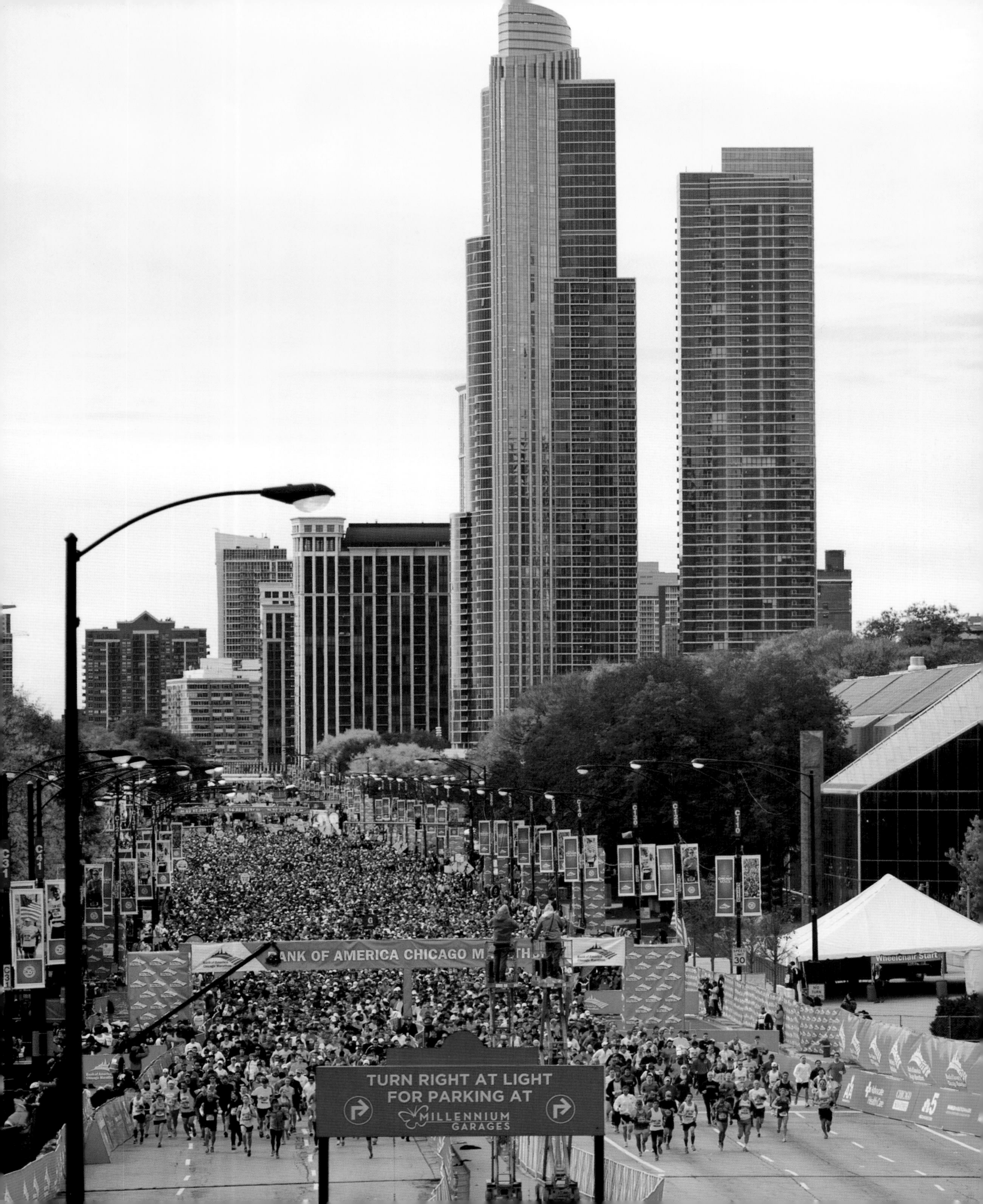

BANK OF AMERICA CHICAGO M
TURN RIGHT AT LIGHT
FOR PARKING AT
MILLENNIUM
GARAGES
Wheelchair Start

THE CHICAGO MARATHON

Fast and flat, with a cheeky incline near the end, the Chicago Marathon is one of the world's most popular. With a city and a course that is steeped in racing history, it should be high on the list of any marathon enthusiast.

While the modern-day Chicago Marathon was first run in 1977, the very first was held in 1905, on 23 September, organised by the newly created Illinois Athletic Club. The original course saw runners start at the Evanston Golf Club, before heading east towards Lake Michigan, into the city and on to Grant Park, finishing in front of a 15,000-strong crowd at the Washington Park horse-racing track.

This first event was reported to have attracted some 100,000 spectators – a crowd that far outweighed the number of athletes taking part. Just twenty runners registered for the event, with fifteen turning up on the day and only seven crossing the finish line. Escorted along the course by cyclists and race officials in cars, the event did not go as smoothly as hoped: during the race, the Rush Street Bridge was forced to open, to allow a steamer to pass along the Chicago River. Only three of the runners had already crossed the bridge before it opened, leaving the remaining entrants momentarily stranded and with no hope of catching the frontrunners.

Despite the fact that the race featured both marathon silver medallist Albert Corey and marathon relay silver medallist Sidney Hatch, who both competed in the 1904 Olympic Games, it was Illinois Athletic Club runner Rhud Mezner who crossed the finishing line first, winning the inaugural Chicago Marathon.

The Chicago Marathon became an annual event until the early 1920s, when challenges of the decade saw it sidelined.

Then, in November 1976, a small group of Chicago running enthusiasts held a meeting at the Metropolitan YMCA on LaSalle Street to plan the revival of the city's marathon, as a rival to the hugely popular New York City Marathon. Despite the objection of the Chicago Parks Superintendent, Ed Kelly, who refused to grant permission for the course to head through any of the parks or along the Lake Michigan lakefront, the proposed marathon was backed by Chicago's Mayor, Richard Daley. Although Daley died shortly afterwards, his successor, Michael Bilandic – a keen runner – was also an advocate, winning Ed Kelly's support and subsequent approval of the race.

The inaugural modern-day Chicago Marathon took place on 25 September 1977. Called the Mayor Daley Marathon and funded by event founder Lee Flahurty, it attracted some 4,200 runners, and Mayor Bilandic and his wife handed out medals to the finishers.

These days, the race is held every October. It has taken place every year since 1977 (except in 1987, when the sponsor pulled out and only a

◀ The modern Chicago Marathon is among the world's biggest races in terms of participation.

▼ A group of marathon runners takes their route through Chicago's Gaelic Park in 1912.

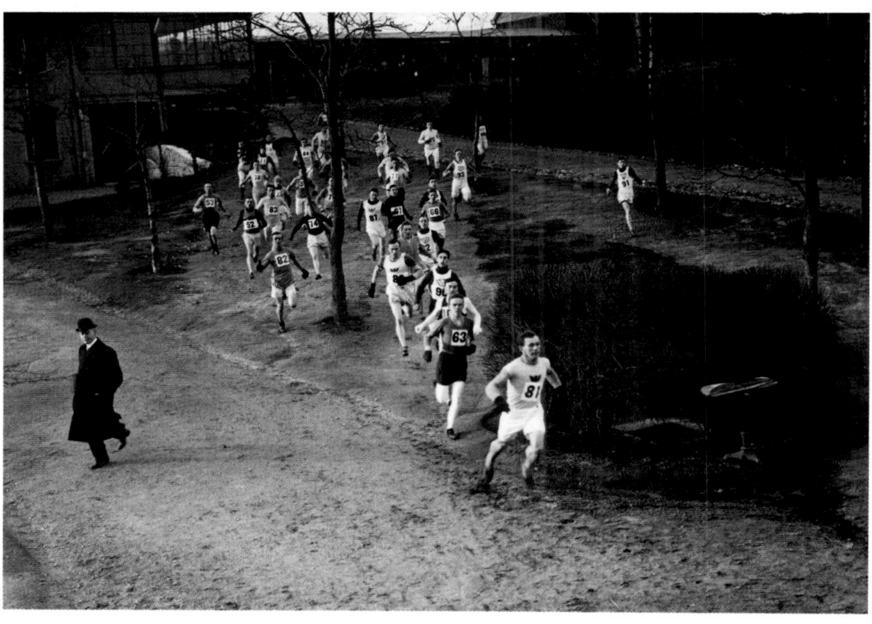

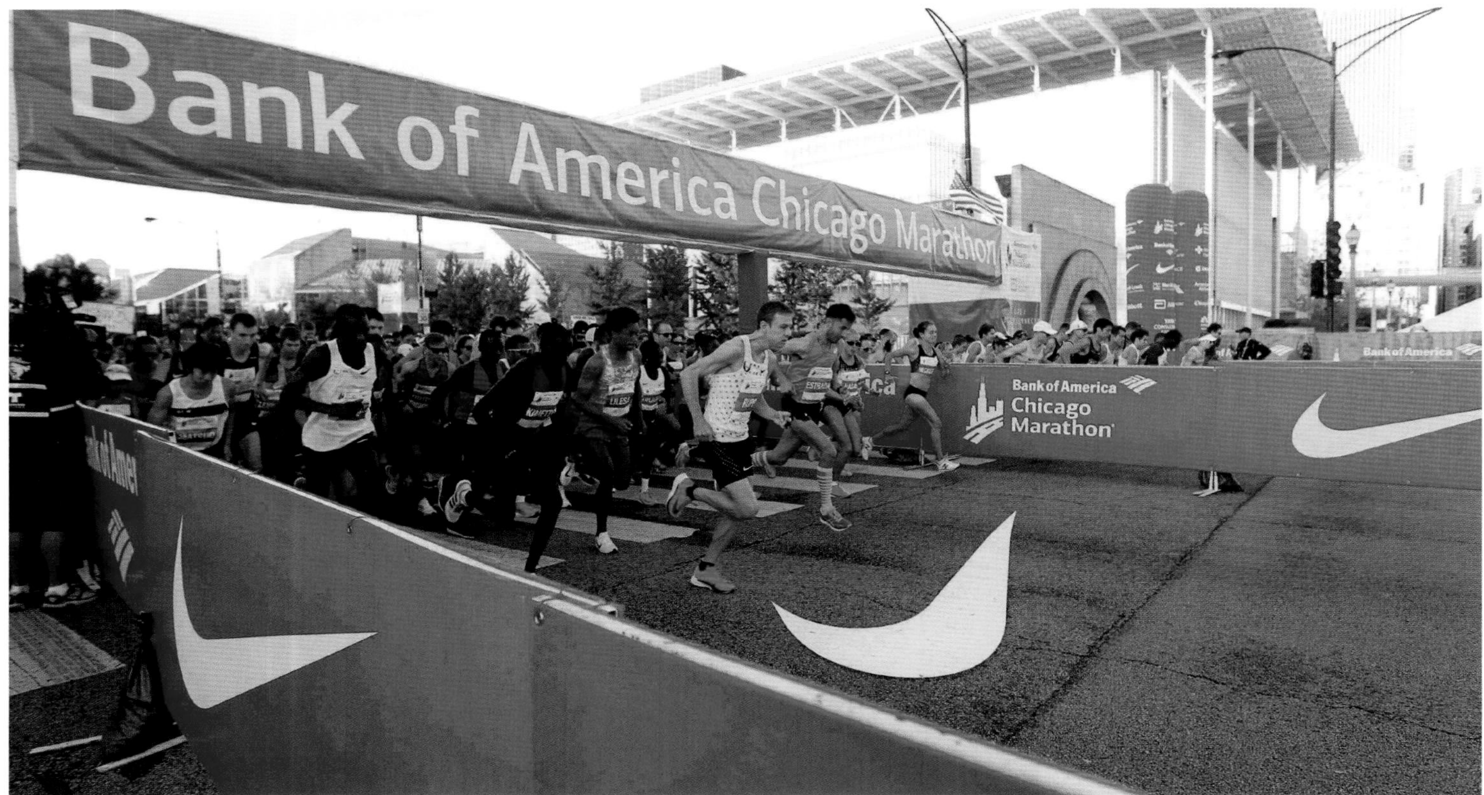

▲ Bank of America first sponsored the marathon in 2008, and has since become closely associated with it.

▶ A finisher's medal from Chicago should be high on the wish list of any marathon runner.

half-marathon took place). Entrant numbers have also steadily grown year on year, and the Chicago Marathon (which has been sponsored by the Bank of America since 2008) now attracts a field of more than 40,000 runners (the largest field size was in 2017, with 44,341) as well as an estimated 1.7 million spectators. This makes it one of the largest and most popular marathons in the world, earning it World Marathon Major status alongside Tokyo, Boston, New York City, London and Berlin.

FAST AND FLAT

One of the factors that make Chicago so popular with elite athletes and fun runners alike is its relatively flat and fast course, making it perfect for a personal best (PB) – and even a world record or four.

The 26.2-mile loop course starts in historic Grant Park (affectionately dubbed Chicago's front yard), in the central business district. The route then takes runners on a tour through 29 of the city's diverse and vibrant neighbourhoods, including Lakeview, Greektown, Little Italy, Pilsen, Chinatown and Bronzeville, before finishing up back where it started in Grant Park. The course offers runners a fabulous scenic tour of the city, allowing them to take in an array of cultures, significant and historic buildings and renowned architecture, not to mention some famous sports stadiums: Wrigley Field baseball park, home to

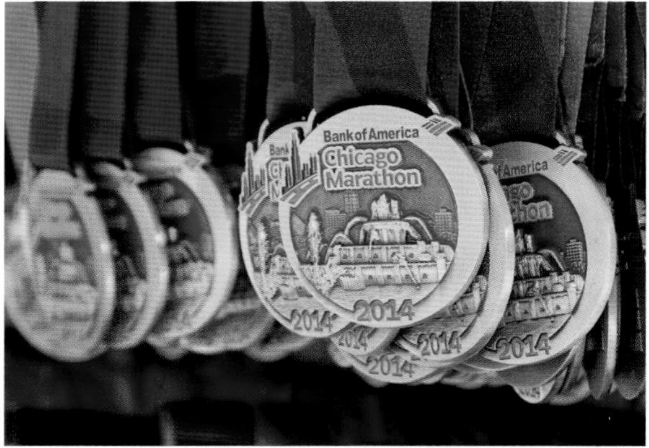

the Chicago Cubs; United Center indoor sports arena, home to the Chicago Bulls of the National Basketball Association and Chicago Blackhawks of the National Hockey League; Guaranteed Rate Field baseball park, home to the Chicago White Sox; and Soldier Field football stadium, home to the National Football League's Chicago Bears.

Of course, the Chicago marathon is popular not only with runners, but with spectators, too. The loop route, plus the abundance of great sights and public-transport options mean that those who come along to cheer are not only guaranteed an eventful and entertaining day, but also often get multiple sightings of their runner. All these factors can account for the fact that so many people come along to support the race.

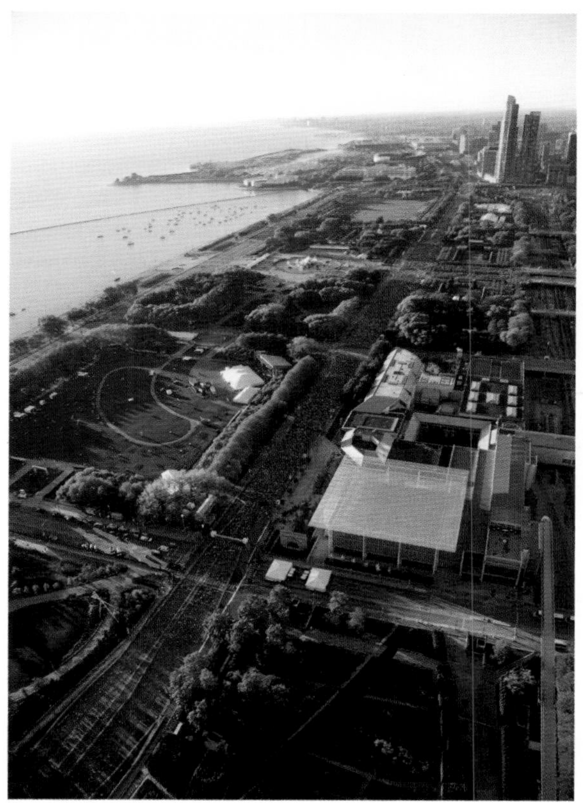

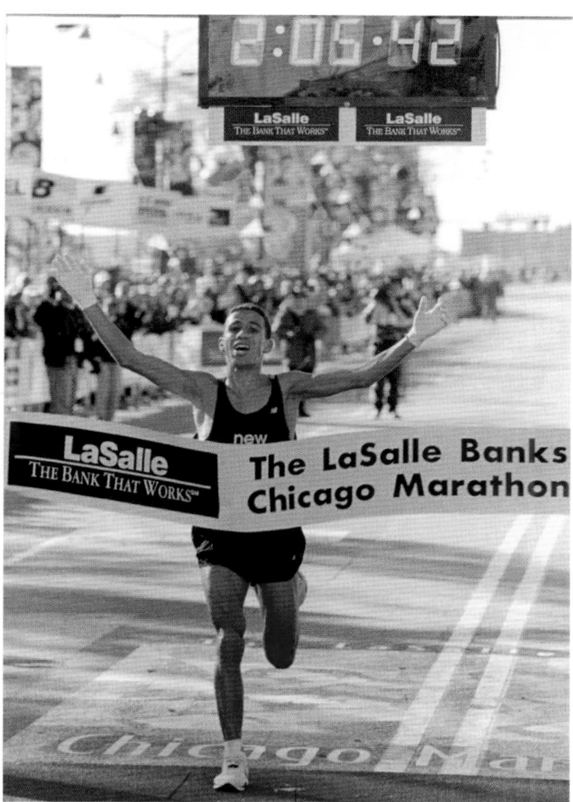

◀ Khalid Khannouchi celebrates winning the Chicago Marathon – and breaking the world record – in 1999.

◀◀ Chicago's mostly flat course and favorable conditions make it a fast race for amateurs and professionals alike.

The course's only slight incline comes during the final mile, but elevation change is minimal throughout. This could account for the fact that, as well as many runners clocking PBs here, the Chicago Marathon has also been the setting for four world records. In 1984, Welsh runner Steve Jones won the event in a time of 2:08:05. It was his first-ever completed marathon (he'd had to drop out the previous year due to injury) and he smashed the previous world record by 13 seconds. Jones again won the Chicago Marathon the following year, achieving his own personal best time of 2:07:13 – a result that was just one second slower than the world record set by Portuguese runner Carlos Lopes at the Rotterdam Marathon earlier that year.

The second time Chicago was home to the world record came 15 years later, in 1999, when Moroccan-American marathon runner Khalid Khannouchi sped into sporting history, becoming the first runner to surpass the 2:06 mark, winning in a time of 2:05:42.

As for the women's race, the world record was broken in two consecutive years. The first, in 2001, was a win by Kenyan marathon runner Catherine Ndereba, who crossed the line in 2:18:47. The following year, British athlete Paula Radcliffe smashed that, winning in a time of 2:17:18 – a course record that, at the time of writing, still stands.

Kenyan distance runner Dennis Kimetto then took the course record in the men's event, when he crossed the line in 2013 in a time of 2:03:45.

While the Chicago Marathon is famed for its flat course and PB potential, and despite the fact that over the years there have been some nail-biting finishes, some participants decide to take on the 26.2 miles at a decidedly slower pace. This was the case back in 1981, but, with a cut-off time of 3.30 p.m., what's to be done? The answer was simple for two Chicago Marathon wannabes: while the rest of the runners that day were most likely still asleep, the two got up and began to tackle the course at 2 a.m. They walked their way to the finish line – joined along the way by the other 5,400 participants, who began the race at the regular starting time.

These days, the entry regulations require everyone to begin at the designated start time, but there is still a marathon cut-off: in order to clock a finish time and bag yourself a medal, you must be able to complete the course in six and a half hours.

"As well as many runners clocking PBs here, the Chicago Marathon has also been the setting for four world records"

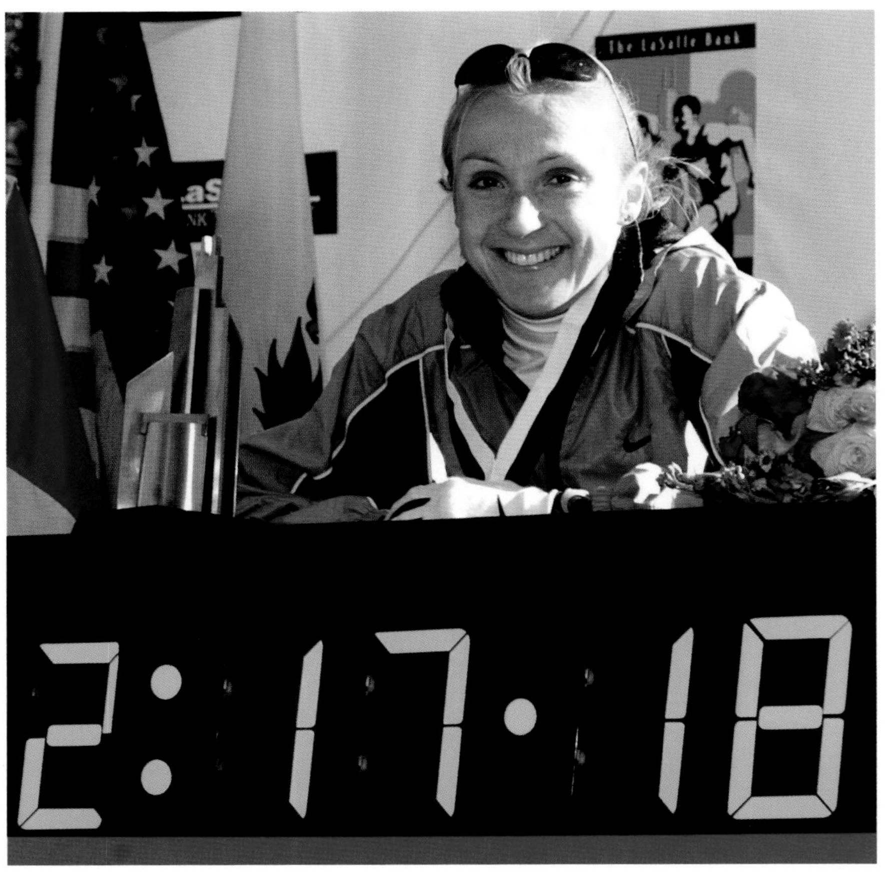

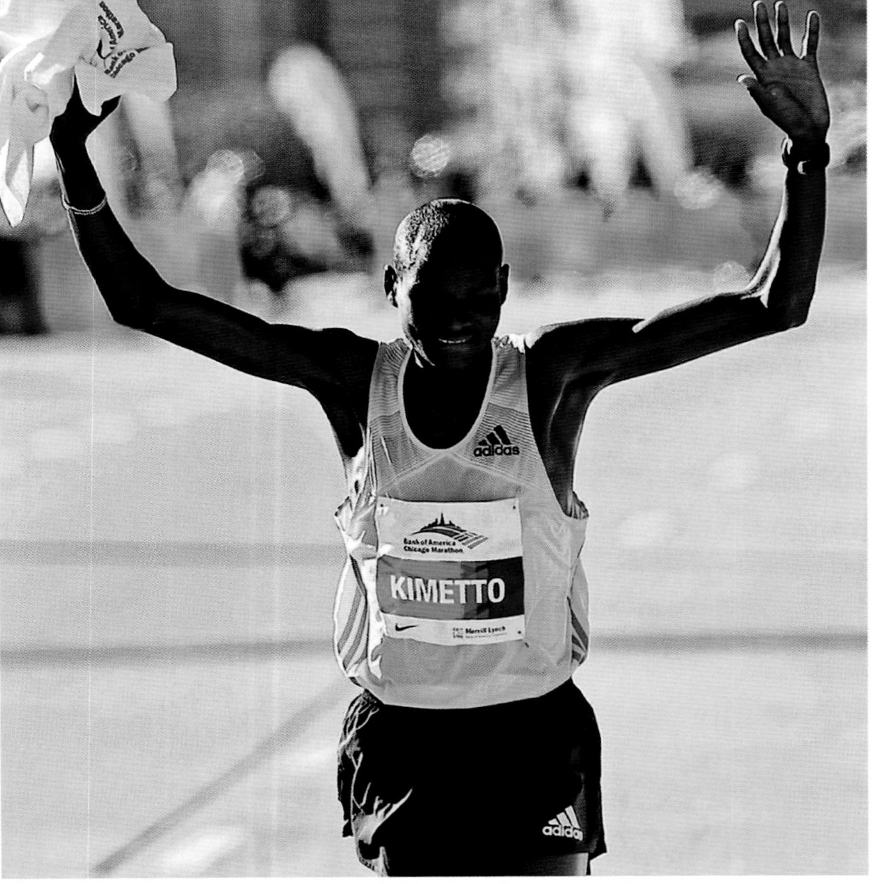

HISTORIC MOMENTS

During its time, the Chicago Marathon has certainly seen its fair share of drama. In 2006, despite winning the men's race in a time of 2:07:35, Kenyan athlete Robert Kipkoech Cheruiyot did not actually break through the tape at the finish line. Instead, he accidentally slipped and fell just before. However, the trajectory of his fall propelled him forwards and he slid under the tape, allowing his timing chip to cross the line. He was ruled as the winner, but he badly injured his head when he hit the ground, suffering a brain contusion and having to be helped from the course with the aid of a wheelchair. He spent the following two days in hospital, for observation.

In 2007, the unseasonably warm weather caused chaos out on the marathon course. The average temperature in the city in October is around 17 °C. However, in that year, the temperature peaked at an astonishing 30 °C. This affected both elite athletes and amateur marathoners alike.

The frontrunners ran a competitive race and the men's finish came down to the wire with Kenyan runner Patrick Ivuti pipping Moroccan runner-up Jaouad Gharib to the post by less than a second. However, Ivuti's finishing time of 2:11:11 was the slowest winning time in 12 years. Female winner Ethiopia's Berhane Adere crossed the line in 2:33:49 – the slowest female winning time in 15 years. Both these results are a good indication of the tough racing conditions.

However, it wasn't only the elite athletes who struggled that day. Some 300 runners required medical attention along the course, and, tragically, one runner died (it was later confirmed the runner had an existing heart condition). When race conditions were deemed too dangerous and many of the water stations ran out of water – officials decided to cancel the event approximately three and a half hours into the race, to ensure runner safety. This resulted in only 25,534 participants making it to the finish line, despite the race welcoming its largest-ever field to the start line (36,867 runners).

◤ British runner Paula Radcliffe made history in 2002 when she set the marathon world record in Chicago.

◥ Legacy finishers who have run in five of the last ten years gain automatic entry.

◀ 2013 Chicago Marathon winner Dennis Kimetto soaks up the crowd's adulation.

▶ Its global appeal and reputation means that Chicago attracts runners from all over the world.

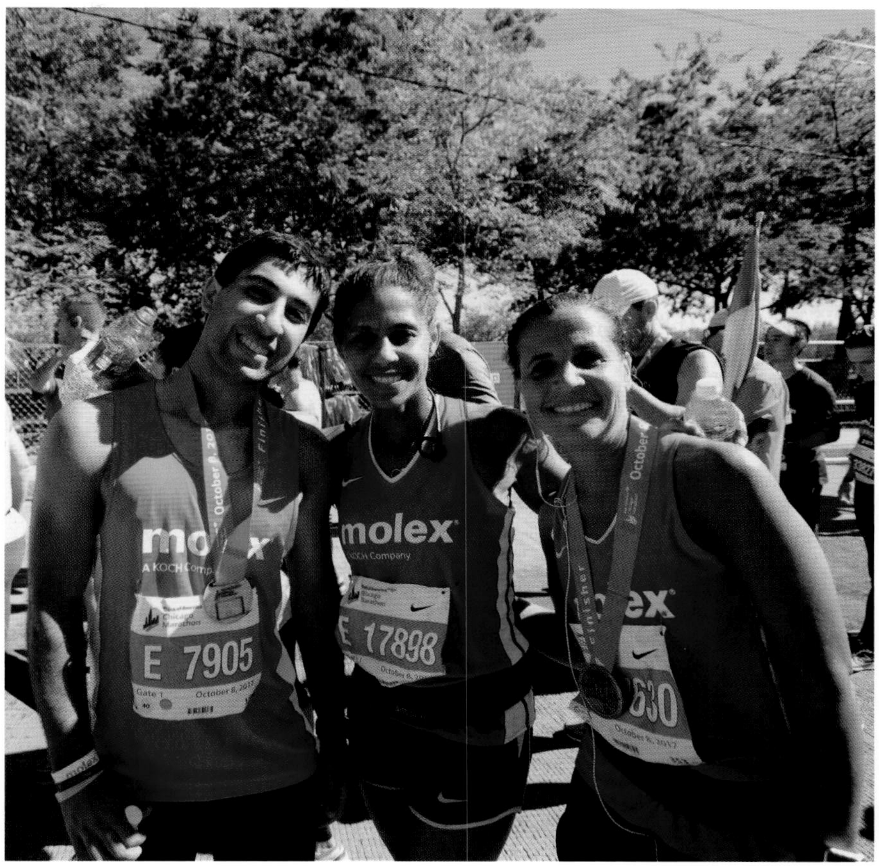

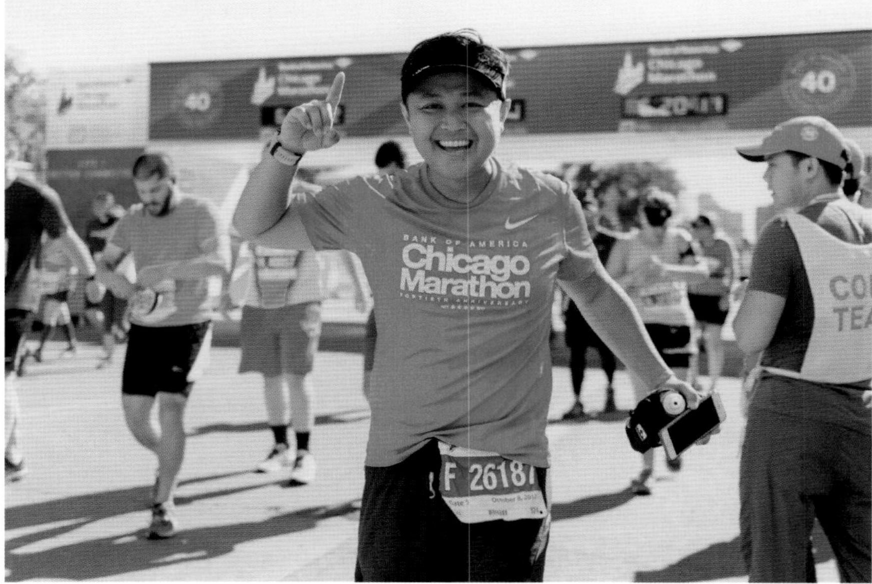

"In 2006, despite winning the men's race in a time of 2:07:35, Kenyan athlete Robert Kipkoech Cheruiyot did not actually break through the tape at the finish line"

RACE ENTRY

There are a few options for entering this marathon, either for guaranteed or non-guaranteed entry. For a non-guaranteed entry, hopeful participants can enter the lottery draw and keep their fingers crossed they win a place.

There are several ways you can get a guaranteed entry into the race. The first is via the charity programme. Each year, approximately 10,000 Chicago Marathon runners decide to do something worthwhile with their marathon place, by raising money for one of the event's registered charities. You will need to apply for your place through your charity of choice. The Chicago Marathon website states that the mandatory fundraising requirements for each charity is $1,000 prior to the entry deadline date or $1,500 after that date, although some charities may set a higher fundraising target.

If you're an international entrant, you can also receive guaranteed entry by purchasing your spot in the race as part of a marathon travel package.

You can also bag yourself guaranteed entry if you've run a qualifying time, based on your age and gender. You must have completed a USATF-certified marathon course within the timeframe from 1 January of the year prior to your application through to the date of your application. A list of qualifying times can be found on the Chicago Marathon website when entries open.

The final way of gaining guaranteed entry is if you qualify as a Chicago Marathon Legacy Finisher: that is, if you have finished the event at least five times during the past ten years.

For all runners, finishing a marathon several times is a huge achievement – and there are six Chicago Marathon runners who have earned the respect of the city, finishing every single race from 1977 up until 2016 – Ron Williams, Joe Antonini, Randy Burt, Henry Kozlowski, Larry Moon and George Mueller (five of the six "alumni" also finished the race in 2017, but Moon had to withdraw after the halfway mark). The six are treated like marathon royalty. Their entry fee is waived and they join the first wave of runners, starting the race just after the elites.

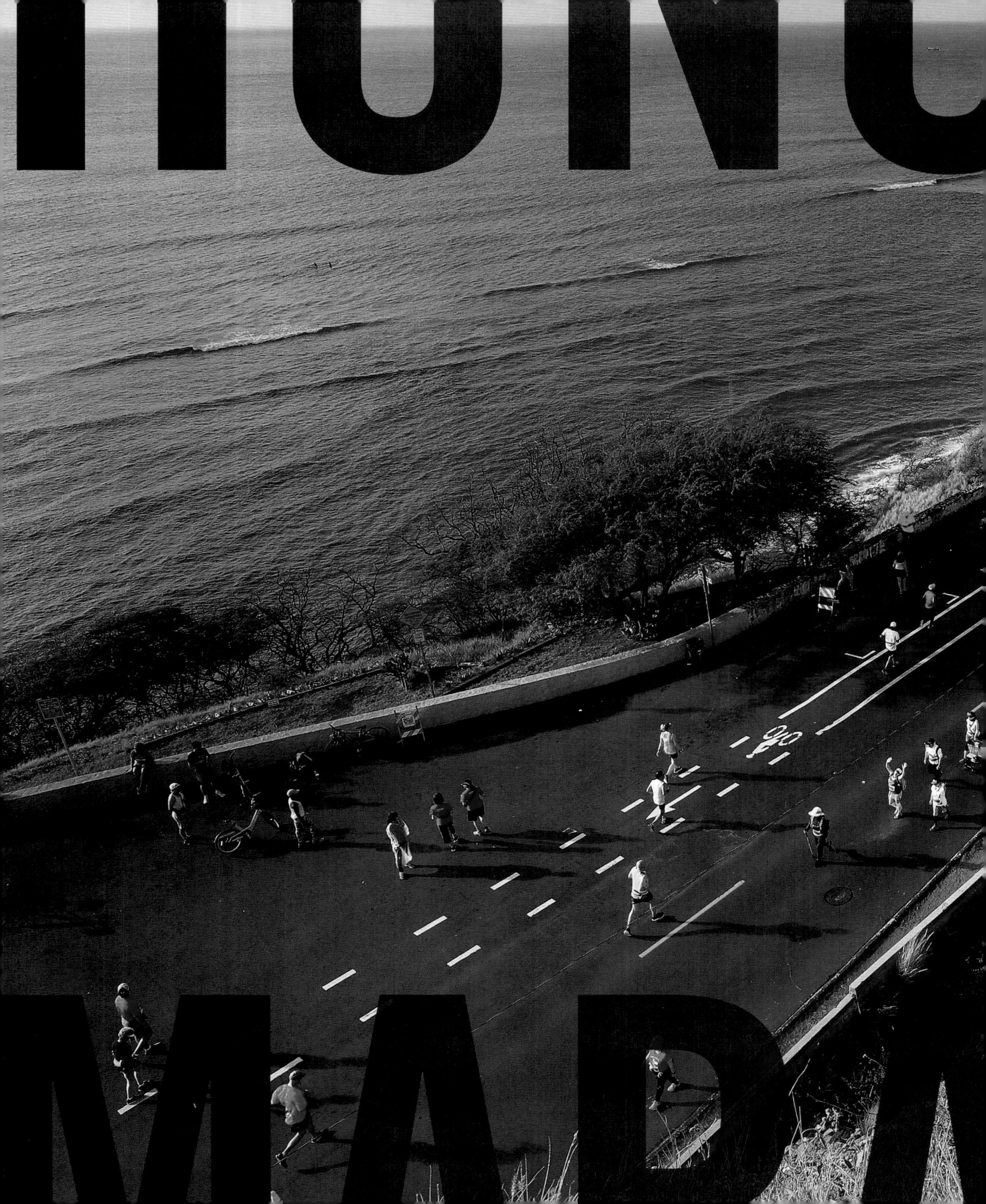

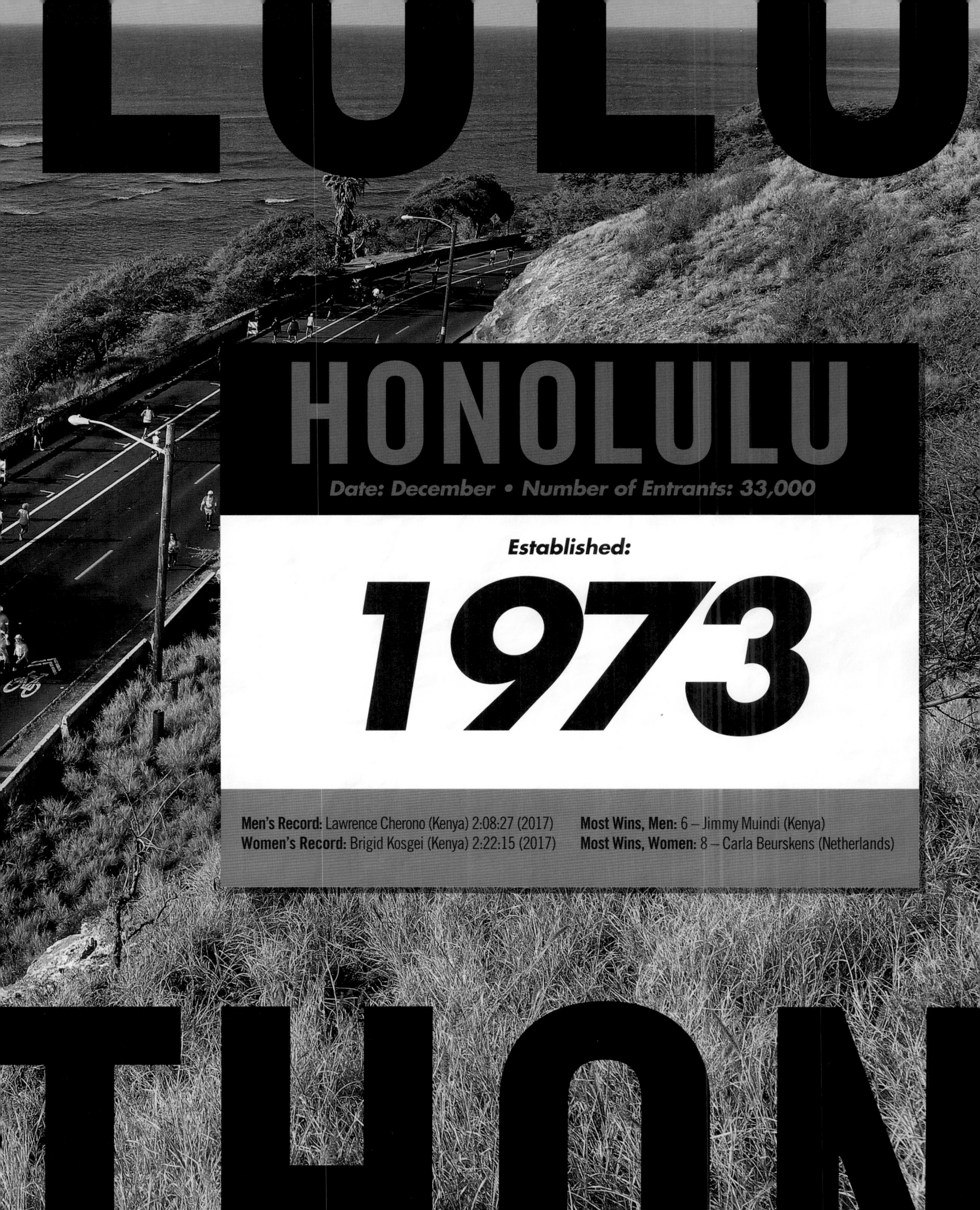
LULU
HONOLULU
Date: December • Number of Entrants: 33,000
Established:
1973
Men's Record: Lawrence Cherono (Kenya) 2:08:27 (2017)
Women's Record: Brigid Kosgei (Kenya) 2:22:15 (2017)
Most Wins, Men: 6 – Jimmy Muindi (Kenya)
Most Wins, Women: 8 – Carla Beurskens (Netherlands)
THON

FINISH
JAL
JAPAN AIRLINES
TOKYO MARATHON 2016
JAL 22853
JAL 3099
JAL 2138
JAL 22727
JAL 18036
JAPAN AIRLINES

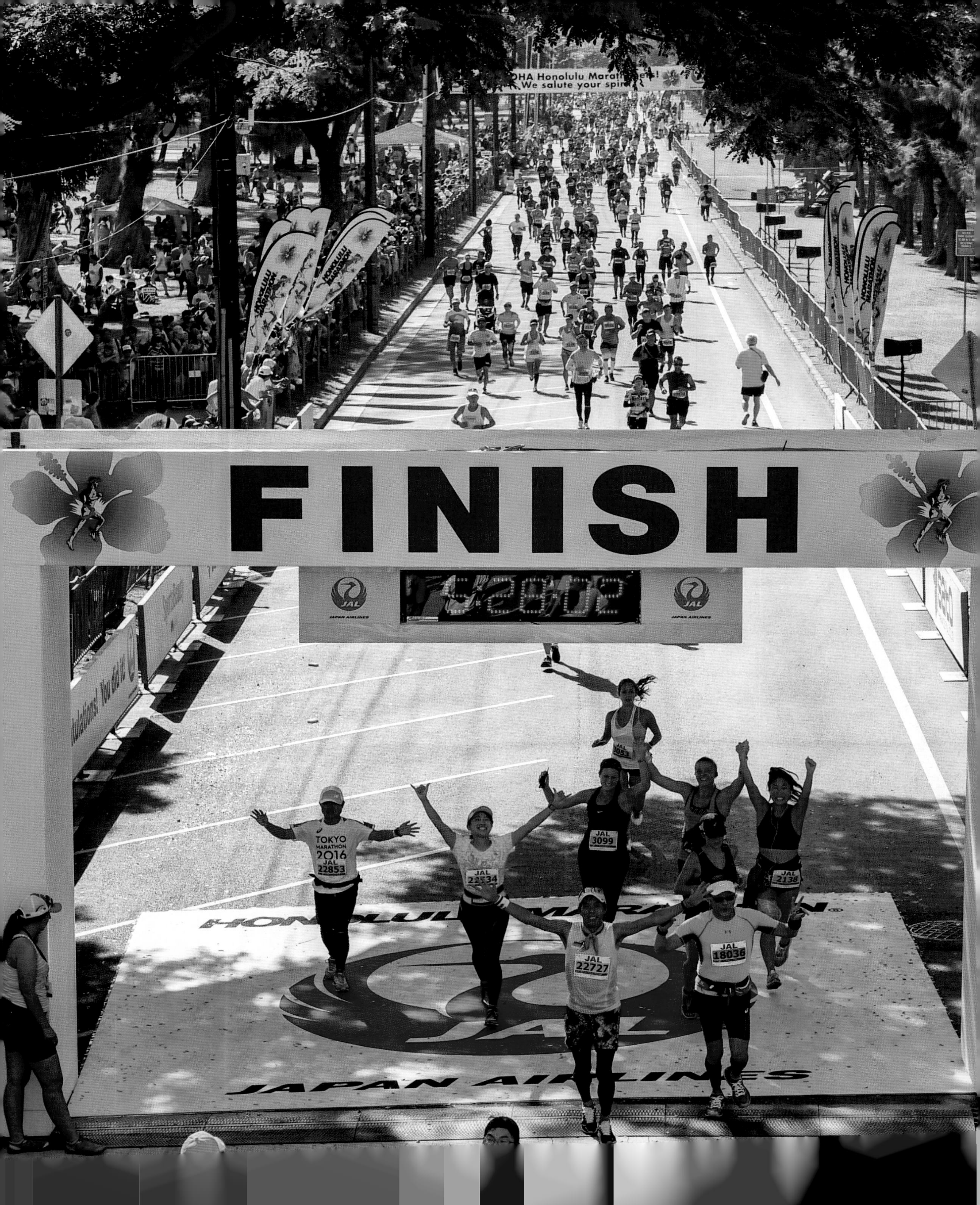

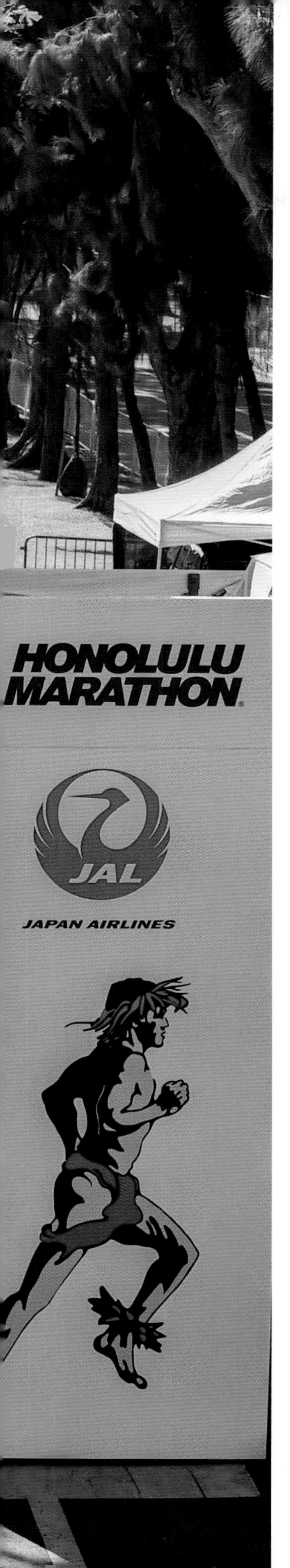

THE HONOLULU MARATHON

A hugely popular marathon with a fun, friendly festival atmosphere, the Honolulu Marathon offers great support and has no time limit for completion. And the setting is one of the world's most spectacular.

This race is currently the fourth-largest marathon in the United States and consistently ranks among the Top 10 largest in the world. It usually takes place annually on the second Sunday of December, amid a fun and friendly weekend festival and beach party. With the time of year clocking an average temperature of 82°F, the race starts at 5 a.m. to help runners avoid the worst of the daytime heat, and, as it starts in the dark, runners are treated to a spectacular fireworks display as they set off on their epic 26.2-mile run.

As well as its beautiful location – the organizers invite you to "run 26.2 miles in paradise" – the Honolulu Marathon's relaxed, laid-back vibe is almost certainly a major factor in its popularity. The welcoming race has no time qualifier to enter and there's also no limit on the number of participants. Instead, it is open to all and, unlike most other large-scale world marathons, it does not set a course time limit. The race stays open until the final competitor has crossed the line, and all finishers are guaranteed a medal and official finisher's T-shirt.

The wonderfully inclusive aspect of the race is most certainly reflected in its statistics. It is a hugely popular event for first-time marathon runners, and, in 2015, approximately 37 per cent of the field had never run a marathon before. It is also a big hit with older generations: in 2014, Honolulu had the largest number of finishers in the 60-plus age category (some 3,326 runners). And, looking back to 2013, it also had the largest number of finishers with a time of six hours or above (10,032) – that's 45 per cent of all finishers. In that year, the final participant crossed the finish line in a time of 19:39:34 – a pace of 45 minutes/mile – and yet the race organizers waited patiently for them to finish. No wonder it's a popular marathon with those who are in no hurry to make it across the finish line.

In fact, the Honolulu Marathon prides itself on supporting and celebrating its final finishers just as much as its frontrunners. In 2017, it was 81-year-old Ayako Hayashi, from Shiki, Japan, who was the final runner across the finish line, at roughly 9.45 p.m. She had been out on the course for a gruelling 16:23:09. While the course was practically empty by 4 p.m., passers-by noticed her and stayed with her for the final five hours of her race, with one fellow runner, Michael Shiroma, turning back and finishing the race with Ayako. It was her seventh consecutive Honolulu Marathon, and she was greeted at the finish line by a crowd of spectators, and rewarded for her mammoth effort with her medal and finisher's T-shirt, plus flowers, a lei (garland of flowers) and a TV interview.

◀ With no time limit for completion, the Honolulu Marathon has a more relaxed atmosphere than many.

"As well as its beautiful location ... the Honolulu Marathon's relaxed, laid-back vibe is almost certainly a major factor in its popularity"

THE HISTORY

The first Honolulu Marathon took place in 1973, founded by former Honolulu mayor Frank Fasi. During the race's first five years, its size doubled annually, seemingly mirroring the increase in the "running boom" of the decade. It has been said that the growth of the Honolulu Marathon – like the growth in the interest in long-distance running itself – came not from a competitive streak, but instead in the pursuit of health, happiness and longevity. In fact, one of the pioneers of the growth of the Honolulu Marathon was cardiologist Jack Scaff – one of the first doctors to prescribe running as a way of both treating and warding off heart disease. This focus on health and happiness for all, no matter what age or ability, is very much reflected in the ethos of the event today, and the marathon prides itself on its inclusivity and support for all entrants.

At the very first race, in 1973, all 167 participants were welcomed and cheered along the course. Some 151 entrants made it to the finish line – including eight-year-old Kris Hilbe. The winner of the inaugural race, Duncan Macdonald, a 24-year-old medical student at the University of Hawaii, crossed the finish line in an impressive 2:27:34, just breaking the state record set back in 1963. The women's division was won by 14-year-old June Chun, who finished in 3:25:51, coming in 47th place overall. It is reported that the crowd of spectators cheered equally for all finishers, from winner Macdonald, right through to the final person to cross the line – a heart-attack survivor who had taken up running to improve their cardiovascular health.

Just five years later, in 1978, the field had grown from 167 to 7,000, with American runners Don Kardong and Patti Lyons winning the men's and women's events, in times of 2:17:05 and 2:43:10, respectively. Lyons actually won the race for four consecutive years, each time beating the women's course record (in 1981, she lowered it to an impressive 2:33:24).

The Honolulu Marathon is a true "destination marathon", and one that's often combined with a holiday for American and international participants alike. Back in 1988, Italian long-distance runner Gianni Poli won the event in a time of 2:12:47 – while on his honeymoon.

As we've already seen, the marathon is popular with first-timers to the 26.2-mile distance, as well as with slower runners due to its lack of cut-off time, but don't be fooled into thinking the race doesn't attract those with a more competitive racing spirit. While the Honolulu Marathon's hilly race profile has excluded it as a setting for world records (something to do with the many volcanic craters), it certainly still attracts a world-class elite field, and many athletes have used it as a springboard to go on to achieve greater feats. In 1993, Korean athlete Bong Ju Lee won the race in a time of 2:13:16. He went on to win the silver medal in the marathon at the 1996 Atlanta Olympic Games.

Kenya's Ibrahim Hussein, who won the Honolulu Marathon three consecutive times,

◢ Spectacular fireworks encourage runners as they make their way around the streets of Honolulu.

▼ 2017 winner Brigid Kosgei (centre) celebrates her victory with Lucy Karimi (left) and Joyce Chepkirui (right).

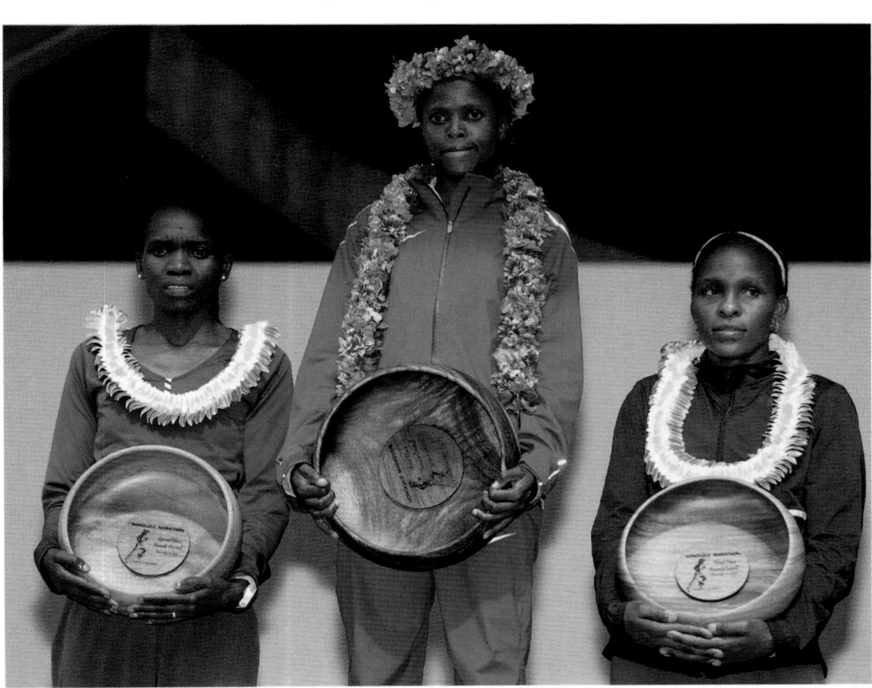

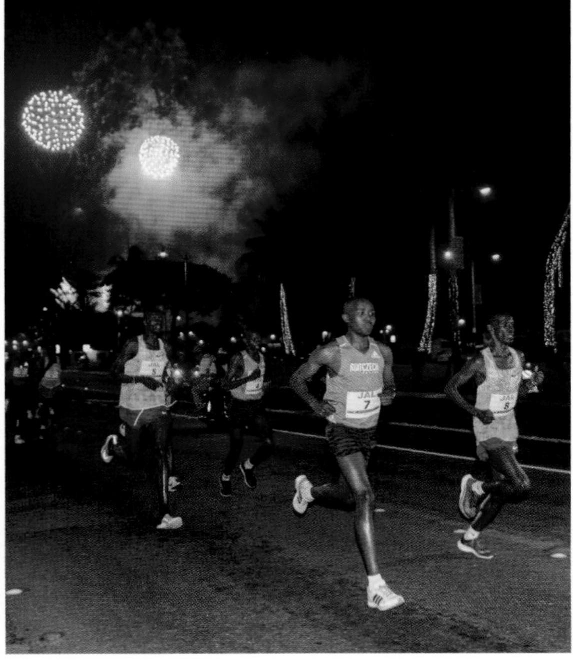

in 1985, 1986 and 1987, also went on to gain success in both World Marathon Majors events and the Commonwealth Games, winning the New York City Marathon in 1987, and coming first in the Boston Marathon an impressive three times, in 1988, 1991 and 1992. He also finished fifth in the marathon at the Commonwealth Games in 1990, in Auckland, New Zealand.

Despite its traditionally challenging race profile, in recent years the Honolulu Marathon's course record has been slashed dramatically. In the 2017 race, both the men's and women's course records were well and truly demolished, with Kenyan athletes Lawrence Cherono and Brigid Kosgei winning in times of 2:08:27 and 2:22:15, respectively. Honolulu Marathon Association's CEO, Dr Jim Barahal, said of the oustanding new course records, "I think we've been seeing . . . that people can run very fast in Honolulu. I think there is a vast talent pool; we are tapping into that next-level pool and people are emerging and [setting] running times that were thought impossible at Honolulu."

THE COURSE

The Honolulu Marathon starts on Ala Moana Boulevard, Hawaiian for "Path by the Ocean" – which is an apt description for the entire marathon. The course heads down to the harbour and past the historic 10-storey Aloha Tower, which was erected in 1926. Runners then turn right into Chinatown and proceed through Downtown Honolulu on South King Street. This historic stretch of the course passes Iolani Palace, the only royal palace on American soil; the gilded statue of King Kamehameha; Kawaiahao Church, built with coral blocks from nearby reefs; Honolulu Hale, city hall; and Mission Houses Museum.

The race forks right onto Kapiolani Boulevard through urban Honolulu and, at Mile 4, turns right down Piikoi Street. The course returns to Ala Moana Boulevard, this time passing Ala Moana Center, a large open-air mall. The bridge spanning the Ala Wai Canal marks the entrance to Waikiki, a concrete jungle of high-rise hotels and condominiums. Just past the Sheraton Moana Surfrider – Waikiki's oldest hotel, built

▼ With more than 30,000 participants every year, the marathon is impossible to ignore if you're in Honolulu.

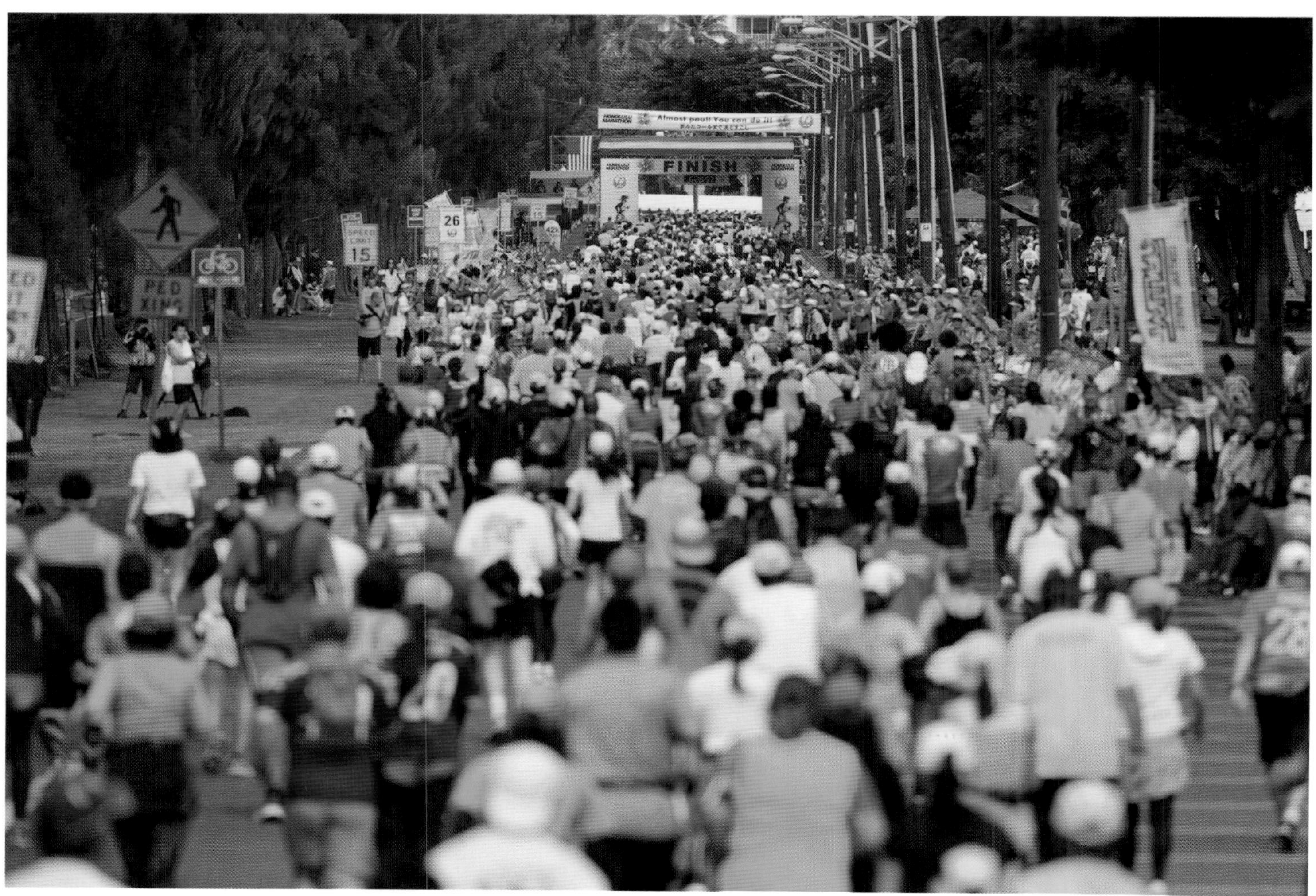

in 1901 – is a spectacular ocean view: world-famous Waikiki Beach. Tourists, sunbathers and surfers flock to this stretch of white sand, often crowding around the statue of Duke Kahanamoku, a renowned surfer and Olympic gold medallist.

Near the sixth mile, the course forks to the left onto Monsarrat Avenue, around the Honolulu Zoo and past the Waikiki Shell. Runners then turn right onto Paki Avenue, which threads around Kapiolani Park, Hawaii's first public park. As the course nears Diamond Head, an extinct volcanic crater some 760 feet high, there are some short, steep inclines. The bonus of this is that runners are rewarded with breathtaking views of Oahu's east coastline. The route circles the crater to the left on Diamond Head Road.

At Mile 10, the race turns right onto Kilauea Avenue, passing through the residential and commercial zone of Kahala, before merging into the Kalanianaole Highway. The coastal route continues for four miles, through the picturesque suburban communities of Waialae Iki, Aina Haina and Niu Valley, with expensive homes often perched on cliffs.

During Mile 16, runners turn left onto Hawaii Kai Drive, with spectacular views of Koko Head ahead – a volcanic crater eroded on one side by the ocean into the popular snorkel spot, Hanauma Bay. The course then turns right back onto Kalanianaole Highway at Maunalua Bay Beach Park, a popular spot for parasailing and outrigger canoes.

For the next four miles, runners double back along Kalanianaole Highway, passing Kawaikui and Wailupe beach parks. At Mile 22, the course turns left onto Kealaolu Avenue along the Waialae Country Club, where the Hawaiian Open PGA Golf Tournament is held. The route then takes in Kahala Avenue, a neighbourhood of luxury homes fronting Kahala Beach and Black Point.

The final mile curves around Diamond Head towards the finish in Waikiki, with the last stretch of the race run along the park past Sans Souci Beach and the Waikiki Aquarium, to the finish line near the Kapiolani Park Bandstand.

"The coastal route continues for four miles, through the picturesque suburban communities of Waialae Iki, Aina Haina and Niu Valley"

▼ Sweeping beaches and panoramic views help the miles fly by for runners.

▶ The dramatic backdrops add a real sense of scale to the Honolulu Marathon.

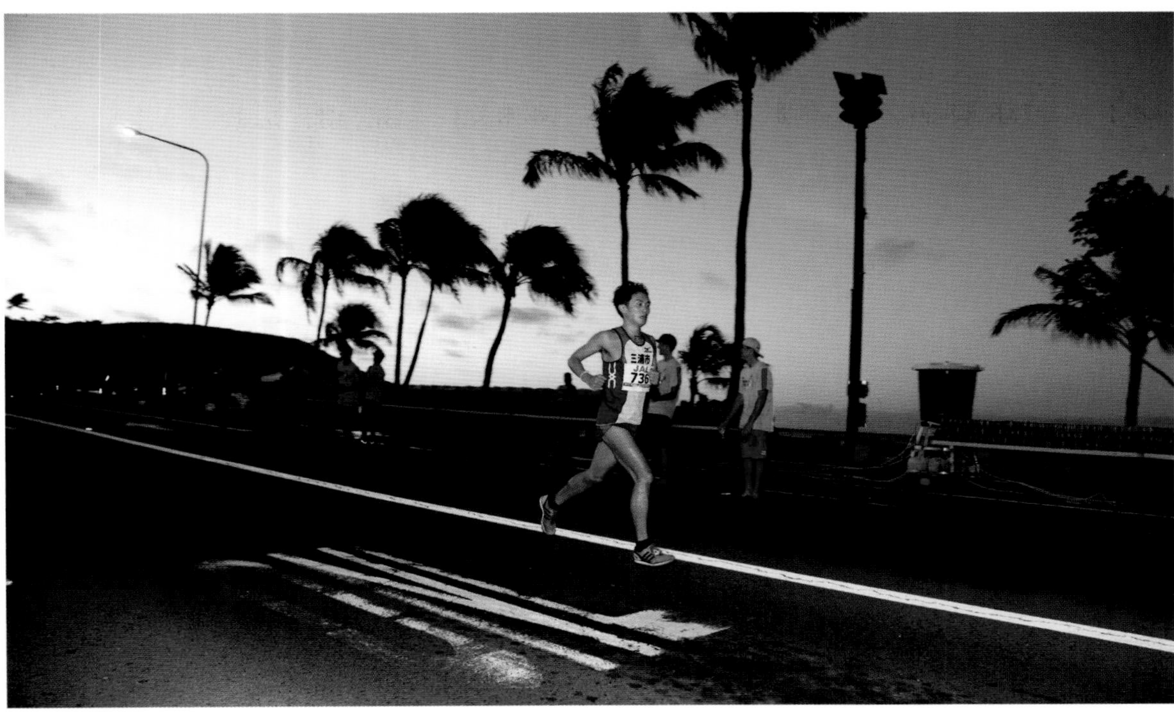

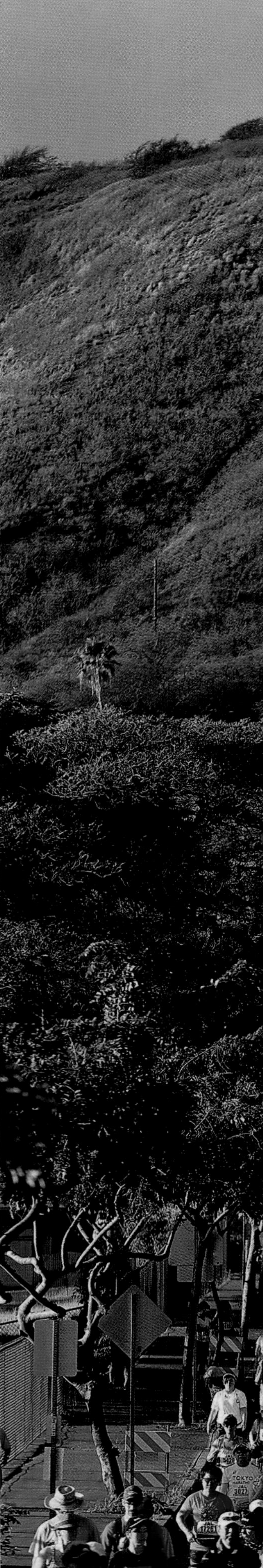

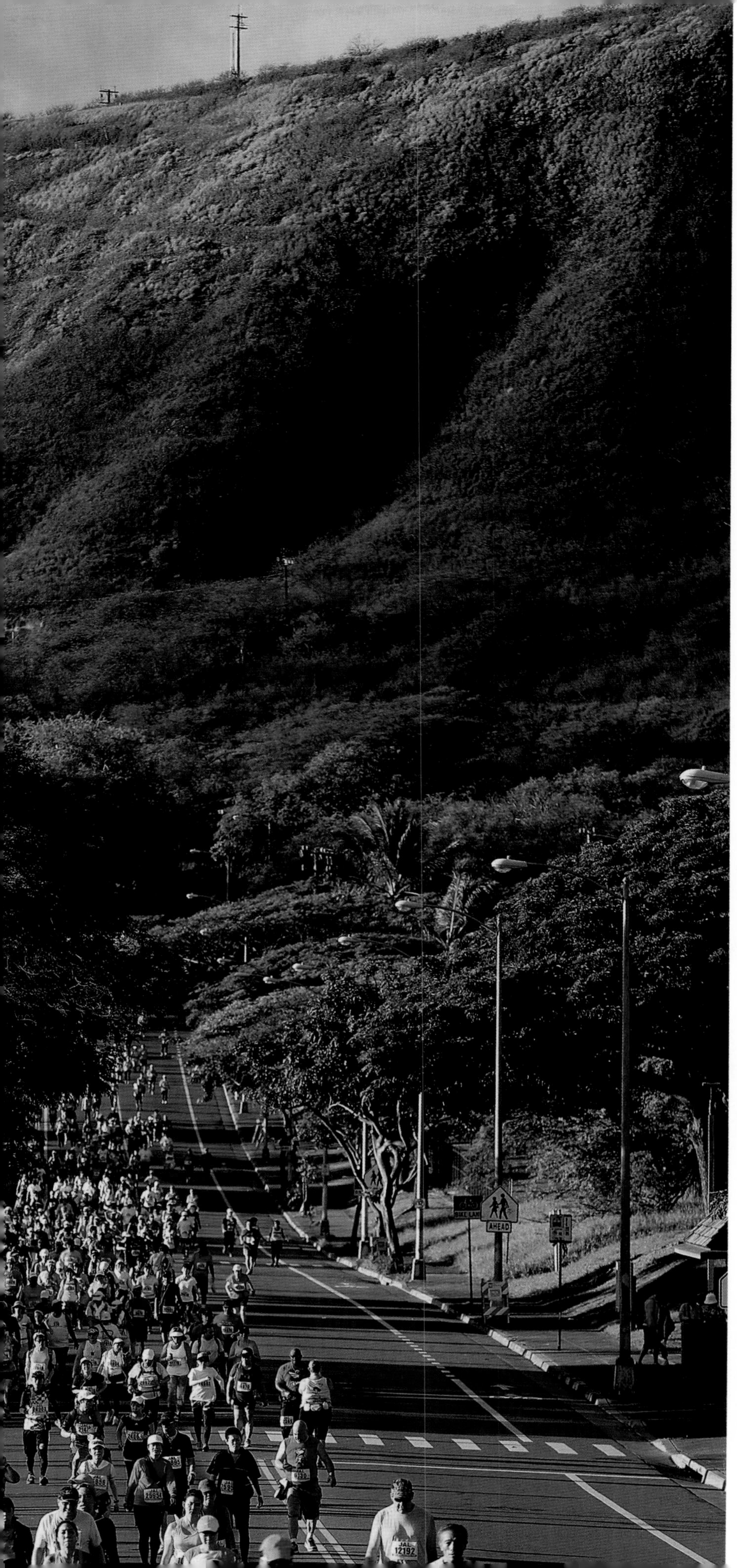

HOW TO ENTER

Since there are no qualifications for the Honolulu Marathon, and there is also no participant limit, there is no need for the usual lottery-style entry system. However, if you would like to fundraise for charity, there is the option of signing up for a VIP Charity Entry. Choosing this option grants free VIP entry into the race, a bespoke fundraising medal, access to the VIP runner lounge at the Marathon Expo, and more.

There is a discounted entry for US active-duty military and their dependents, and due to the fact that there is always such a high number of entrants from Japan, there is a designated Japanese Honolulu Marathon registration system.

If you'd like the experience of running in Honolulu, but don't quite fancy the full marathon distance, a 10km option is available – the "Start to Park 10K" – which has the same start time as the Sunday marathon, and also the Kalakaua Merrie Mile, which takes place on the Saturday morning before the main event. This one-mile fun run is open to all marathon and 10km entrants, as well as family and friends, and children of all ages, and culminates in a party on Queen's Beach.

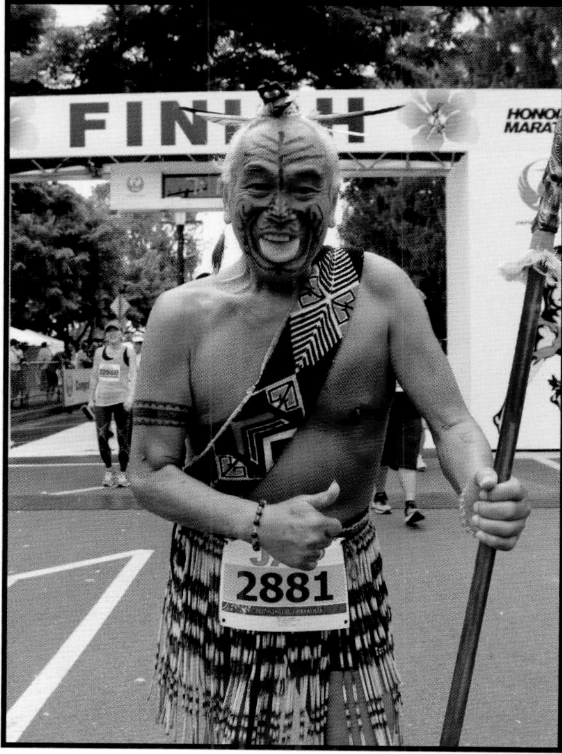

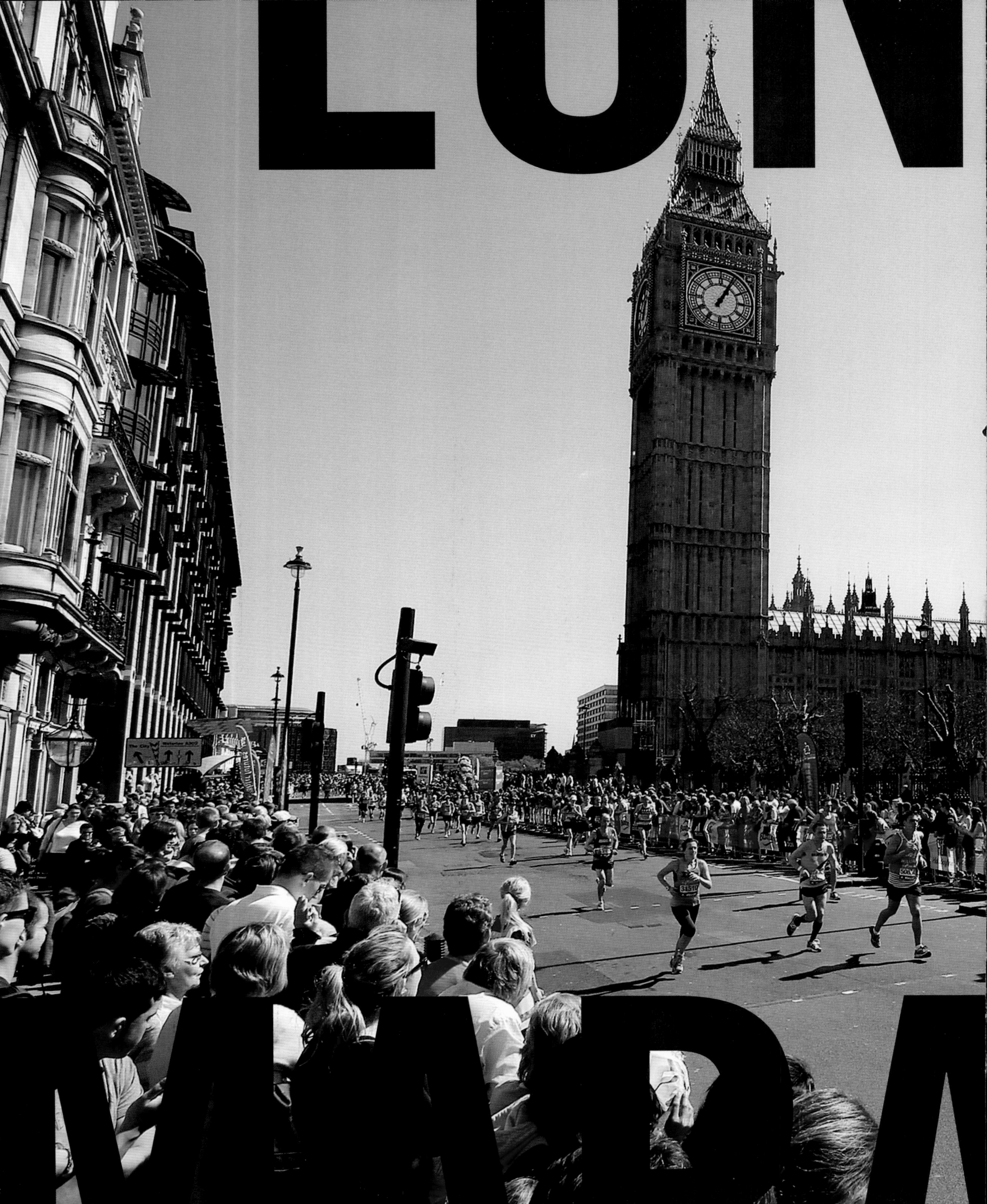

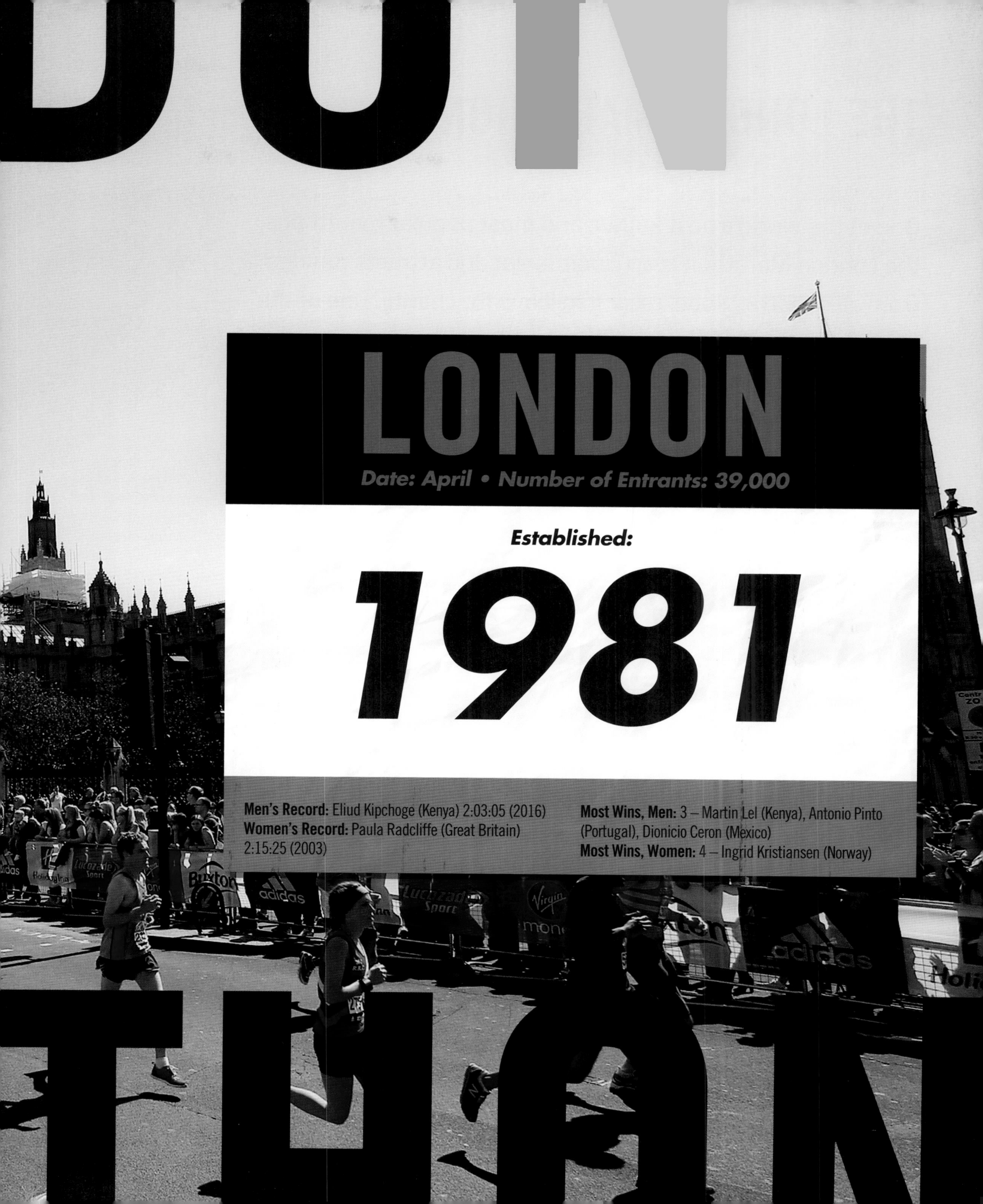

LONDON
Date: April • Number of Entrants: 39,000
Established:
1981
Men's Record: Eliud Kipchoge (Kenya) 2:03:05 (2016)
Women's Record: Paula Radcliffe (Great Britain) 2:15:25 (2003)
Most Wins, Men: 3 – Martin Lel (Kenya), Antonio Pinto (Portugal), Dionicio Ceron (Mexico)
Most Wins, Women: 4 – Ingrid Kristiansen (Norway)

THE LONDON MARATHON

One of the world's best known and most popular marathons, the London Marathon is an iconic event and attracts runners from all over the globe, raising millions for charity. One of the largest fundraising events in the world, it has reportedly raised a massive £770 million since launch.

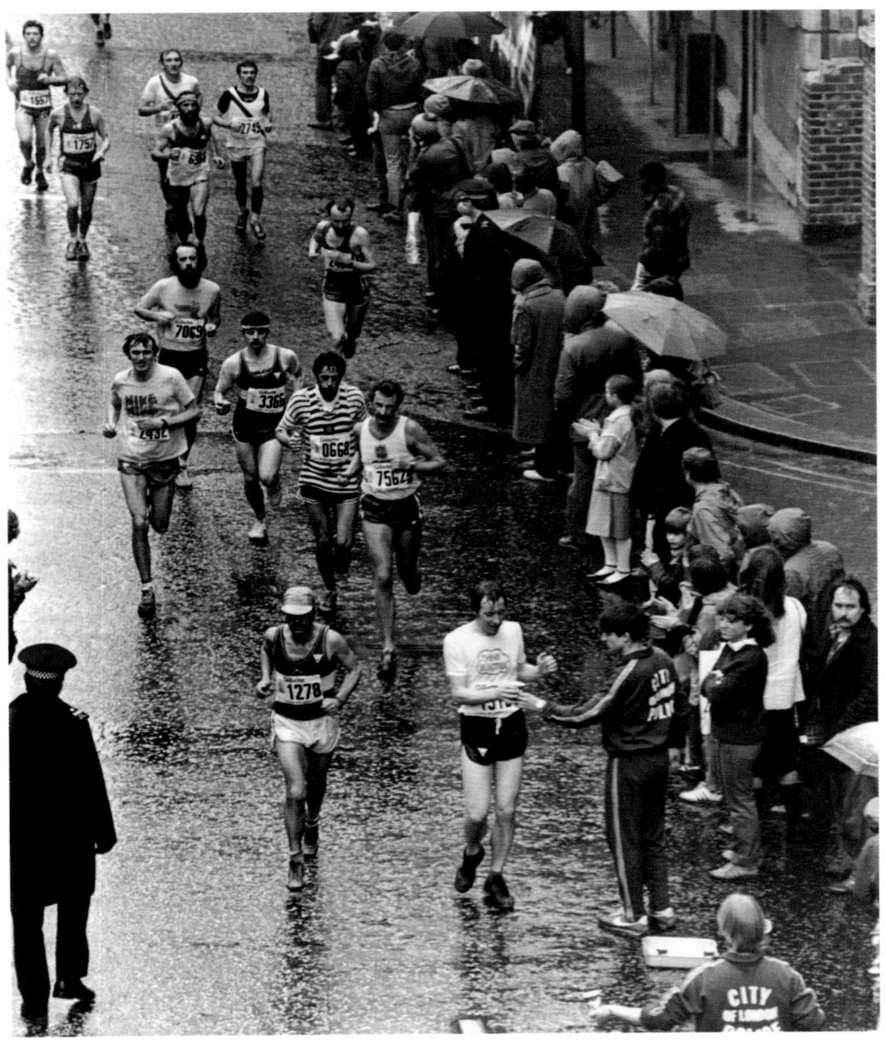

▲ Unsurprisingly for it's location, it rained heavily during the first ever London Marathon in 1981.

▶ These days the sun is more often than not shining on the runners as they cross over Tower Bridge.

THE HISTORY

The London Marathon is clearly a huge success story and has come a long way since it was first held way back at the start of the eighties. When the very first London Marathon took place in March 1981, more than 20,000 runners applied to take part but only 7,747 were accepted, so, even then, it was a popular choice for many. The race was the brainchild of former Olympic champion, Chris Brasher, who was also a journalist, and his friend, John Disley. Both were inspired after entering and completing the New York Marathon in 1979, which Brasher described in an article for the *Observer* as "The World's Most Human Race".

Brasher concluded his article by saying he wondered "whether London could stage such a festival". Disley was equally inspired. He returned from New York, raving about the "laughter", "cheers" and "suffering" during the New York marathon and referred to it as the "greatest folk festival the world has ever seen". The pair returned together to America to find out more about how the big marathons were organized and began to devise the course for the London Marathon.

They designed a route for the very first marathon using the Thames as what they called a "handrail", which would involve closing just two bridges. One of them was Tower Bridge, which was closed on Sundays anyway. A course that took in many sights, including Cutty Sark, Tower Bridge, the Embankment, Big Ben and Buckingham Palace was approved by the police, but the chairman of the Greater London Council (GLC) warned the pair that ratepayers would never bail the race out. It had to be self-sufficient. So Brasher turned to his

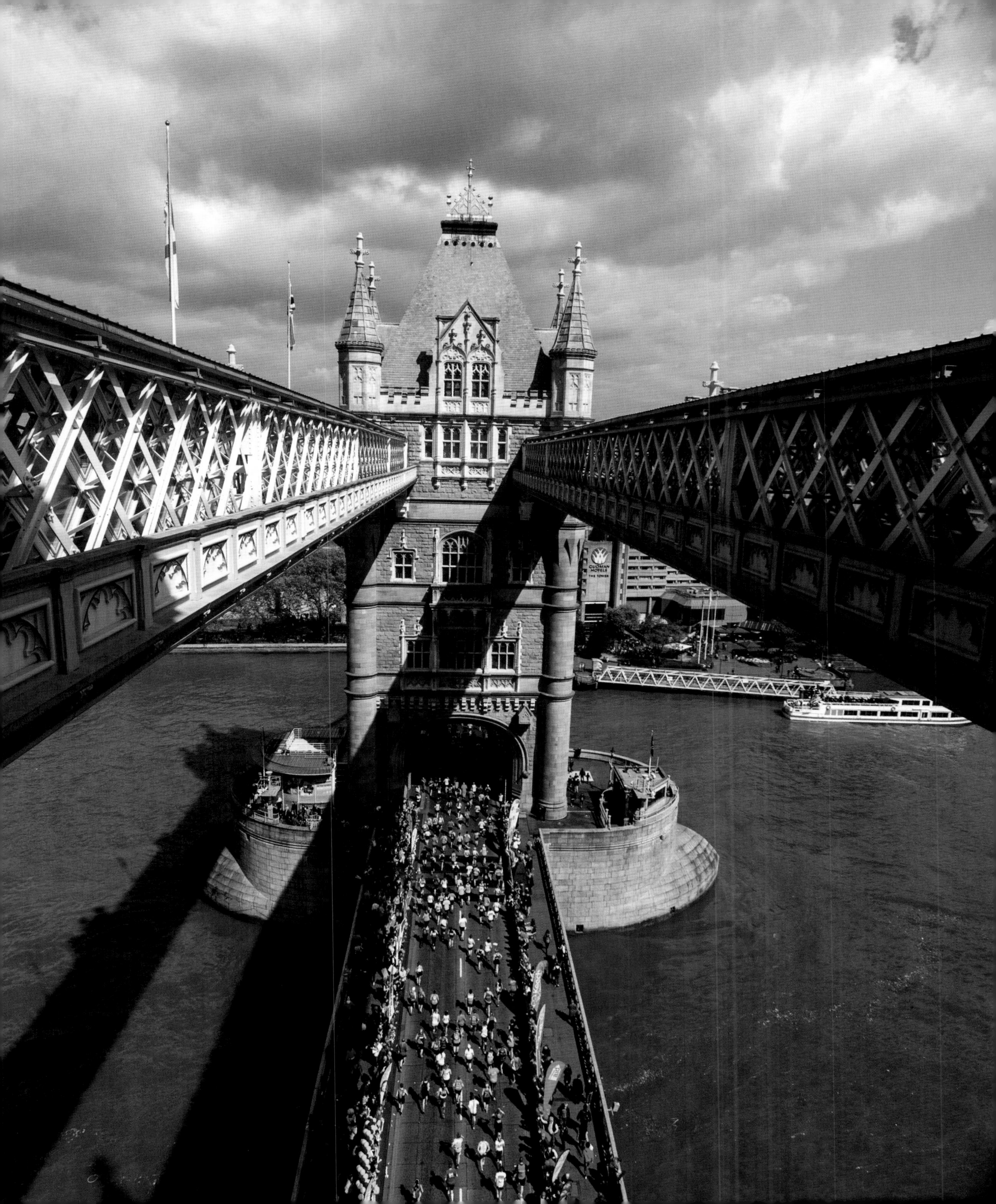
GUOMAN HOTELS
THE TOWER

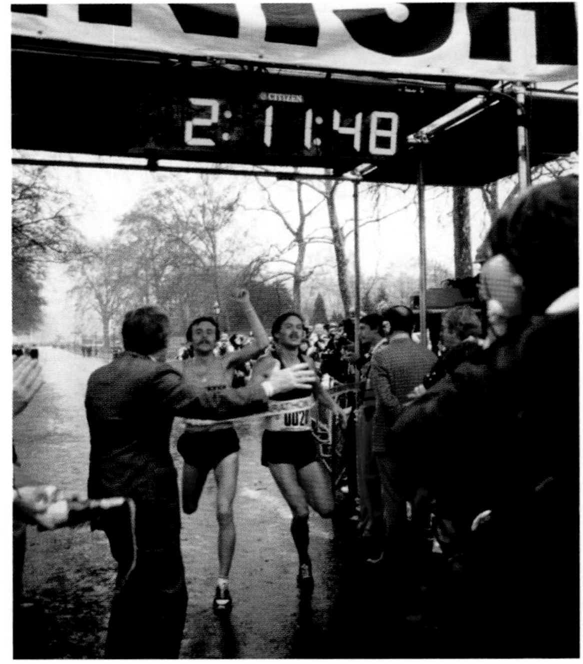

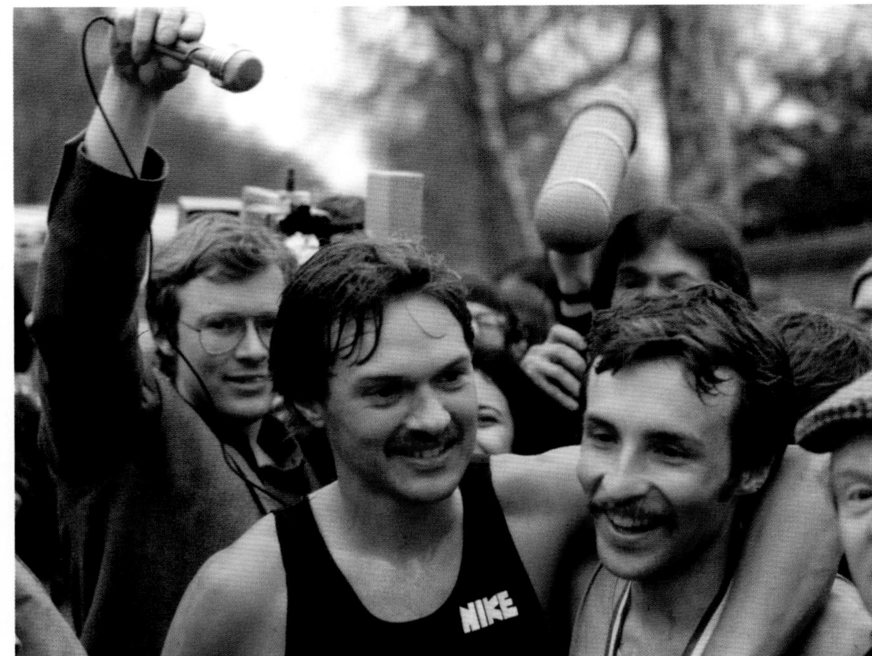

▲ Inge Simonsen, (left) and Dick Beardsley (right) celebrate becoming the joint winners of the inaugural London Marathon.

◤ Simonsen and Beardsley cross the finish line at exactly the same moment, in a time of 2:11:48.

wife and asked if they could take out a second mortgage on their house.

Thankfully, they didn't need to do this, as sponsorship was secured from Gillette, who had just pulled out from a cricket sponsorship; the initial race budget was £75,000. Disley and Brasher had a vision for the London Marathon, and they knew what they wanted it to stand for. They wanted the marathon to have a fast, flat course; to raise money for local sporting facilities in London; and to boost tourism, putting Britain on the map for organizing major sporting events.

Five months later, the first-ever London Marathon took place on 29 March 1981. Out of the 7,747 entrants, there were 6,255 finishers. Incredibly, and perhaps fittingly given what the Marathon was to become, there was a dead heat between American long-distance runner Dick Beardsley and Norwegian distance runner Inge Simonsen in the men's category (finishing in 2:11:48). The pair even held hands as they crossed the finish line in joint-first place. In the women's category, 43-year-old mother-of-two Joyce Smith came first with an impressive time of 2:29:57.

Another notable entrant was former long-distance runner David Bedford, who had enjoyed considerable success as an athlete in the 1970s. Bedford made a snap decision to enter the first London Marathon while drinking in a Luton nightclub. He bet a friend that he would be able to complete the race the next day, then rang his friend Chris Brasher, to ask him for a race number. Brasher replied that it was too late, but Bedford turned up anyway, having had a curry on the way home from the nightclub in the early hours. He ran the London Marathon after just 15 minutes of sleep, throwing the curry up at the halfway point, a sight that was captured on television cameras worldwide. Bedford went on to be the race director for the London Marathon for 19 years, eventually stepping down in 2012.

THE COURSE

The London Marathon course has changed only very slightly over the years. It's a largely flat course around the River Thames and has markers at one-mile intervals. It begins at various points in different waves – the "red" start is in Greenwich, the "green" start is in St John's Park, and the "blue" start is on Shooter's Hill Road. The route heads east through Charlton and the three courses come together after nearly three miles in Woolwich.

At the 10K mark, the course goes past the Old Royal Naval College and Cutty Sark, before moving into Deptford and Surrey Quays. Then it goes through Bermondsey and crosses the halfway point at Tower Bridge, a popular spot for those watching the marathon, and one that TV viewers will know plays host to cameras, where many charity and celebrity runners are accosted by a TV presenter and interviewed about their progress. At Tower Bridge, the noise from the crowds is deafening but the entire course offers incredible crowd support, with spectators yelling at runners to continue, even if they stop to tie a shoelace or take an energy gel. The noise and cheering can become overwhelming at times,

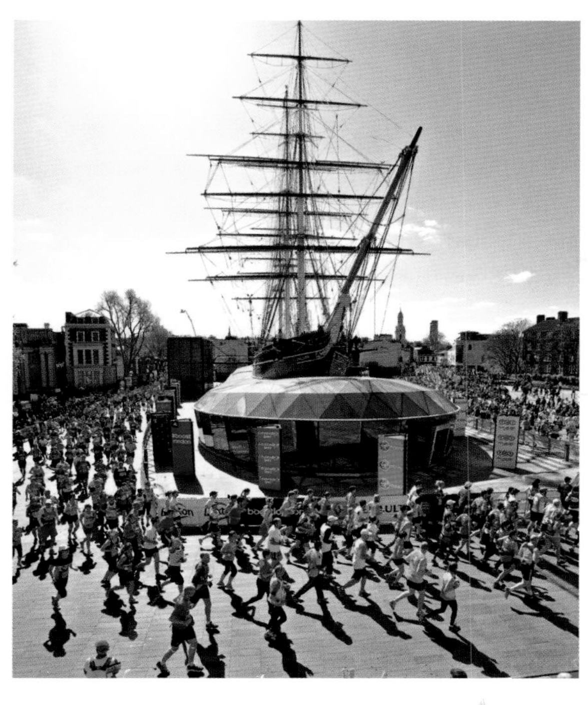

▲ London Marathon runners get a panoramic view of the Cutty Sark on their route.

▼ Support outside the Houses of Parliament is particularly strong.

but the support is most welcome during the later stages of the race.

Later stages go through Blackfriars, Victoria Embankment and Temple, before turning into Westminster. The final stage of the course covers St James's Park and the finish line is located at The Mall on the approach to Buckingham Palace, where the cheering is again overwhelming.

The London Marathon is not just a marathon, but a great example of human spirit and camaraderie, as exemplified in 2017 when club runner David Wyeth's legs were beginning to give way. He was battling to reach the finish line in the final stages, when fellow runner Matthew Rees slowed down and gave up his own race time to support him to the finish line.

A huge part of the London Marathon's appeal is the stories of the runners who enter to fundraise, and the array of outrageous costumes. Expect to see any type of costume you can think of, from superheroes to rhinos, birds, pantomime horses and cows. Previous entrants have included a woman with her face protruding through a Mona Lisa picture frame and another woman running as a giant toilet roll.

In 2012, Lloyd Scott, a 40-year-old former professional goalkeeper from Rainham in Essex, walked the London Marathon wearing an antique diving suit that weighed around 130lb. It took him six days and he raised over £100,000 for the charity CLIC – Cancer and Leukaemia in Childhood, a condition he had himself as a child. Scott had already previously completed the London

Marathon, making his debut in 1989, just three weeks after having a bone-marrow transport for leukaemia. Amusingly, Scott also set the record for the slowest-ever marathon time. After that, the London Marathon organisers reviewed the rules and decided that the marathon had to be completed by 6 p.m. the same day.

Celebrities are a huge part of the London Marathon story. Triumphs have included boxer Michael Watson, who had spent 40 days in a coma and suffered brain damage after being struck during a boxing match in 1991 by Chris Eubank. Watson was forced to use a wheelchair for six years while recovering, and had endured six operations to remove a brain clot, yet he completed the London Marathon in 2003. It took him six days and two hours, and Chris Eubank completed the last mile with him.

Former rower and double Olympic medallist James Cracknell first ran the London Marathon in 2006 in a formidable time of three hours, finishing an hour ahead of his former rowing teammate, Matthew Pinsent. Four years later, he suffered brain damage when he was struck by a lorry in the US, while attempting to cycle, run and row across the country in 18 days. After recovering, he has since gone on to run the London Marathon several times. He completed it in 2:50:43 in 2015, narrowly beating Formula 1 racing driver Jenson Button, who ran it in 2:52:30, and raising money for the brain-injury charity Headway.

There have been many older runners who have completed the London Marathon. Jenny Wood-Allen completed the race in 2002 in 11 hours and 34 minutes at the age of 90, while the oldest male finisher remains Fauja Singh, who completed the course at the age of 93 in a time of 6:07 in 2004. His best marathon time is 5:40 at the age of 92. He went on to run the Toronto Waterfront Marathon at the age of 100.

The marathon also attracts many of the world's best athletes. Paula Radcliffe not only set a women's world record in 2003, when she ran the London Marathon in 2:15:25, but also knocked 1:53 off her marathon time in October the previous year. Athlete Mo Farah was only 15 when he ran the Mini Marathon for the first time and went on to run it another two times. In 2014, he ran the London Marathon for the first time and finished eighth, with a time of 2:08:21.

But you don't need to be an athlete to run the London Marathon. If you can secure a ballot place, or obtain a place via a charity close to your heart, you can be assured of endless, almost deafening crowd support on virtually every stage of this flat, fast course, as well as an experience that will stay with you for a lifetime. Just don't get too demoralized if you get overtaken by a purple Rhino!

▼ London is an extremely inclusive race, welcoming runners of all abilities and from all walks of life.

▶ When runners reach Buckingham Palace and The Mall, they know the end is in sight.

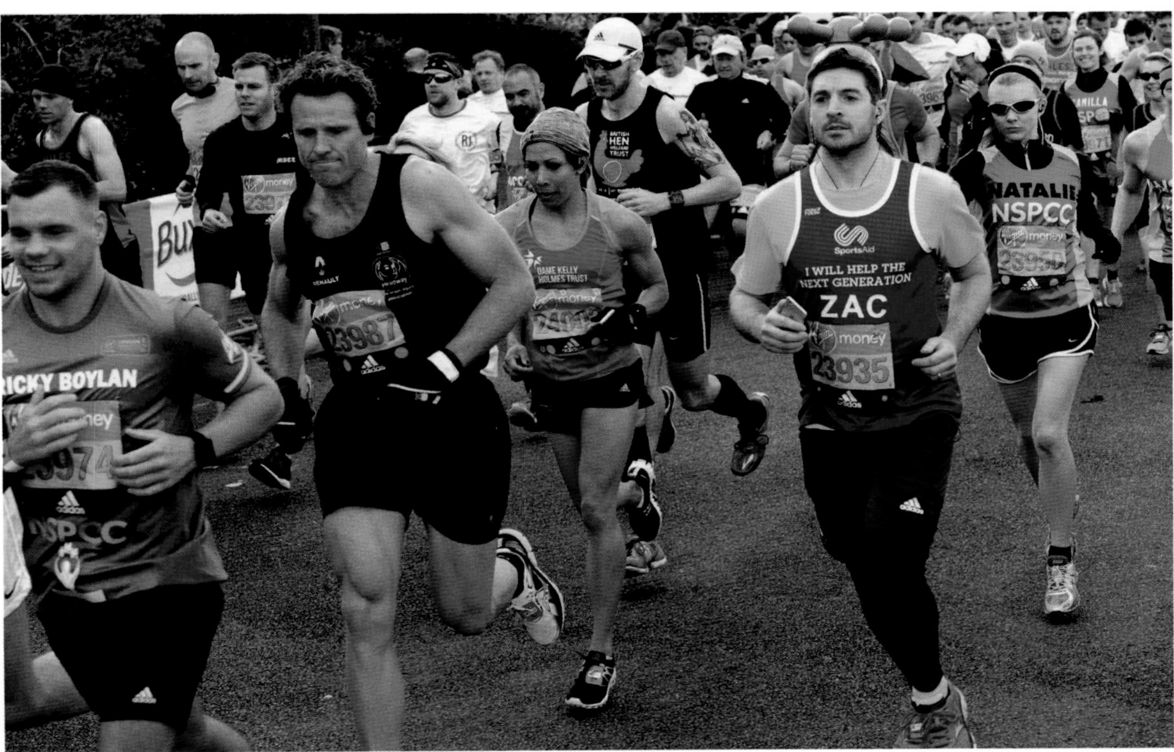

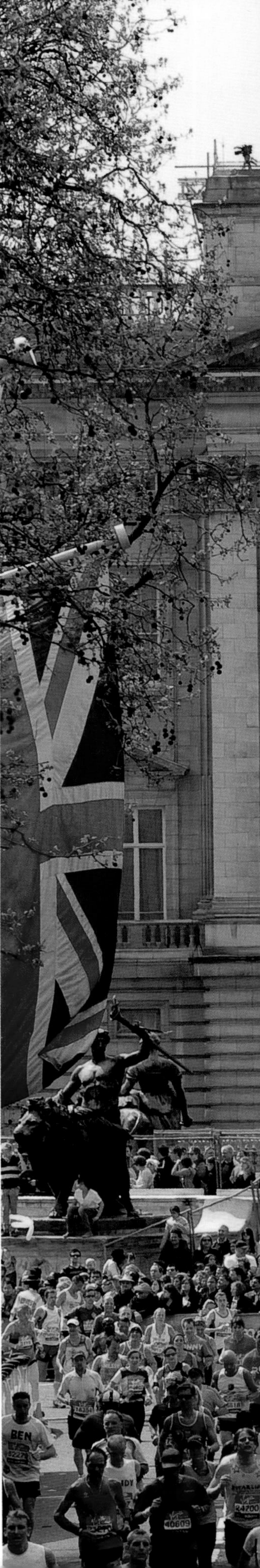

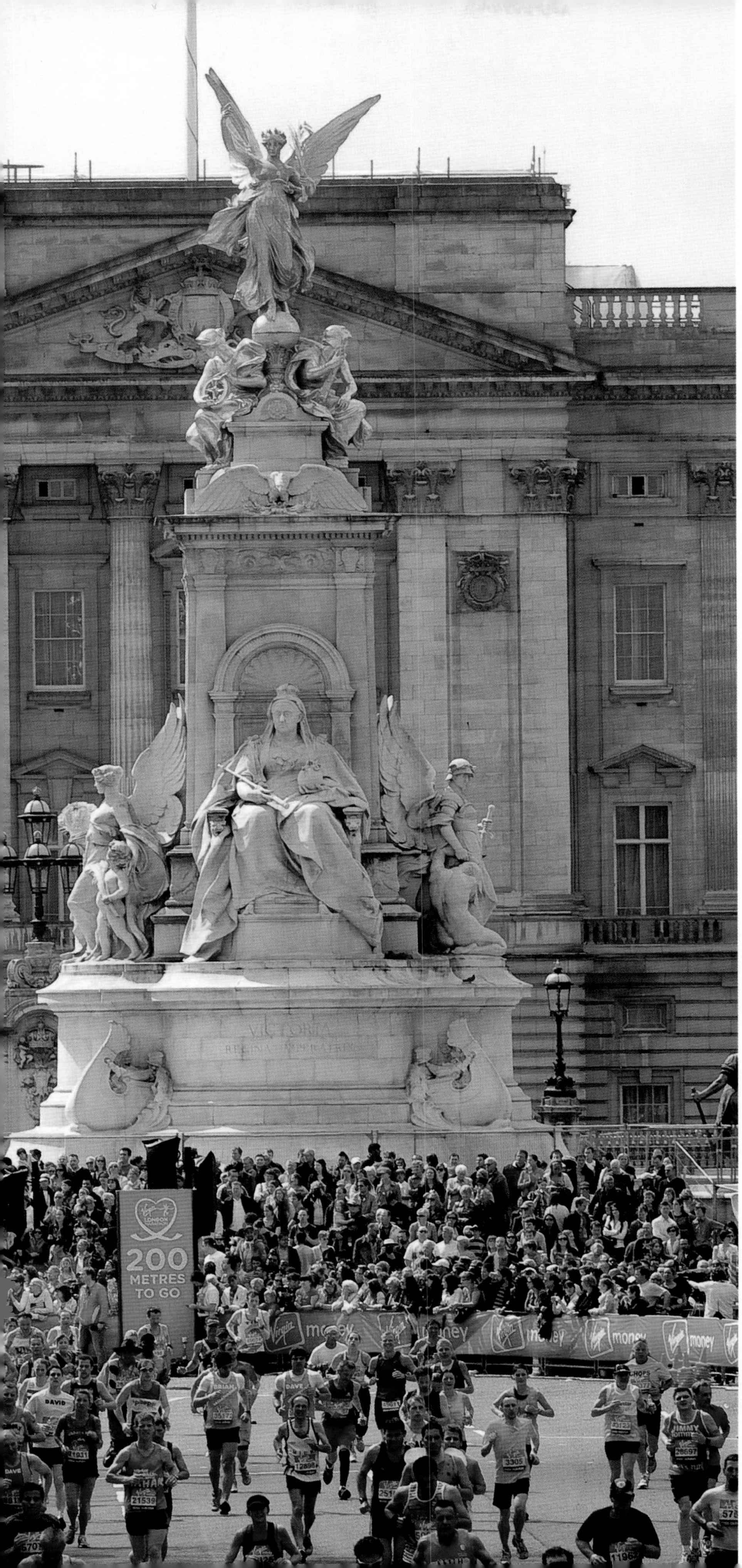

THE BALLOT

The London Marathon can be a notoriously difficult race to get into, as it has a ballot that is entirely random. Around 17,500 runners are accepted from the ballot; in 2018, more than 386,000 runners applied for a ballot place. The ballot usually closes in early May, with applicants notified by October as to whether they have been successful or not.

If you're not fortunate enough to secure a place in the ballot, you may be able to get a Golden or Silver Bond place through a charity, which entails contacting the charity directly and applying for a place. If you are accepted by the charity, you will be expected to raise a considerable sum of money, usually around £2,000 to £2,500. Many people use the marathon as a chance to fundraise for causes close to their hearts, knowing that having a strong, personal reason to complete the race will motivate them to get out and train during the cold winter months. When you don't feel like doing that long three-hour pre-race training run, you'll be sure to find the motivation if you're fundraising for a cause you truly believe in.

Another way to gain entry into the London Marathon is to obtain a "Good For Age" entry. In the men's category, a male runner aged 18–40 will need to have completed a marathon in sub-3:05; a runner aged 41–49 will need to have completed one in sub-3:15; and a runner aged 50–59 will need to have completed a sub-3:20-hour marathon. In the women's category, a female aged 18–40 will need to have run a marathon in sub-3:45; a female aged 41–49 will need to have run one in sub-3:50; and a female aged 50–59 will need to have run a marathon in sub-4:00.

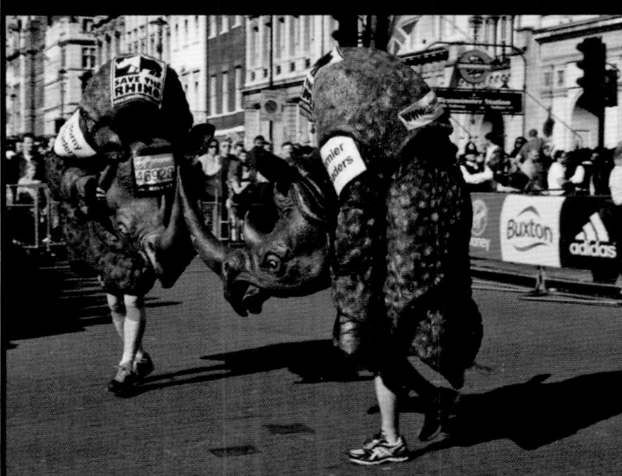

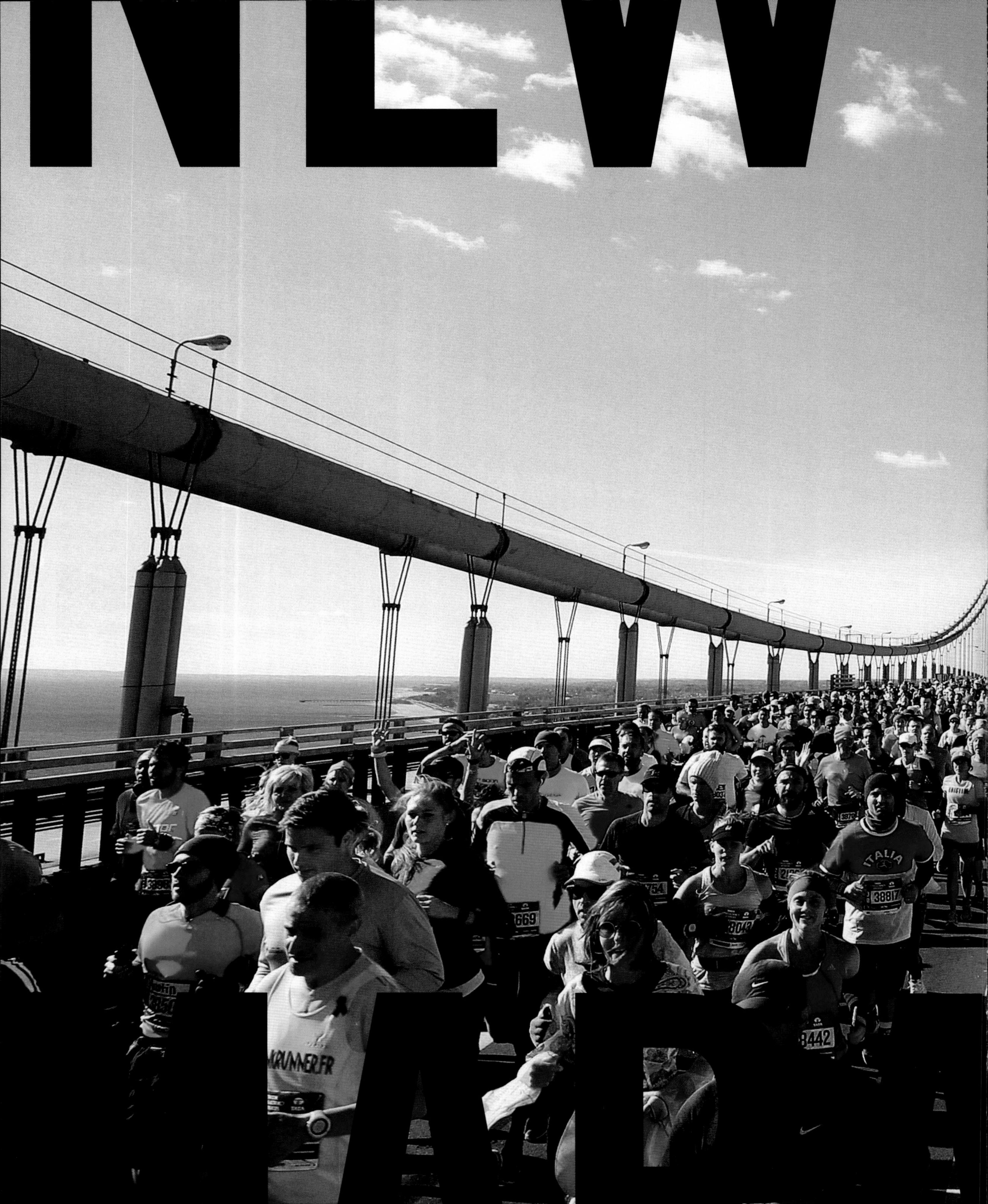
ITALIA
38817
8442

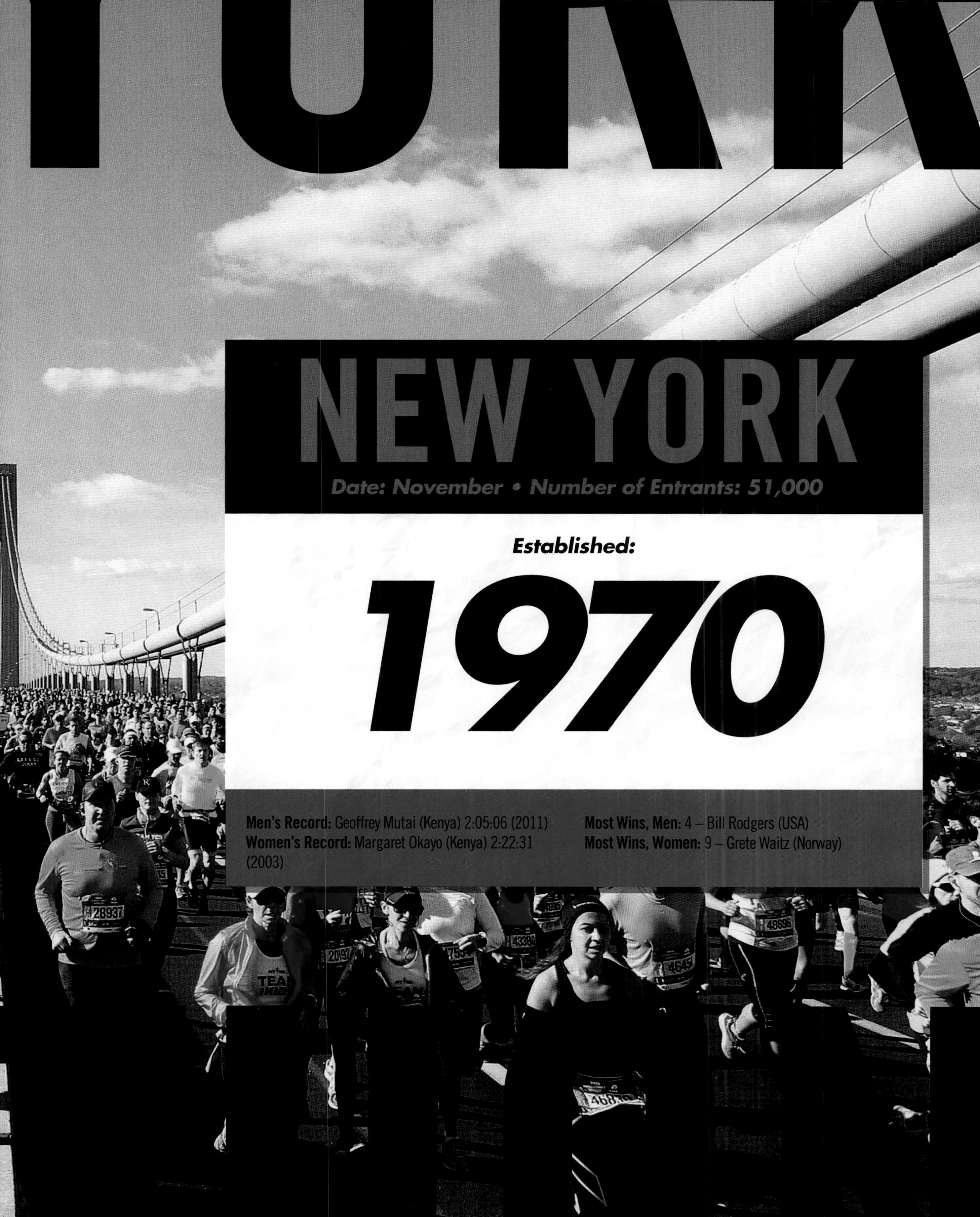

NEW YORK

Date: November • Number of Entrants: 51,000

Established:

1970

Men's Record: Geoffrey Mutai (Kenya) 2:05:06 (2011)
Women's Record: Margaret Okayo (Kenya) 2:22:31 (2003)

Most Wins, Men: 4 – Bill Rodgers (USA)
Most Wins, Women: 9 – Grete Waitz (Norway)

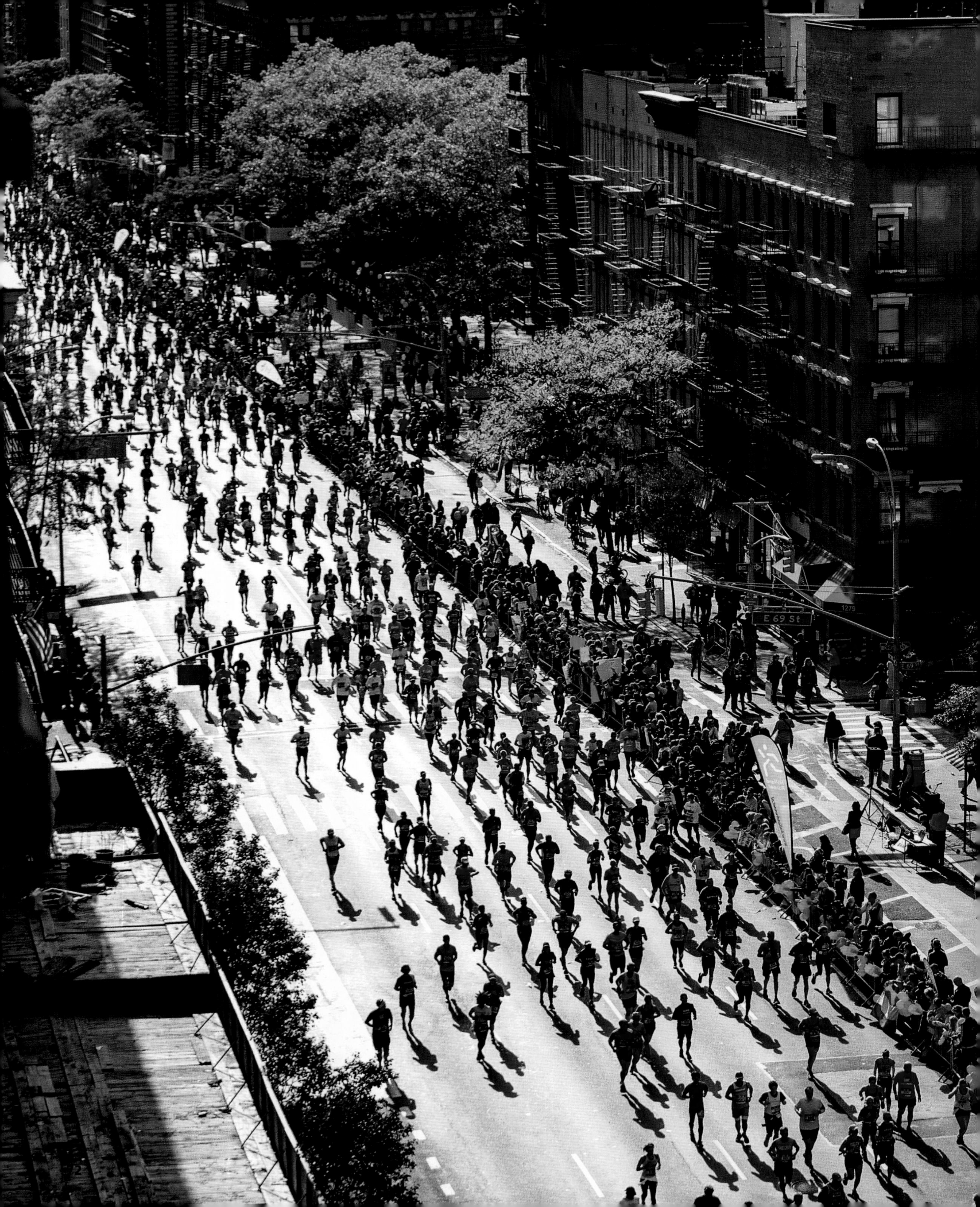
1279
E 69 St

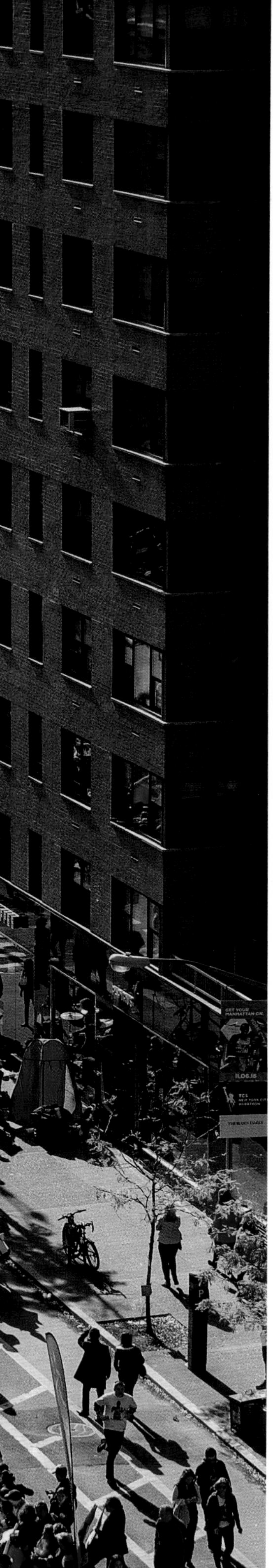

THE NEW YORK CITY MARATHON

A World Marathon Major that takes in all five of New York City's iconic boroughs, this hugely popular race has been running since 1970. In the decades since, it has come to be seen as a true symbol of the pride and strength of New York's huge, but tight-knit community.

The New York City Marathon is big and bold. One of the six World Marathon Majors, it officially gained its bragging rights as the world's largest marathon when, in 2016, 51,388 participants crossed the finish line. But, despite the fact that it's claimed its place as one of the top marathons in the world, the New York City Marathon had humble beginnings – and its history has encompassed everything from women's-rights protests, to world records, to displays of human resilience and solidarity.

TOUR OF THE BOROUGHS

The inaugural New York City Marathon took place in 1970, organized by New York Road Runners' presidents, Fred Lebow and Vincent Chiappetta. On a total budget of $1,000 – $300 of which was self-funded by Lebow – 127 competitors gathered in Central Park on race day, having paid their $1 entry fee. A far cry from today's course, which takes runners on a tour of New York City's five boroughs, the route consisted of loops around Central Park. Just 55 male participants crossed the finish line (the only female entrant had to withdraw mid-race, due to illness), with American runner and New York City fireman Gary Muhrcke winning the event in a time of 2:31:38, watched by a crowd of just 100 spectators. What makes his win even more impressive is that he'd worked a busy night shift at the fire station in Far Rockaway the night before the race.

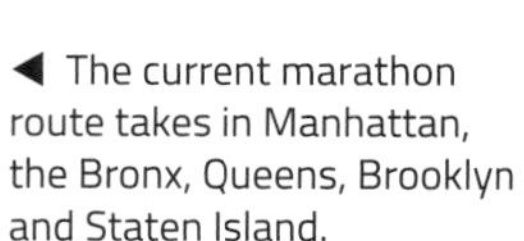

◀ The current marathon route takes in Manhattan, the Bronx, Queens, Brooklyn and Staten Island.

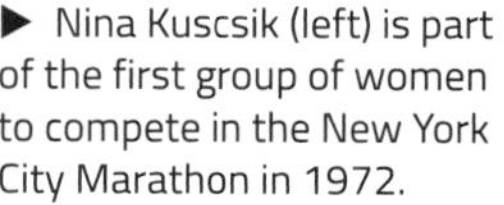

▶ Nina Kuscsik (left) is part of the first group of women to compete in the New York City Marathon in 1972.

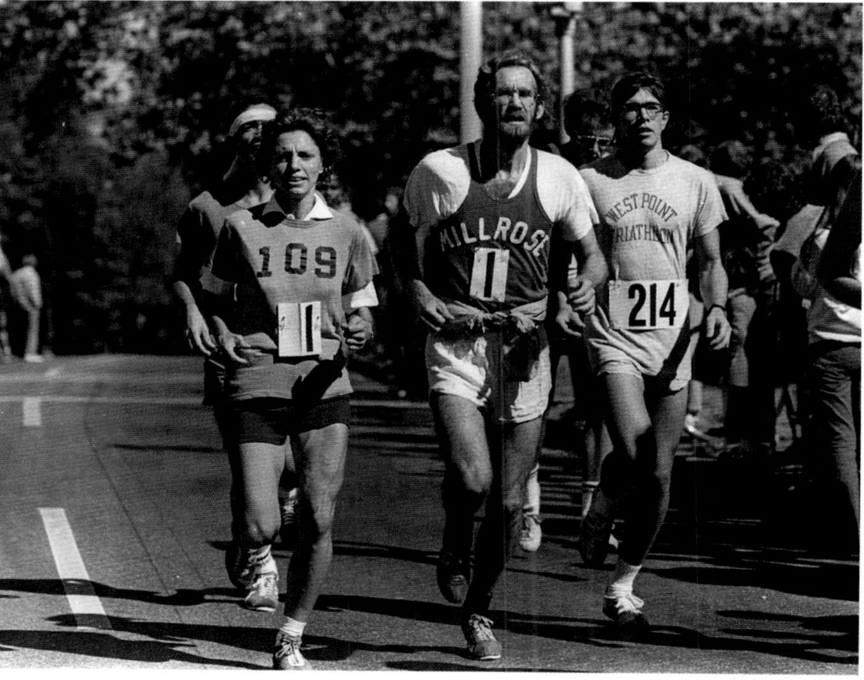

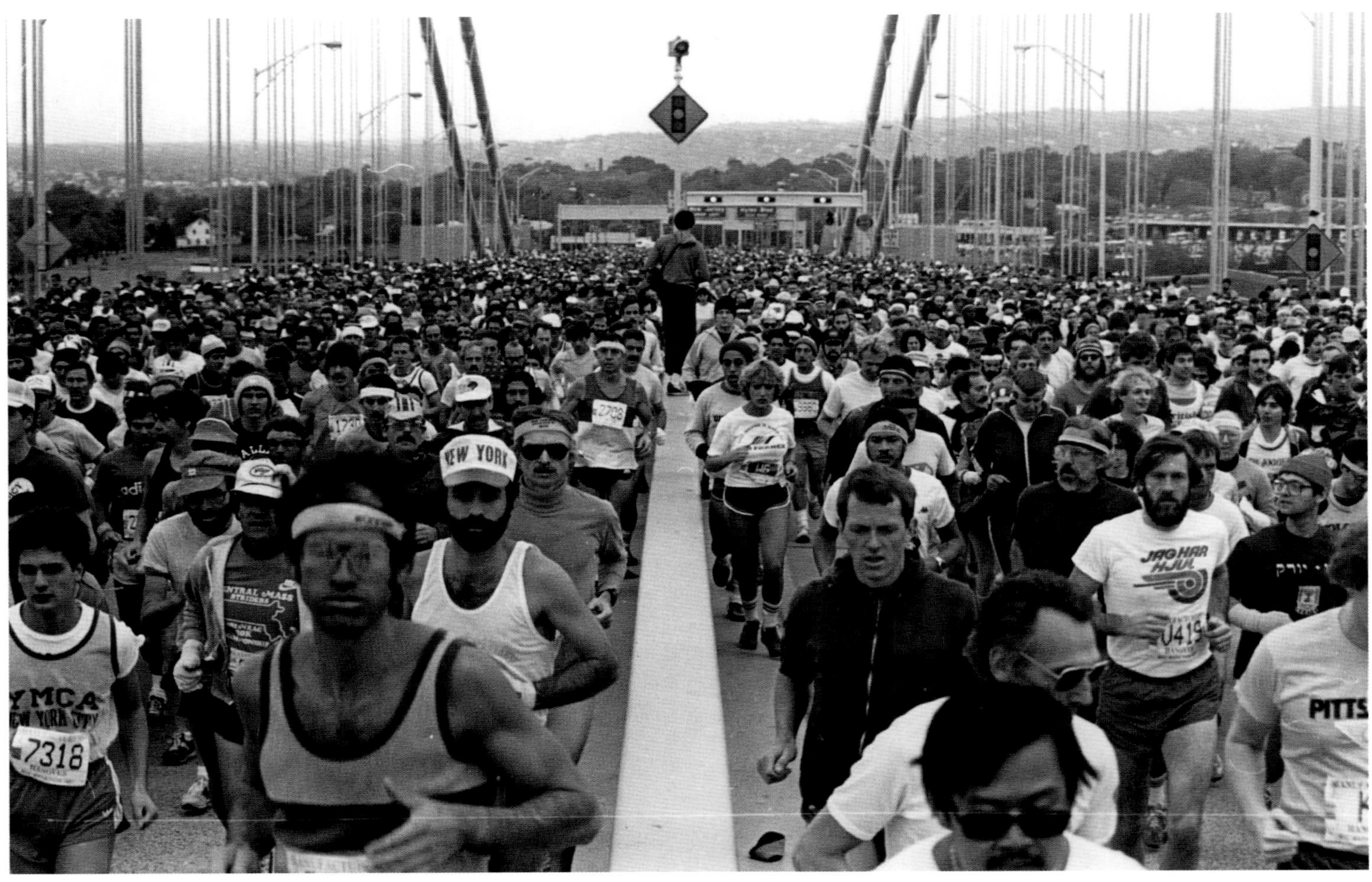

▲ A packed field at the NYC marathon in 1972 includes women for the first time.

Two years later, the race made history before even a single step had been run. In 1972, there were six female competitors registered for the race, in a field of 278. But the Amateur Athletic Union (which had previously banned women from running marathons, on the grounds of unfounded "research" that claimed women risked infertility from long-distance running) had imposed a rule. Female competitors needed to start the race 10 minutes before the men and from a different start line, in an act that meant women were "separate but equal". However, many male and female runners of the time viewed this as simply another form of discrimination, in a bid to keep women on the sidelines of sport.

And so, when the starting gun went off for the women's race at 11 a.m., the six women – Lynn Blackstone, Jane Muhrcke, Liz Franceschini, Pat Barrett, Nina Kuscsik and Cathy Miller – calmly sat down cross-legged on the floor. They then held up handwritten signs with slogans such as 'Hey AAU, this is 1972. Wake up!' and 'The AAU is archaic'. When the start gun went off for the men's race 10 minutes later, the women got up and ran alongside their male counterparts. They incurred a 10-minute time penalty, but their actions helped to change the face of running, allowing men and women to compete alongside each other.

This "sit-in" has not been the only time women have made history at the New York City Marathon. In 1974, Kathrine Switzer (of Boston Marathon fame) became the first (and only, to date) New York City resident to win the event, crossing the finish line in 3:07:29.

In 1976, the New York City Marathon saw its most significant change and, in celebration of the US bicentennial, it moved out of Central Park and was instead run through the streets of the city, traversing all five boroughs. The change proved popular and what was intended to be a one-time celebration course became the annual route.

NEW COURSE RECORD

Two years later, in 1978, Norwegian long-distance runner Grete Waitz won this marathon, setting a new course record and world record of 2:32:30. It was her first marathon: she had previously never run further than 12 miles. The following year, Waitz went on to win again, smashing her own

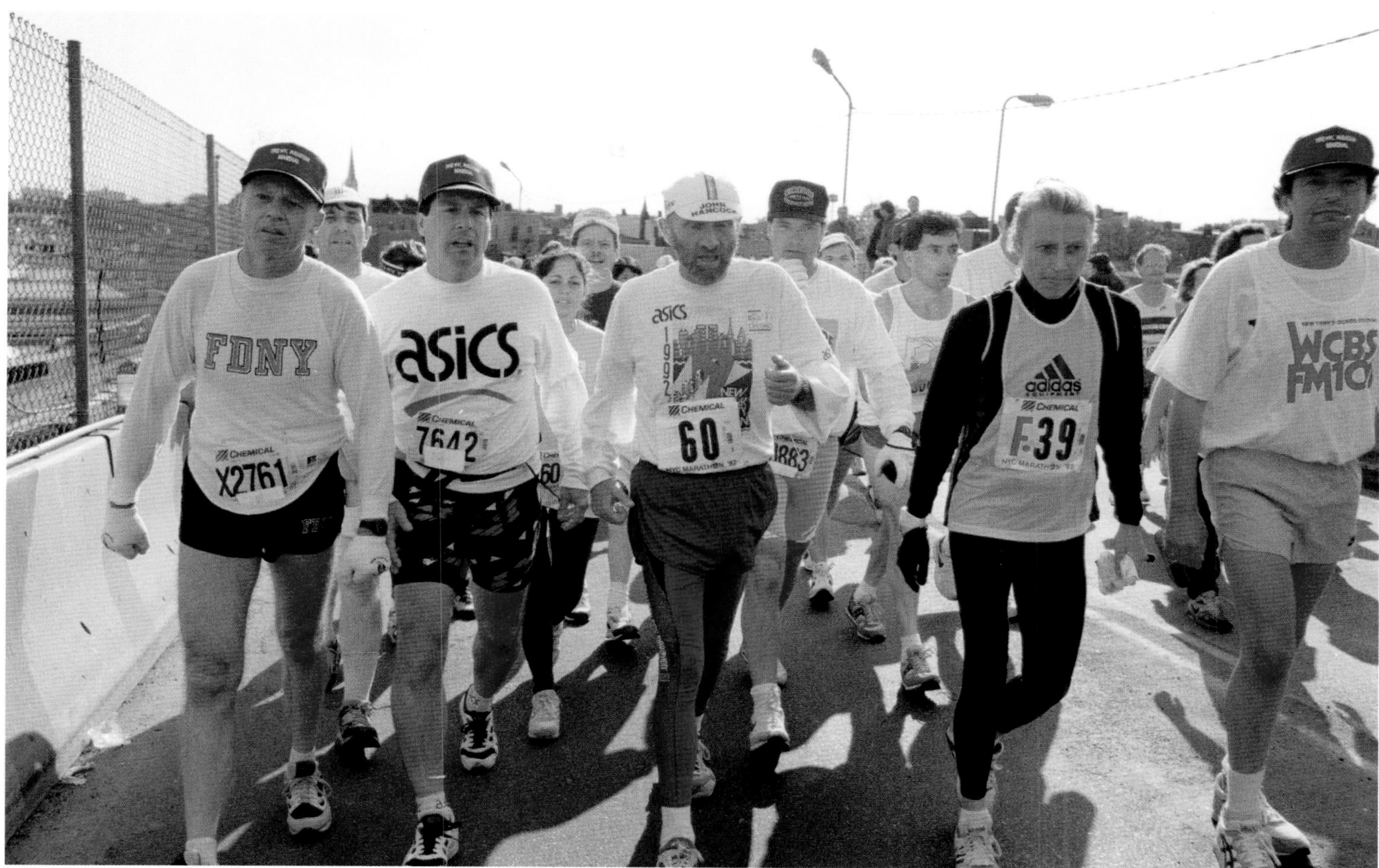

▲ Grete Waitz and Fred Lebow, both legends of the NYC Marathon, compete in an emotional race in 1992.

world record and becoming the first woman to break the 2:30:00 barrier, in a time of 2:27:33.

Waitz won the marathon nine times in total, taking the world record down to 2:25:41 in 1980. However, it was her final New York City Marathon that was her most poignant. Race cofounder Fred Lebow had been diagnosed with cancer in 1990 and two years later, in 1992, the pair ran the marathon together in celebration of Lebow's 60th birthday, crossing the finish line side by side in a time of 5:32:35. He died two years later. In 2011, Waitz herself passed away due to cancer, but has gone down in history as a sporting legend, with the New York Road Runners sponsoring an annual 10km – Grete's Great Gallop – in her name.

The New York City Marathon has grown in popularity over the years, and is a true symbol of the pride and strength of New York City's community. This vibe shone through in 2001, when the marathon took place on 6 November, almost two months after the 9/11 Twin Towers terrorist attack. Despite the evident heartbreak, as runners acknowledged the altered Manhattan skyline and remembered those who had lost their lives in the attack, participants ran with positivity, hope, spirit and determination, with the slogan "United We Run" at the forefront of their minds. A phenomenal 23,648 runners crossed the finish line that year.

Since 1970, the New York City Marathon has been cancelled only once, in 2012, in the wake of Hurricane Sandy. The late-season post-tropical cyclone swept through the Caribbean and up the East Coast of the United States in late October that year, killing 42 people in New York and causing floods and fires throughout the city. Skyscrapers swayed, gas stations were forced to close due to power shortages and a tanker ran aground on Staten Island. The New York City Mayor's Office estimated that the storm caused $19 billion worth of damage and losses.

The New York City Marathon was initially intended to go ahead as planned that year, but the staging of the race became increasingly controversial in the days prior to the event. While some called for the event to take place, in the hope that it would boost morale and the economy, others felt staging the race would be insensitive, especially in light of the fact that the race was due to start on Staten Island – the borough that was hardest hit by the superstorm. In the end,

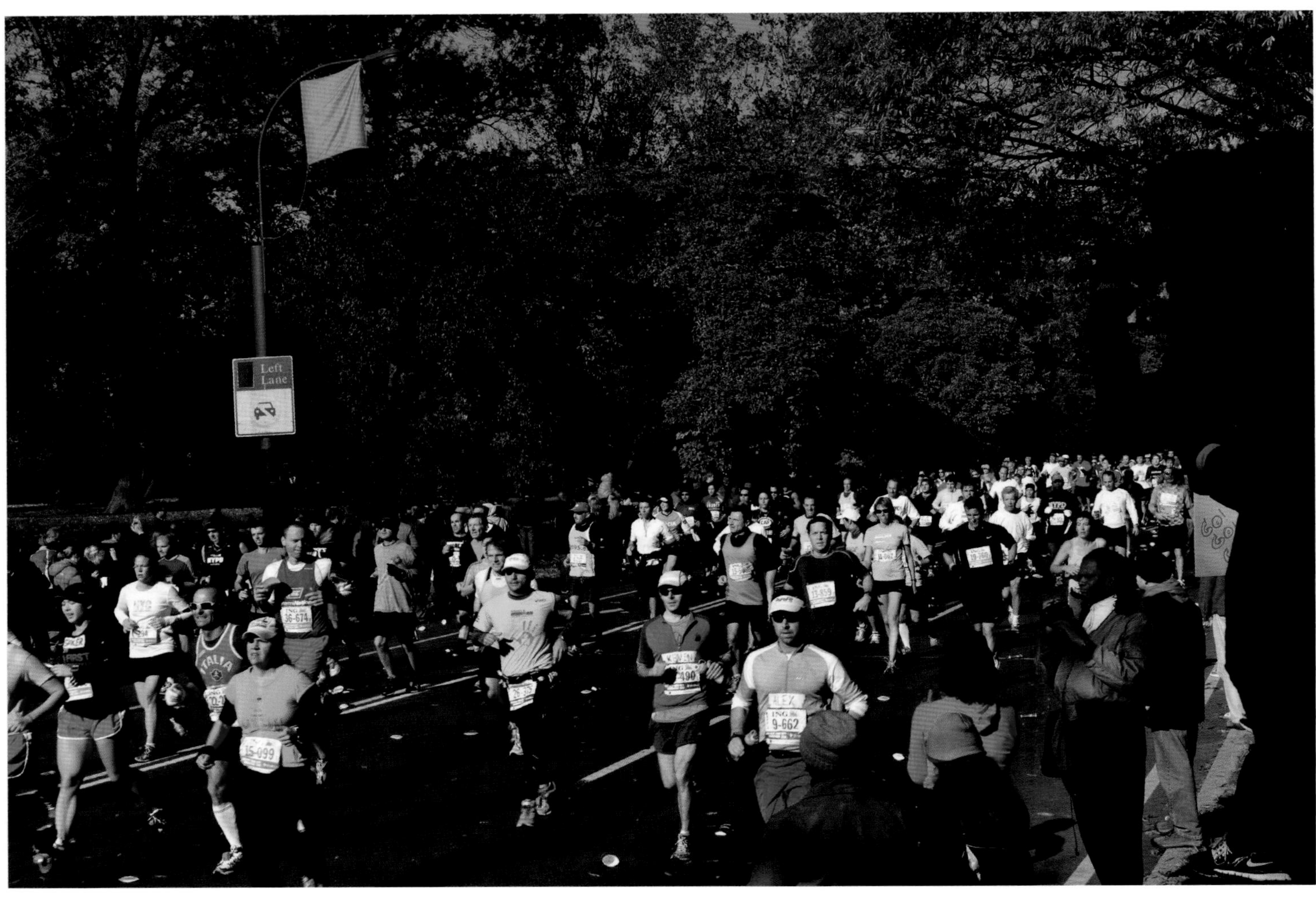

▲ A record year in 2016 saw the NYC Marathon become the biggest in history in terms of participation.

the event was cancelled just 40 hours before it was due to go ahead. Mayor Michael Bloomberg explained: "While holding the race would not require diverting resources from the recovery effort, it is clear that it has become the source of controversy and division."

Because of the late cancellation of the race, many runners had already arrived in the city. Some used their time to help the clean-up effort, while others assembled in Central Park on the morning the race had been due to take place, and ran an informal 26.2 miles instead. All entrants were offered either a full refund, or entry into a future NYC Marathon or the 2013 NYC Half-Marathon.

From its small beginnings back in 1970, which saw just 55 finishers, the New York City Marathon now attracts more than 50,000 participants annually – a tribute to its popularity. In 2016, it broke the record for the largest marathon field in history, with 51,388 runners crossing the finish line out of 51,995 participants who started the race – an impressive 98.8 per cent completion rate.

THE COURSE

While there have been a few changes over the years, much of the route remains faithful to the original course set out in 1976, when the marathon first took to the New York City streets.

It's an inspiring route, which takes runners through all five of New York City's boroughs. Starting on Staten Island, the first two miles of the race is spent crossing the Verrazano-Narrows Bridge across to Brooklyn. At the halfway point, participants enter Queens, over the Pulaski Bridge, before the Queensboro Bridge sees them arrive at First Avenue in Manhattan during Mile 15. Crossing the Willis Avenue Bridge, runners do a short stint in the Bronx at around Mile 20, before re-entering Manhattan and heading down Fifth Avenue, hitting Central Park and Mile 23. Mile 25 sees them leave the park for a section along Central Park South, before heading back into the park and running the last 600m to the finish line.

Due to its five bridge crossings (which all involve inclines), plus a series of (sometimes steep) undulations in Central Park, the marathon

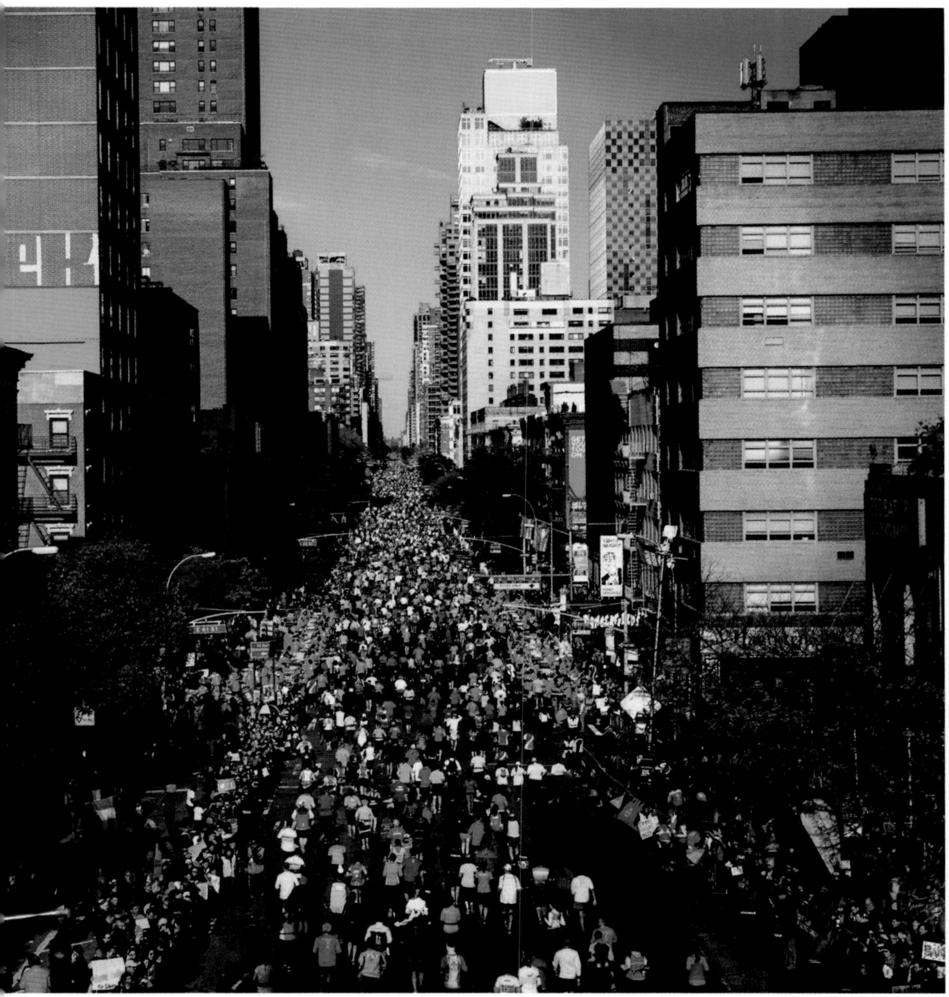

▲ New York City might not be the place to set a PB, but its atmosphere simply has to be experienced.

is not considered to be especially fast, although the course records are speedy: 2:05:06 in the men's race, set by Kenya's Geoffrey Mutai in 2011, and 2:22:31 in the women's race, set by Kenya's Margaret Okayo in 2003.

The course is also popular with spectators, with more than 1 million people lining the route to cheer on the runners. New Yorkers are famed on marathon day for their tireless support and creative signs ("An Uber from here to the finish line costs $40.15!"), and the roar of the crowds – especially the noise as you arrive in Manhattan on First Avenue, and as you hit Central Park near the finish – will help to keep your spirits up, even when your feet are feeling well and truly punished.

"In 2016, it broke the record for the largest marathon field in history, with 51,388 runners crossing the finish line out of 51,995 participants"

SECURING A PLACE

As with other World Marathon Majors, there are several ways to secure a guaranteed place in the New York City Marathon. First, you can secure a place via NYRR Team For Kids or another Official Charity Partner, if you pledge to meet their minimum fundraising requirements.

Second, members of New York Road Runners can take part in the club's 9+1 or 9+$1K programme. To do this, they must have completed nine scored, qualifying NYRR races throughout the year before they wish to run the NYC Marathon, as well as one volunteering shift for the club (a monetary donation of $1,000 can substitute for the volunteering shift). Third, runners who have already completed 15 New York City Marathons are eligible for guaranteed entry in future years.

Then there are the Time Qualifiers, which are based on age and gender, a full list of which can be found on the New York City Marathon website. You can also get a qualifying time if you've taken part in one of the following recent NYRR races: NYRR Fred Lebow Manhattan Half, United Airlines NYC Half, 2017 SHAPE Women's Half-Marathon, Airbnb Brooklyn Half, NYRR Staten Island Half or the TCS New York City Marathon. Finally, if you live outside the USA, you can book your place in the marathon through an International Travel Partner.

For non-guaranteed race entry, you can enter the lottery draw and keep your fingers crossed. As with places in other highly coveted marathons, competition is stiff – for the 2017 New York City Marathon, 98,247 hopefuls entered the draw for just 16,211 places – an acceptance rate of 16.5 per cent. However, as the saying goes, you've got to be in it to win it.

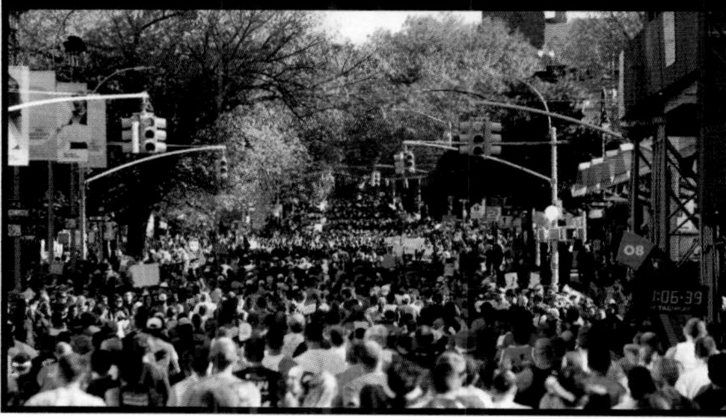

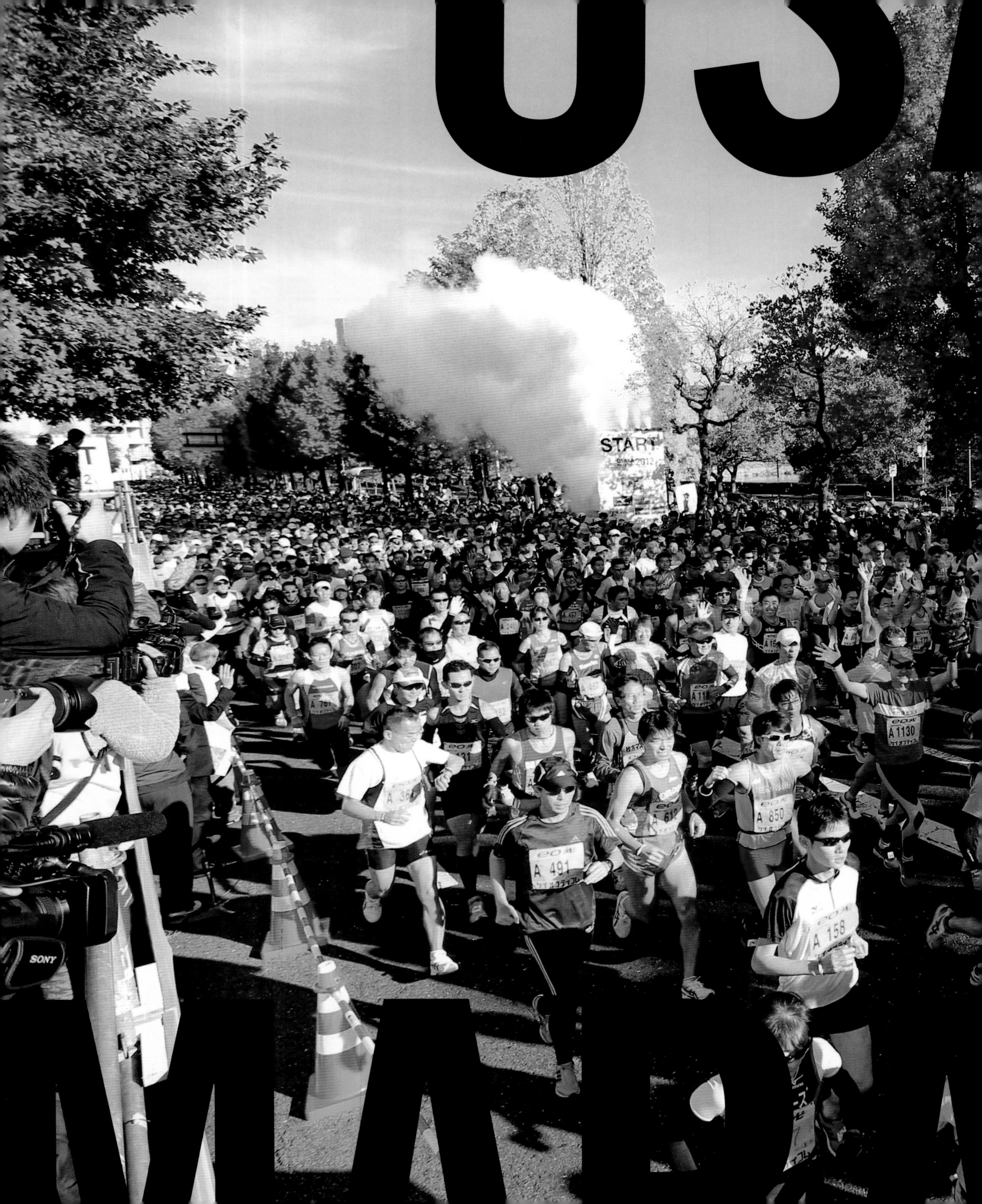
START
A 1130
A 850
A 491
A 158

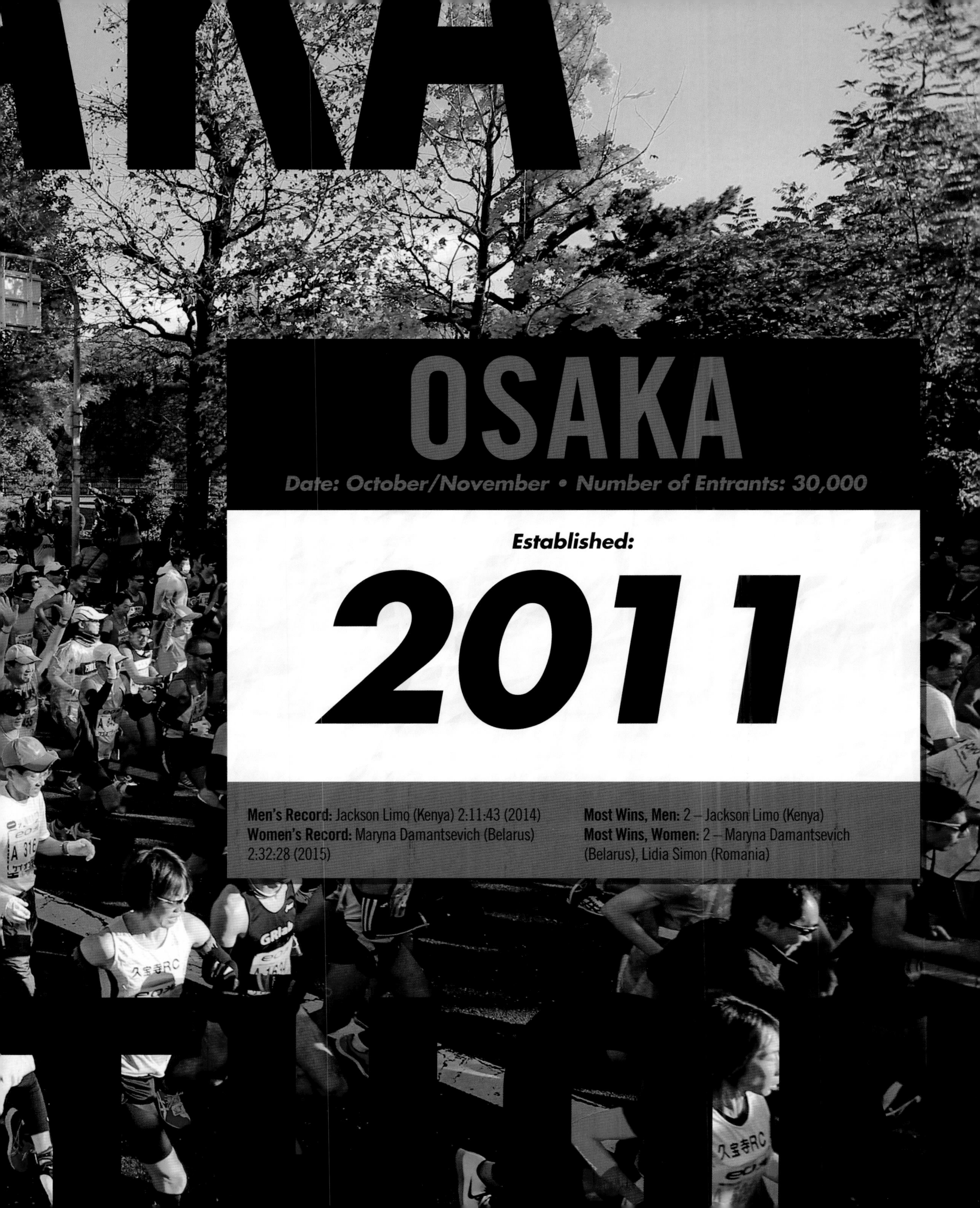

OSAKA

Date: October/November • Number of Entrants: 30,000

Established:

2011

Men's Record: Jackson Limo (Kenya) 2:11:43 (2014)
Women's Record: Maryna Damantsevich (Belarus) 2:32:28 (2015)

Most Wins, Men: 2 – Jackson Limo (Kenya)
Most Wins, Women: 2 – Maryna Damantsevich (Belarus), Lidia Simon (Romania)

THE OSAKA MARATHON

A friendly marathon that, despite its massive scale, runs like clockwork. Add to that a city with a fascinating cultural heritage and a country that just loves running, and the Osaka Marathon has a lot to offer.

▶ Osaka Castle makes for an imposing landmark that can be seen consistently throughout the route.

The people of Japan are famously keen on their running. It's a country that's often considered to be the most running-obsessed culture in the world, so it's something of a surprise to consider that the very first Osaka Marathon took place as recently as October 2011. It now typically takes place in late November and is a road race, mainly on flat tarmac, offering a great atmosphere. Anyone who signs up for a race in Japan can be sure of an incredible amount of support from local crowds. The whole town will come out and cheer the runners on when there's an event taking place, so a warm welcome from the locals and a great deal of encouragement can be guaranteed if you decide to take part in this well-organized marathon in an extraordinary country.

Osaka is Japan's second-largest metropolitan city after Tokyo and has many appealing tourist spots, such as Universal Studios, Osaka Castle and a shrine called Sumiyoshi Taisha. It also has a Buddhist temple called Shitenno-ji, which is the oldest officially administered temple in Japan. There's no shortage of things to see and do and it could be a good opportunity to combine a race experience with some sightseeing.

"I didn't really expect to see how much they had closed down all of the roads within Osaka... It was like the London Marathon on acid! Locals were proud to support Osaka as a city. They were there to support everyone taking part."

A SEAMLESS EXPERIENCE

If you're the type of person who likes to plan and organize everything, this is a marathon you'll love. Despite the long flight to Japan, the experience on arrival is seamless. Organized, prompt, efficient and extremely polite, the Japanese welcome runners from all over the world and are keen to showcase the delights of their country.

However, if this is a marathon you fancy adding to your bucket list, make sure you allow yourself plenty of time to recover from jetlag. You'll want to arrive in Japan at least a week before the race, to enable your body to adapt and for you to get into a regular sleep pattern.

The marathon event is jointly hosted by the Japan Association of Athletics Federations and *Yomiuru Shimbun*, a national Japanese newspaper. In its very first year and despite minimal marketing and promotion, the race attracted 170,000 entrants, of whom 27,161 started the race and 26,175 completed. The first Osaka Marathon was sponsored by sports brand Mizuno, whose staff were encouraged to experience (i.e. run!) the marathon, and had at least 60 members of staff taking part, clearly demonstrating their commitment to the event.

John Hooper, who was the European sports promotions coordinator for Mizuno at the time, ran the event that year. He had previously completed seven marathons and was impressed with the organization of this particular race. "I didn't really expect to see how much they had closed down all of the roads within Osaka," he recalls. "If that happened in London it would have caused chaos, but virtually every road was closed here. It was like the London Marathon on acid! Locals were proud to support Osaka as a city. They were there to support everyone taking part."

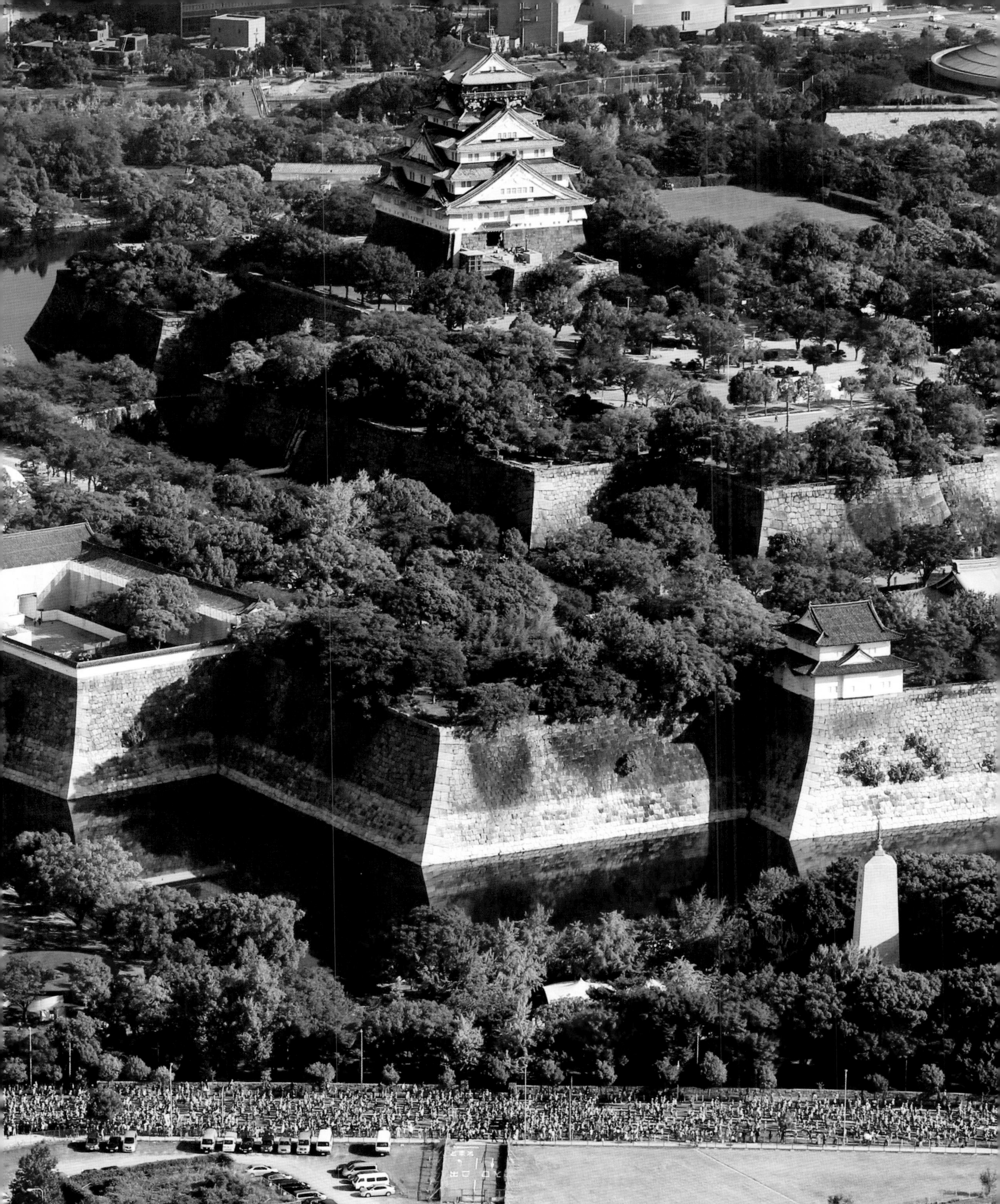

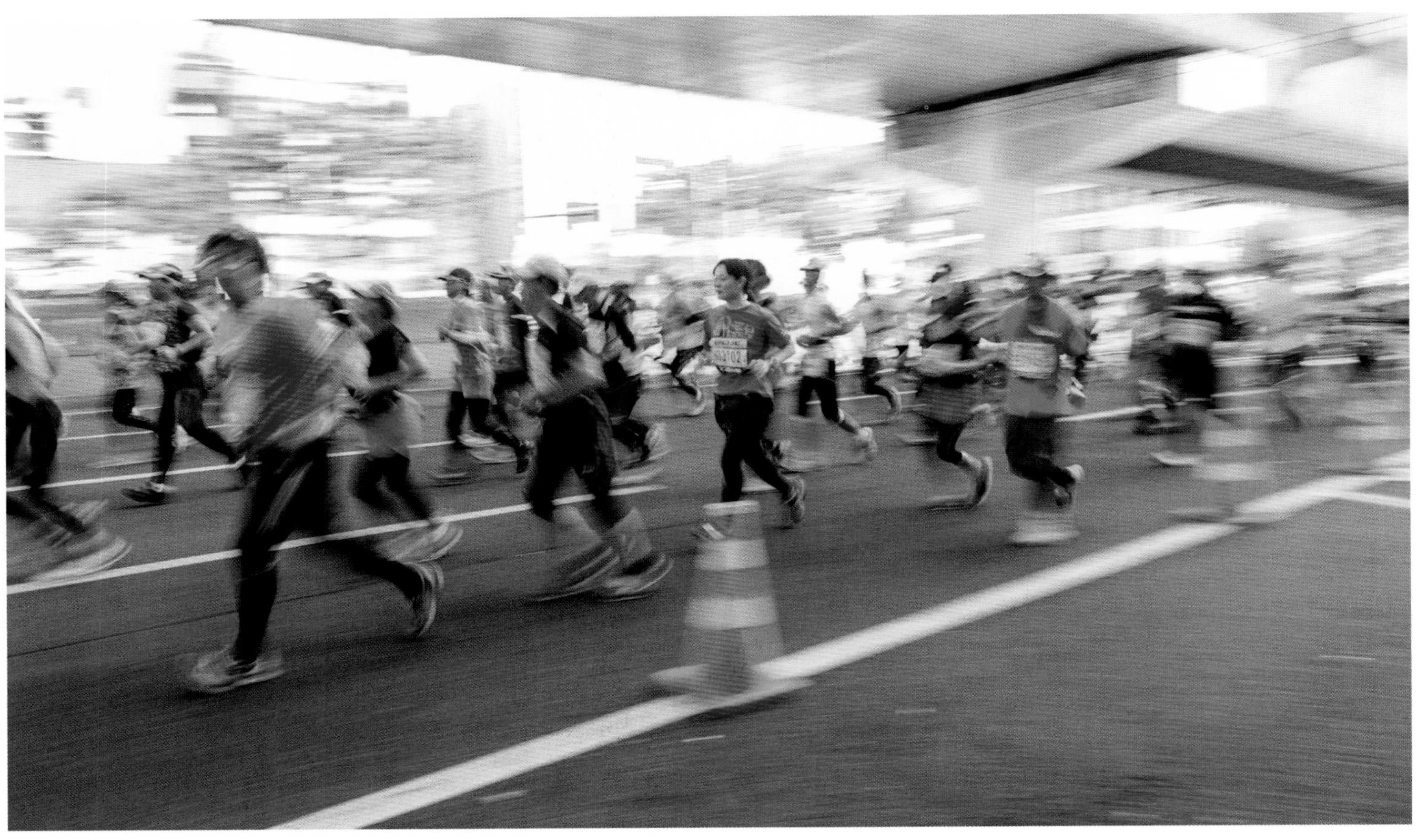

▲ During the marathon, the entire city of Osaka effectively shuts down to accommodate it.

A FESTIVAL OF RUNNING

The race is preceded by a busy expo, where runners collect their race numbers and get to shop for last-minute race-day essentials or anything they may have left behind. The Osaka Marathon is an urban road race offering good personal-best potential. It now starts at the 400-year-old Osaka Castle Park and finishes at INTEX Osaka, a large international exhibition hall where the expo is held. It's a flat course and passes through Sennichimae (a shopping arcade), Nakanoshima, Kyocera Dome Osaka (used for sporting and musical events) and various other sights before finishing at the INTEX. It also takes in the Osaka Prefectural Government office building, Midō-suji Boulevard (a popular street lined with a fabulous border of gingko trees), the centre of economic and cultural activities in Osaka and Osaka City Central Public Hall.

During the race, women like to dress up in style. You won't find many of them running in boring black fitness-wear or trying to blend in with the other runners. Participants are noted for their outrageous and flamboyant costumes, "skorts" (a combination of shorts and skirts), and the brighter the colour choices, the better, with runners tackling the course while wearing fuchsia pink and an array of other bright, neon colours. There are many costumes to be seen in this race too, with a former participant dressed as a Power Rangers hero and another participant dressed as a caveman. During the very first race in 2011, one man was spotted dressed up as the World Cup, while another ran in drag with huge legs and fake boobs. The spirit of the race is good, too: local runners didn't stop smiling and seemed to enjoy every minute of the marathon.

The race is intended to be fun and centres on seven charity themes with organized colour codes representing causes. Red supports your hopes to live, orange is meant to assist your dreams, yellow is to support your family, green is to conserve the natural environment, aqua is to provide clean water, navy blue is intended to brighten your children's future and purple is to preserve the city of Osaka.

RACE COMPETITION

The Osaka Marathon has an unusual twist. Everyone who enters it is taking part in a competition, even if they don't realise it, courtesy of the Nanairo (rainbow colour) Team Competition. Entrants are divided into seven teams and the team with the best average time among all finishers is the winner. Charity is also a huge part of this race and the event organizers encourage runners to make donations to the various causes they support.

Getting around Japan in the lead-up to the race or afterwards is fairly straightforward, despite the language barrier. Japan has a culture distinct from any other country on Earth, and it's certainly worth taking your time to explore the area while you're there. That said, one similarity is the subway system, which is easy to navigate and follows a fairly universal map system. Lines are colour-coded and each of the stations is numbered, so, if you want to get around and see the sights, you should be able to navigate public transport without any major issues. It also helps that friendly station staff speak basic English and the subway trains are immaculate, entirely free from litter. The transport system also offers women-only carriages. After an earthquake in the northeast wiped out two power stations, electricity is in limited supply, so the tube trains have their lights on only when underground, and even the large department stores have air conditioning turned off.

As for the marathon itself, if you choose to do it, you won't be sorry. The Osaka Marathon is hugely popular and has been called one of the best sporting events in the world. Even if you don't fancy doing the full marathon, but you like the idea of visiting Osaka, note that there's also an 8.8km race you can take part in on the same day.

Once you've completed the marathon, there are plenty of fascinating sights to see, including various temples, one of which is the Hōzen-ji, said to have been founded in 1637. There's also a stone-paved alley called Hōzen-ji Yokocho, which used to be the grounds of the Hōzen-ji temple and offers many restaurants and bars. It's a busy, dynamic area and features stone tablets with inscriptions from a famous novelist. There's also another Buddhist temple called Isshinji, said to have been built in 1185. The belief is that the ex-Emperor Goshirakawa, in search of a happy life, repeated the name of the Buddha while the sun was setting.

There are also various shrines you can visit, including the Sumiyoshi Taishi Shrine, founded in the third century, which is one of Japan's oldest. It was founded even before Buddhism was introduced and offers amazing architecture. Another shrine you may wish to visit is the Tenmangû Shrine, built in 949, which has been burned several times. The building and door were rebuilt in 1845 and this shrine plays host to the Tenjin Matsuri, a festival held in July, which is 1,000 years old and is one of Japan's greatest festivals. Around 3,000 people who attend the festival dress up in clothing from the eighth and twelfth centuries and march beside portable shrines. There's also a procession of boats.

While you're in Japan, you may wish to sample the local dishes, though you may prefer to steer clear of anything too spicy or radically different from your usual food choice the night before the marathon. Osaka is well known for good food. The word "kuidaore" ("eat till you drop") is heard so frequently here that it's practically the city motto. Delicacies from okonomiyaki (see description below) to conveyor-belt sushi were invented here and continue to thrive.

Make sure you sample some delicious food after the marathon, too. There are various tasty local dishes on offer. These include takoyaki – dumplings with batter or eggs and flour with sliced octopus, ginger, spring onions and tempura crumbs. Or you could try the aforementioned okonomiyaki, a savoury pancake made from eggs containing grated yam and shredded cabbage. You can add anything you like – cheese, tomato, pork.

Going to Japan is an experience of a lifetime. The marathon is great fun, and the locals are polite and friendly. You really couldn't ask for more in the way of a race experience and, more than that, a life experience that will stay with you forever.

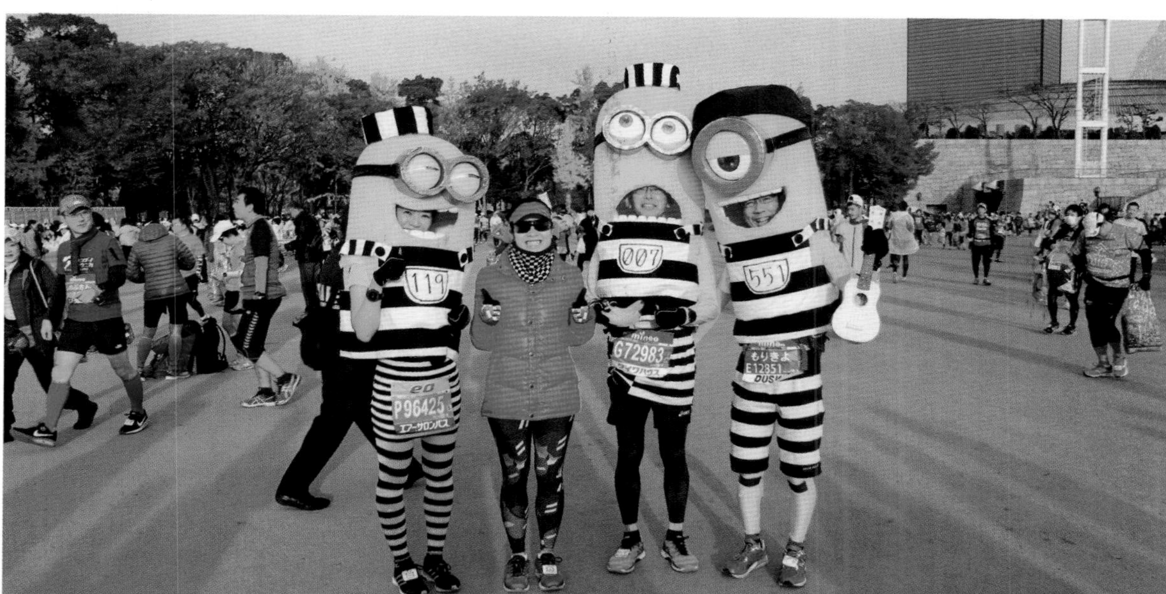

▶ Fancy dress isn't an exception in Osaka, it's practically the norm.

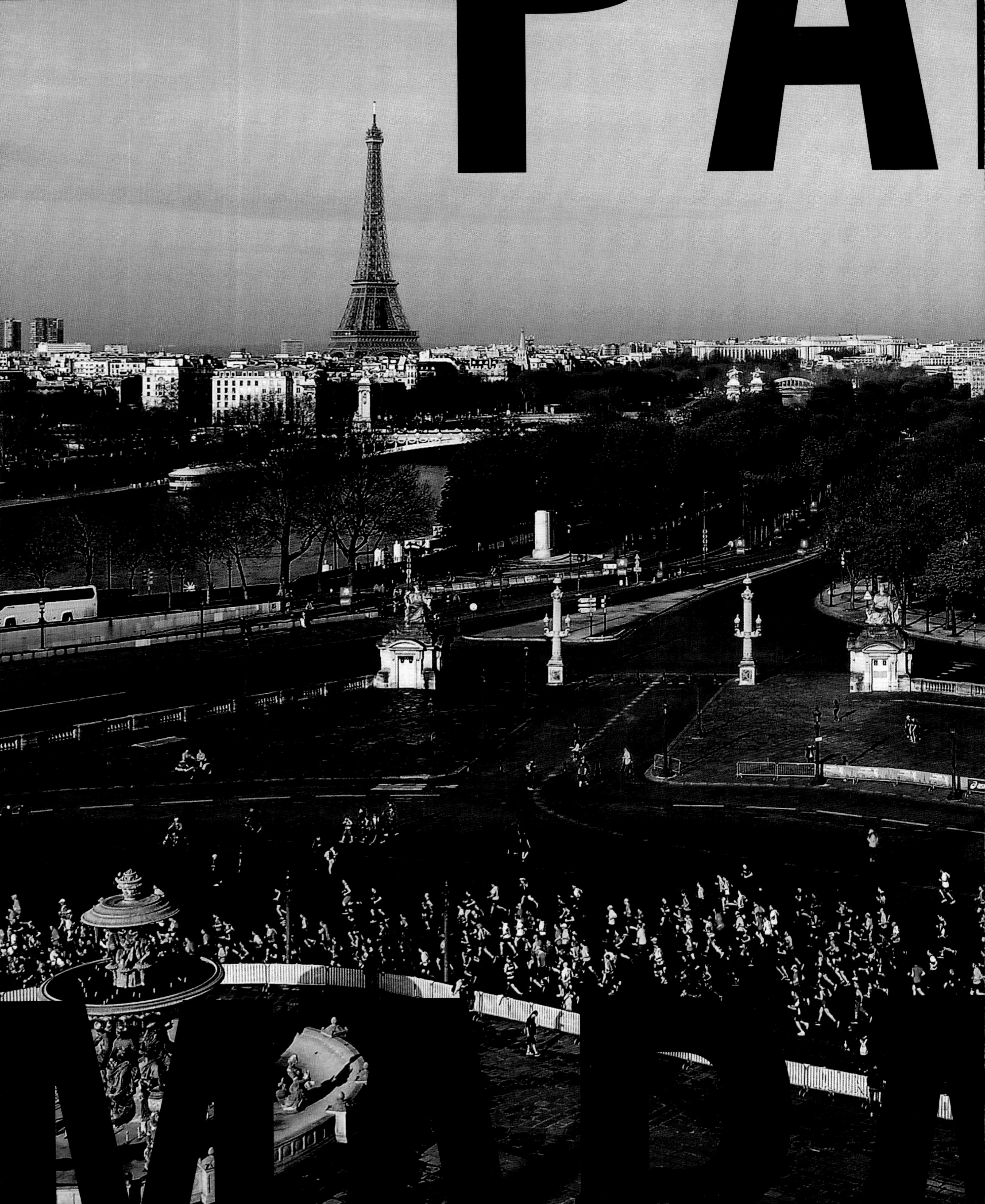

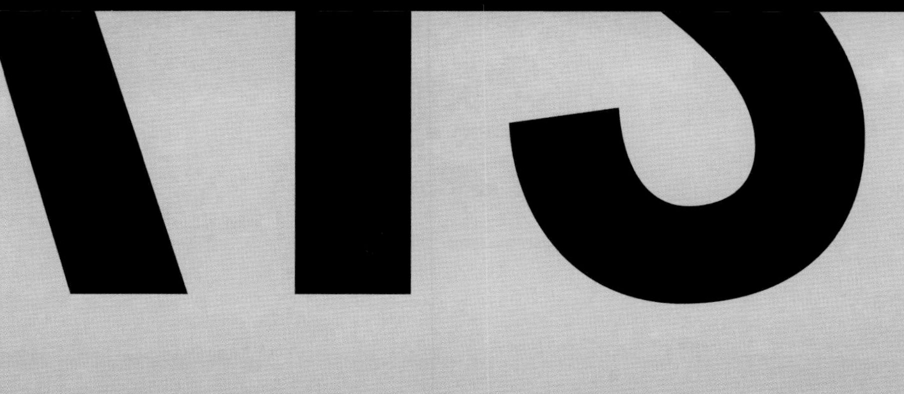

PARIS

Date: April • Number of Entrants: 17,000

Established:

1976

Men's Record: Kenenisa Bekele (Ethiopia) 2:05:04 (2014)
Women's Record: Purity Rionoripo (Kenya) 2:20:55 (2017)

Most Wins, Men: 2 – Paul Lonyangata (Kenya), Steve Brace (United Kingdom), Ahmed Salah (Djibouti)
Most Wins, Women: 2 – Atsede Baysa (Ethiopia)

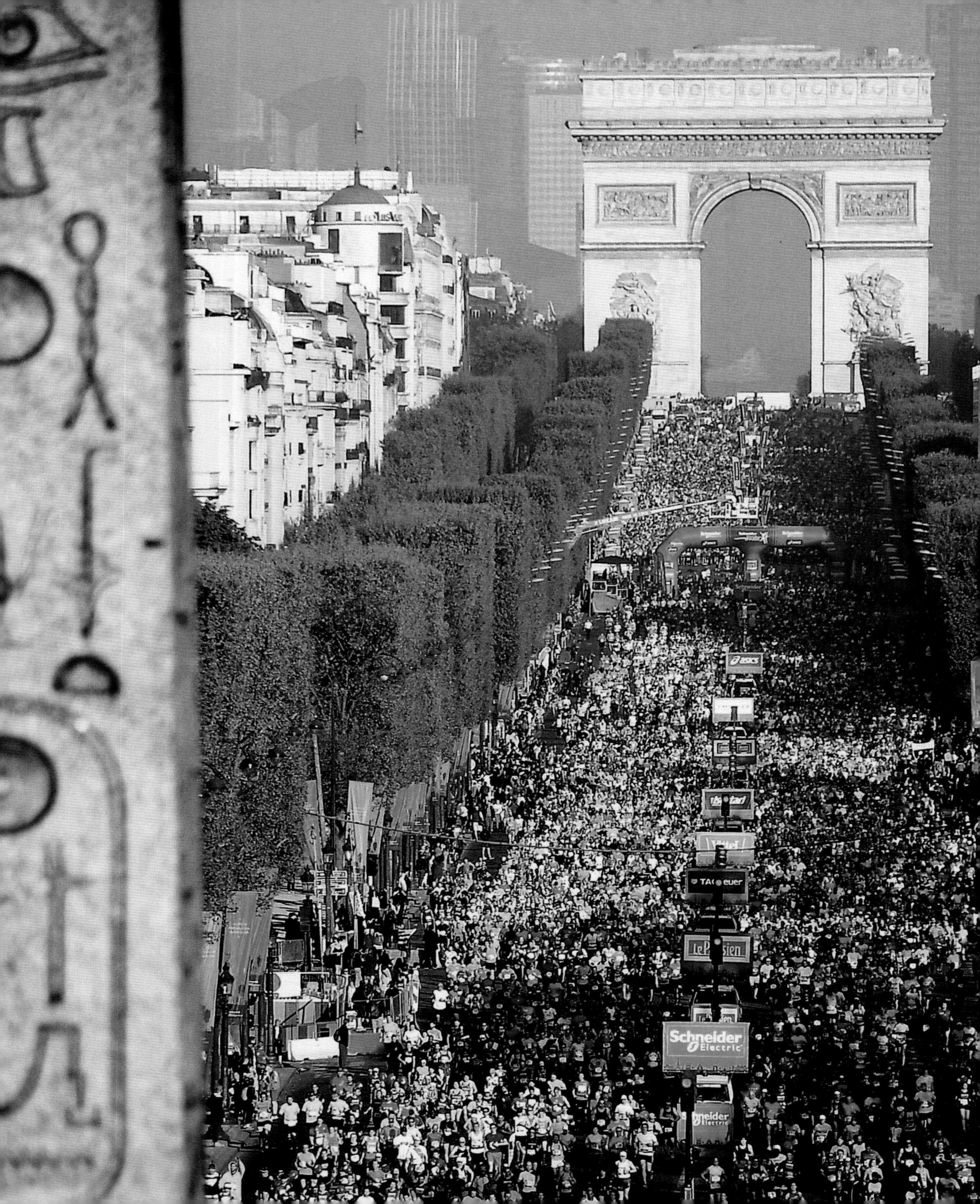
asics
Schneider Electric

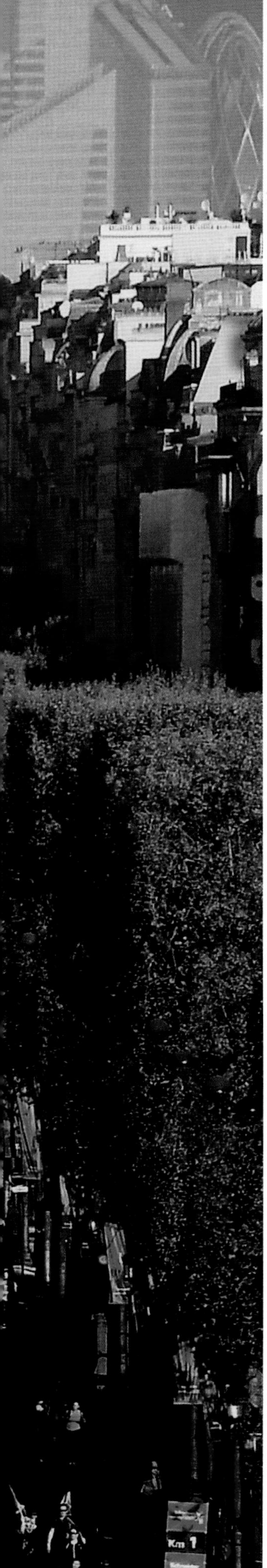

THE PARIS MARATHON

Run the premier race in Paris and you'll see all the sights that any tourist would want to take in. With a winding route around the City of Lights, this marathon is a popular choice for many good reasons.

The Paris Marathon usually takes place in early April and starts at the Champs-Élysées. It's one of the most popular distance marathons in Europe and attracts around 57,000 runners from all over the world. The great thing about the Paris Marathon, apart from the amazing sights and scenery, is its accessibility. Flights and rail links are plentiful throughout Europe, and transatlantic routes are available from most major North American cities as well.

This popular marathon is one you should add to your bucket list, and, if you want to run only one or two marathons, Paris is definitely one to consider. Be mindful of the weather, though. Paris in April can be wet or very hot, so make sure you've got a variety of running kit to choose from. Take waterproof kit and plenty of layers, so that you're prepared for whatever the weather throws at you on race day.

SCENIC COURSE

Famous for offering a fantastic, scenic course that takes in all the sights you would want to see while in Paris, the very first Paris Marathon took place on 19 July 1896. During that first event, 191 runners completed a 40km course from Paris to Conflans-Sainte-Honorine via Versailles. That race was won by a British man, Len Hurst, who ran it in 2:31:30. He was given 200 francs for his efforts. Large crowds came out to witness the first event and all runners who finished the race in less than four hours were awarded a medal.

◀ Runners make their way down the Avenue des Champs-Élysées during the Paris Marathon.

The modern Paris Marathon was inaugurated in 1976, the year that the New York Marathon became a mass-participation event. The winner was a Frenchman, Jean-Pierre Eudier, who completed the course in 2:20:57. In 2003, a new record was set for the Paris Marathon by Kenyan Mike Rotich, who finished in a time of 2:06:33.

But it's not just elite athletes who flock to Paris to run this marathon. The race is also famed for the high volume of recreational runners it attracts. Around 50,000 people usually take part in the Paris Marathon these days. It's easy to see why. The course has everything you'd possibly want. In fact, the best way to describe its route is to list every single landmark you can think of and link them in a huge loop that spans the entire city. The race starts on the Avenue des Champs-Élysées, with a downhill route, and circles around the Place de la Concorde. A long loop takes runners into the heart of Paris. The race has been praised as the world's most scenic marathon, and is virtually flat all the way around the course.

MILES FLYING BY

The halfway point of the course is at Rue de Charenton. The sights you can see on your way around the course will make the miles go by quickly, – though be careful to avoid slipping on one of the banana skin lying around the race stations. There are some narrow streets to contend with, but it's well worth it. The Place de l'Opéra is an astonishing sight, and the course passes the Louvre and then you'll see the Eiffel Tower, before you head along the Seine and through the Alma tunnel, where Princess Diana tragically died in 1997. At the end of the race, you can enjoy a cold beer outside Gare du Nord before heading home. It really is the perfect marathon experience.

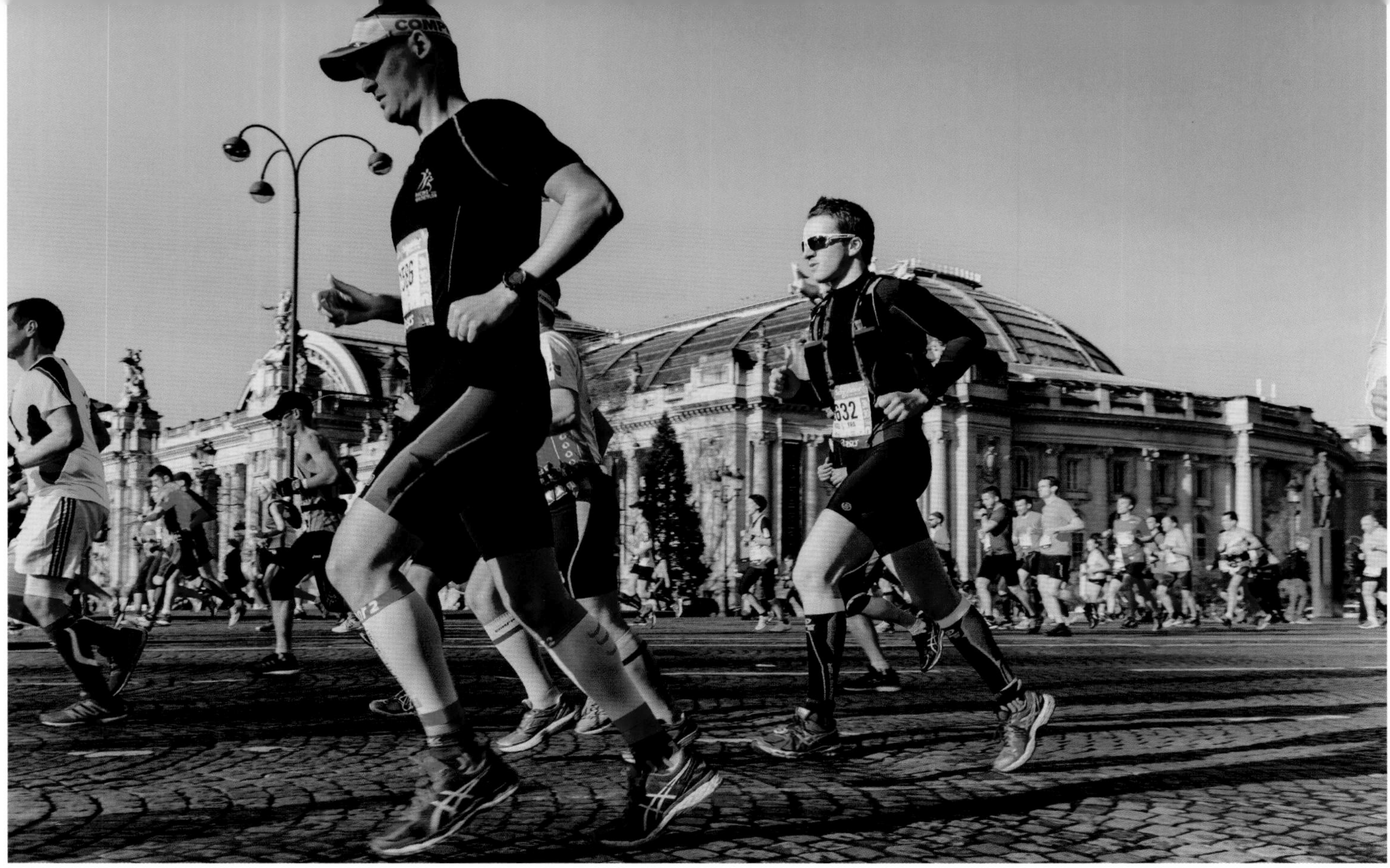

▲ In terms of historical sights and points of interest, there are few marathons in the world that can top Paris.

Aid stations offering dry and fresh fruit, water and sugar are located at every 5km of the race, so you can be sure you won't go hungry. In fact, the race is famed for its fuel stations. You can grab a handful of apricots, nuts, sugar cubes, raisins, apples and orange slices, if you need the energy.

REPEAT THE EXPERIENCE

Those who have run the Paris Marathon usually end up doing it again, and it is often referred to as "unforgettable". It is a crowded event, with space often limited along the sections of the course that go through various parks, but it's worth it for the incredible views and is likely to give you the experience of a lifetime. The crowd support in Paris is good but some participants who have also run the London Marathon have claimed that the London crowds can be more supportive.

However, the crowd support is not to be dismissed. *Women's Running*'s contributing editor, Lisa Jackson, ran the Paris Marathon several years ago while battling with a knee injury. The atmosphere and support during the race helped her make it to the finish line. "Having passed the Louvre, spotted the Eiffel Tower and run along the *quais* [public path] next to the Seine and through the Alma tunnel, we finally entered the leafy Bois de Boulogne park, where we were greeted first by a troop of transvestite pom-pom-waving cheerleaders and then by supporters offering us cups of red wine. Only in France! By this time, I was starting to feel elated – my knee felt fine and each step made me more convinced I was going to finish as I'd felt in control the entire time. As the end drew near, I sped up and actually sprinted the final 5km."

Lisa adds, "The Paris Marathon was so unforgettable that, when I wanted a special race to mark my tenth marathon, I chose to return. And so, once again, I lined up at the start with my trusty aunt, plus a school friend I hadn't seen for 20 years who'd got back in touch after reading my book, *Running Made Easy*. All three of us were dressed as bumblebees – complete with yellow-and-black face paint and pipe-cleaner antennae. The look on my friend's face as she excitedly scanned the sea of runners stretching out in front of us on the Champs-Élysées was enough to tell me she knew she'd chosen the perfect venue for her first marathon. And unlike five years before, I was grinning from ear to ear at the start, not just the finish. Perhaps it was the knowledge that I was once more about to experience one of the world's most spectacular marathons."

ELITE APPEAL

The Paris Marathon also attracts a strong field of athletes. In 2014, male winner Kenenisa Bekele from Ethiopia broke the course record with a debut time

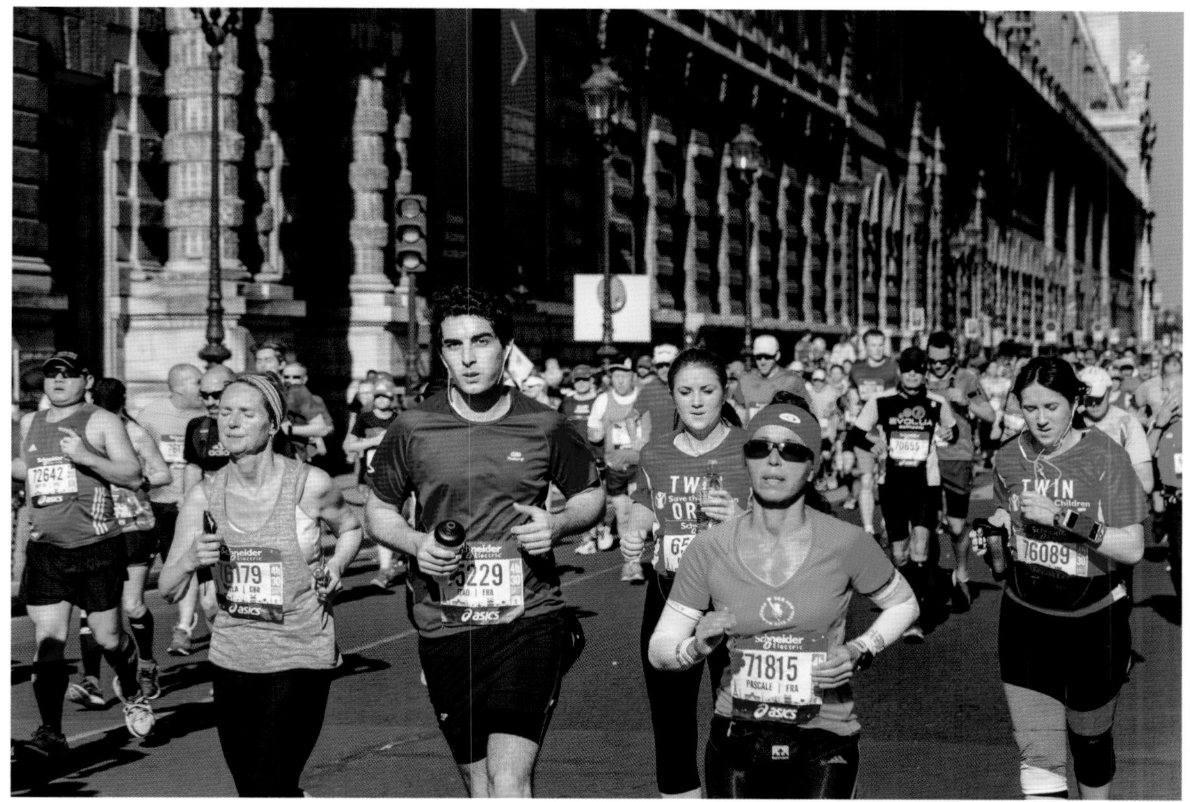

◀ The Paris weather can vary in April, but severe heat is always a possibility.

▽ Runners passing the Eiffel Tower get a dose of much-needed refreshment.

of 2:05:04. It was the fastest-ever debut by a runner over the age of 30. That same year, the women's winner, Flomena Cheyech, finished in 2:22:44.

In 1989, the Paris Marathon was won by a Brit, Steve Brace, a former long-distance runner from Wales, who completed the course in 2:13:03. He won it again the following year in a slightly slower time of 2:13:10. The Paris Marathon wasn't held the following year, in 1991, due to the Gulf War.

These days, runners flock from overseas to take part in the race, with around 23,000 participants coming from abroad, which makes up around 40 per cent of the field. Many participants from overseas describe the course highlights as Notre-Dame Cathedral and the Eiffel tower.

Bear in mind that to run this race you're required to get a medical certificate from your doctor stating that you're fit enough to participate. Registration for the Paris Marathon normally starts in September and you'll save money by registering early. Your predicted race time will determine the colour of the race bib you'll be given: the first two zones of red and yellow will require you to prove you've run a qualifying time from a race in the past two years – you'll need to have run from 3:00 to 3:15 for a marathon.

If you are unable to secure a place directly through the organizers, you can apply for a charity place, which will entail raising a certain amount for your chosen charity. Travelling to the race is a doddle: just hop aboard Eurostar in London and in just over two hours you'll be at the Gare du Nord station in the heart of Paris. Return tickets cost from about £125. (Flying is also an option but, with long check-in times and the fact that the airports are some way outside the city, isn't nearly as convenient.) Getting to the start is easy, too, as Paris's extensive Metro system deposits you right at the start. Paris is extraordinarily scenic, with plenty of must-see sights to keep you occupied, masses of crowd support to keep your spirits up and no nasty hills or bridges to slow you down. Being a top city-break destination, Paris has a host of hotels to choose from. Stay at one of the many budget options near the Gare du Nord and you'll be able to ask if they'd mind your having a quick shower after the race before you collect your luggage and head off home.

"The Paris Marathon was so unforgettable that, when I wanted a special race to mark my tenth marathon, I chose to return."

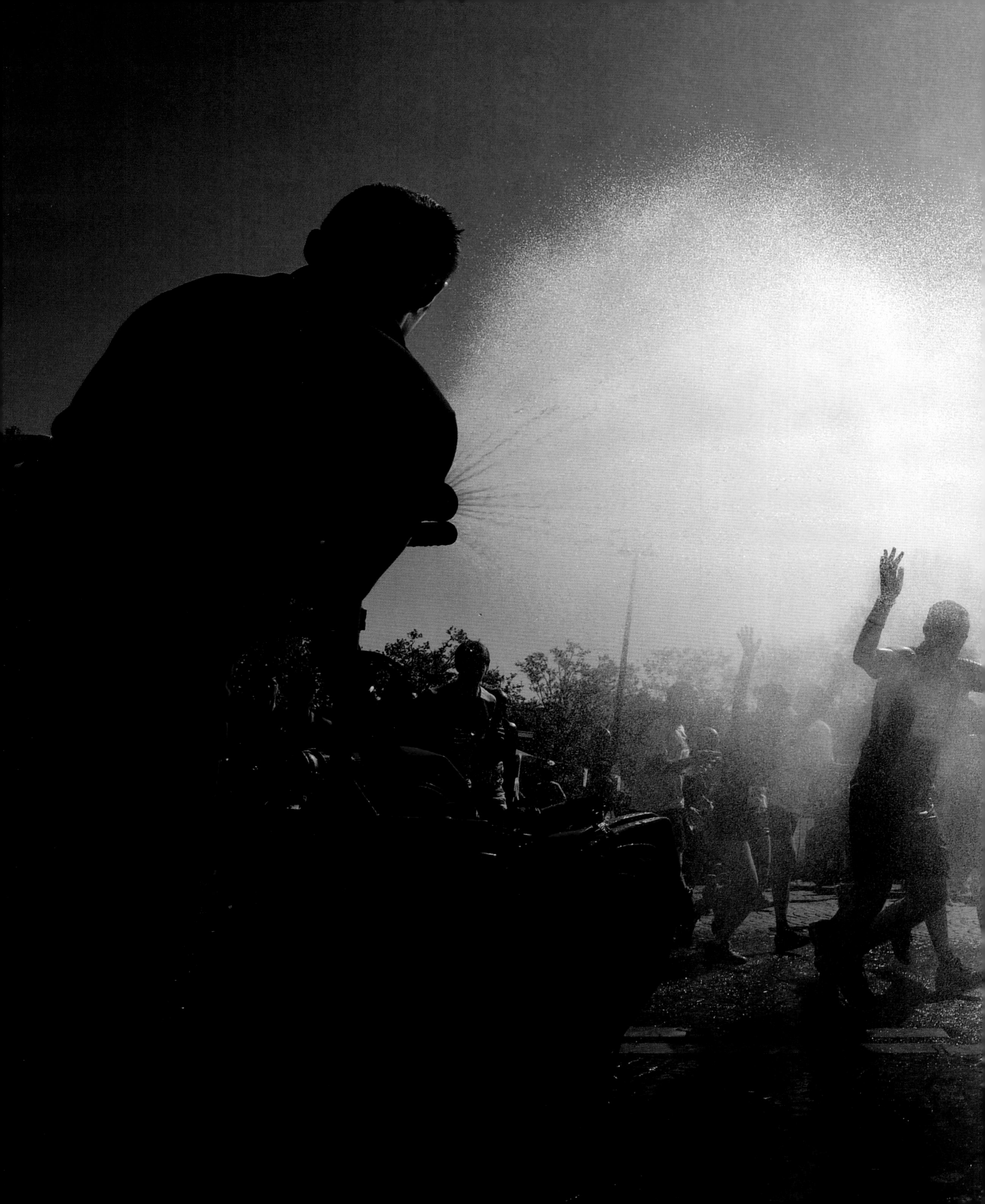

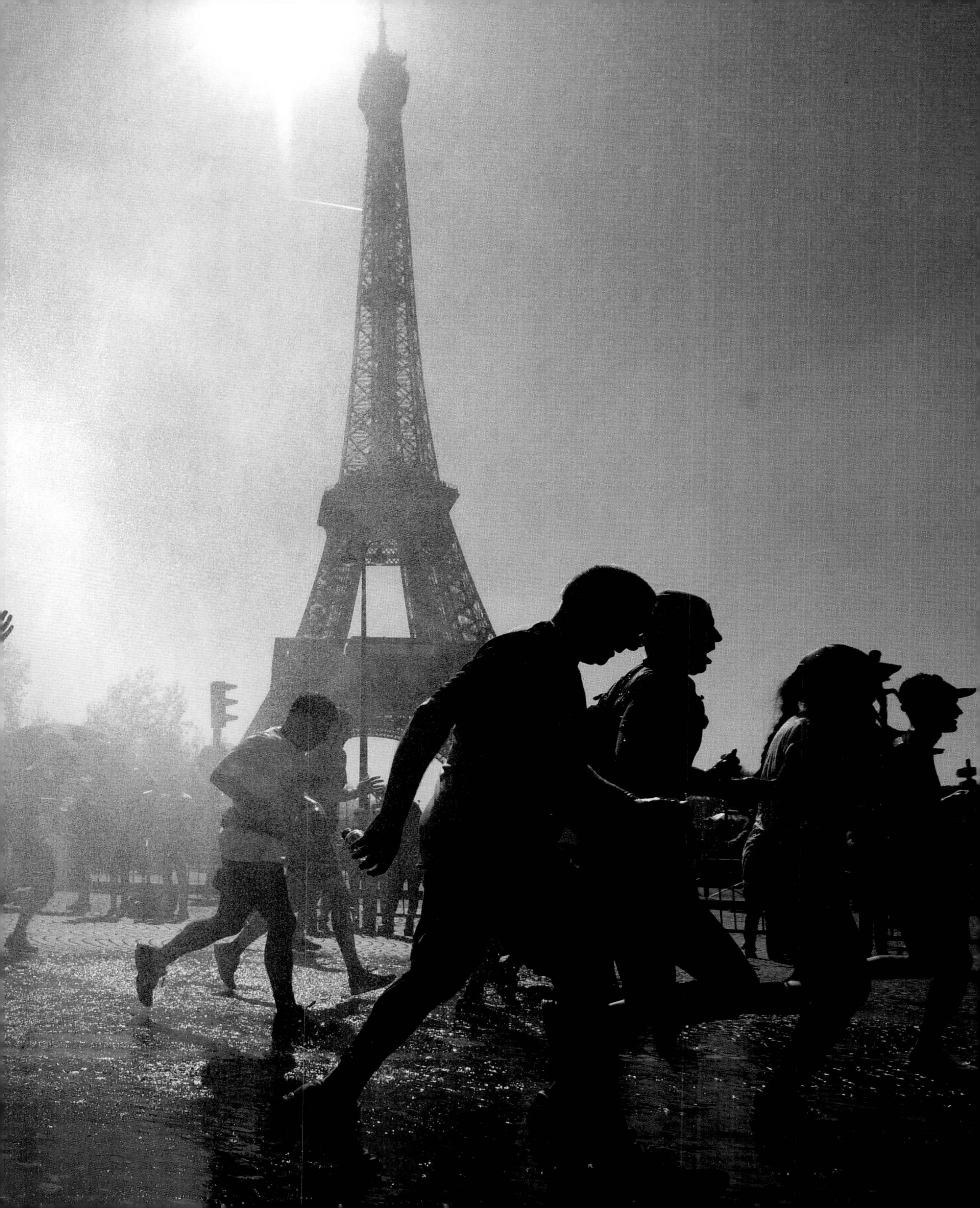

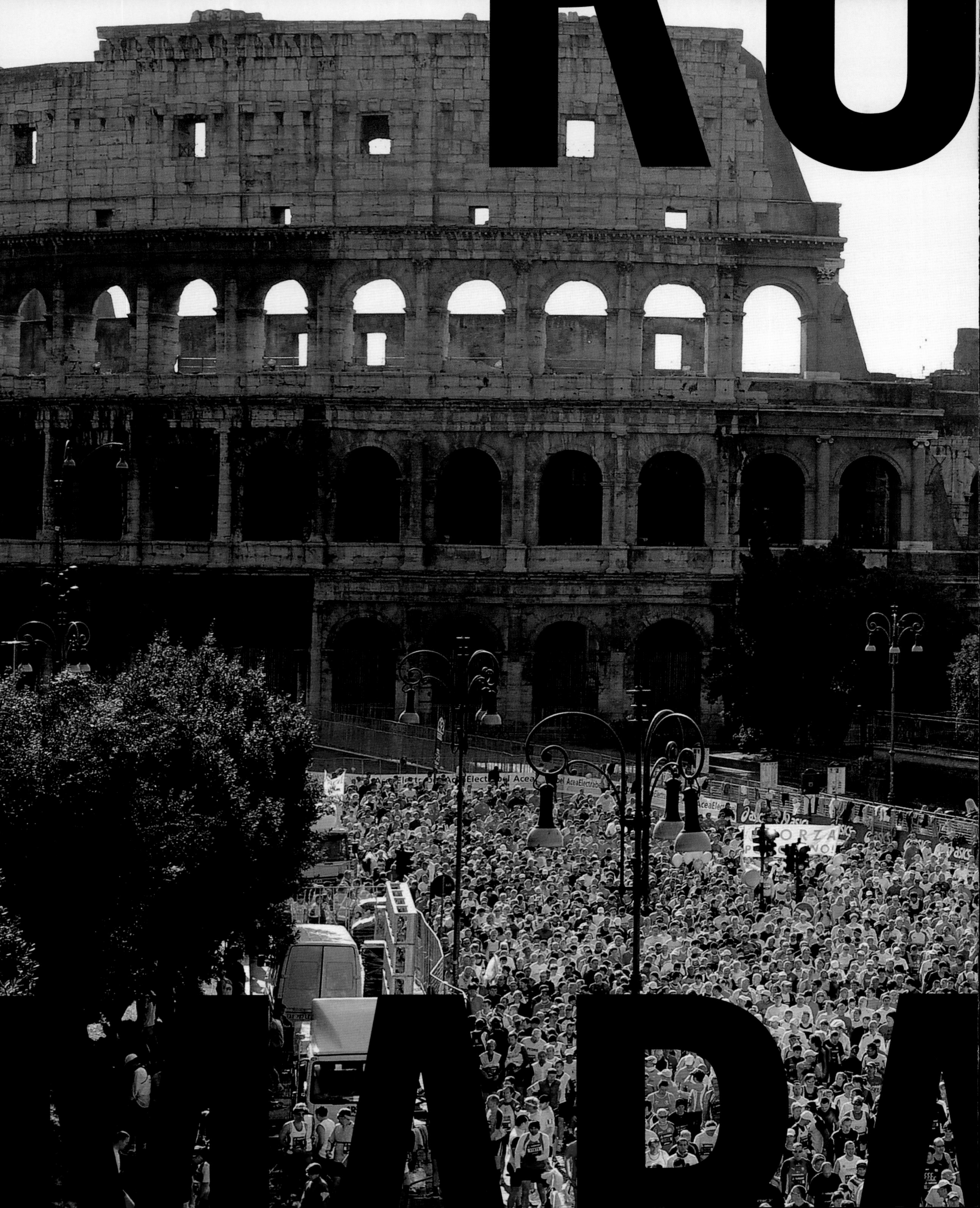

ROME

Date: March • Number of Entrants: 15,000

Established:

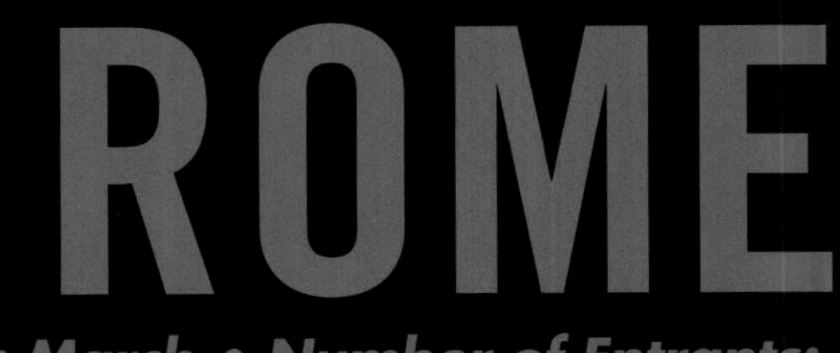

Men's Record: Benjamin Kiptoo (Kenya) 2:07:17 (2009)
Women's Record: Galina Bogomolova (Russia) 2:22:53 (2008)

Most Wins, Men: 1 – Various
Most Wins, Women: 3 – Rahma Tusa (Ethiopia), Firehiwot Dado (Ethiopia)

THE ROME MARATHON

Wonderful pre-race food, a great deal of history and amazing support are three good reasons why you may wish to put the Rome Marathon on your bucket list, as is a great course that is mostly flat.

The Rome Marathon offers runners the chance to combine their love of running with the opportunity to experience one of the most visited cities in Europe. Known as the Eternal City, Rome has a great deal of history to offer, from the historic fountains to the modern Olympic Stadium.

In ancient times, Romans celebrated their victories over their foes by holding huge games there: when Trajan conquered Dacia in 107 AD, for example, 11,000 animals and 10,000 gladiators fought to the death. And it's incredible to think that, even today, Rome knows how to stage a breathtaking spectacle – even if in this case the celebrations last only seven hours (the official cut-off time) instead of 123 days, as Trajan's Games did.

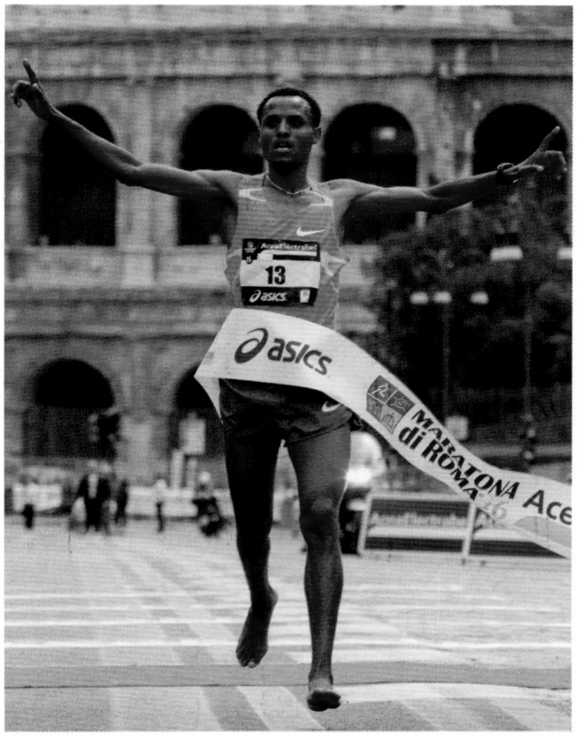

▶ Siraj Gena crosses the finish line barefoot in 2010, as a tribute to Abebe Bikila.

▶▶ The route through Rome passes many stunning and historic churches, but St Peter's Basilica is easily the most spectacular.

The very first Rome Marathon was held in 1982 and the men's winner was Belgian athlete Emiel Puttemans, in an impressive time of 2:09:53. The women's winner was Italy's own Laura Fogli, who completed the race in a time of 2:31:08.

The race doubled as the Italian Marathon twice – in 1983 and 1986. In 2000, the typical race month was switched from March to 1 January to celebrate the start of the new millennium. The IAAF Rome Millennium Marathon was supported by Primo Nebiolo, president of the Worldwide Athletics Federation, and national federation president Gianni Gola. The race began in St Peter's Square, where Pope John Paul II gave a short speech in approval of the event and to encourage the runners. The bells of St Peter's were rung instead of using the normal pistol at the start of the race.

The male winner in 2000 was Josephat Kiprono from Kenya, who ran the race in 2:08:27, while the women's winner was Tegla Loroupe, also from Kenya, who ran the race in 2:32:03.

ANNIVERSARY RACE

In 2010, the Rome Marathon was held to commemorate the 50th anniversary of Abebe Bikila's barefoot win at the 1960 Rome Olympic Marathon. The 2010 men's winner of the Rome Marathon, Siraj Gena, earned a bonus for crossing the line barefoot to pay homage to Abebe Bikila's style. He completed the race in 2:08:39.

In 2013, the year that marked the 29th edition of the race, the organizers faced a particularly tough challenge, as the event coincided with the election of Pope Francis. There were fears that the marathon would have to start at 4 p.m. if he were to be enthroned on race day, meaning everyone bar the elite athletes would've finished in the dark. As things turned out, the race started at 9.30 a.m.

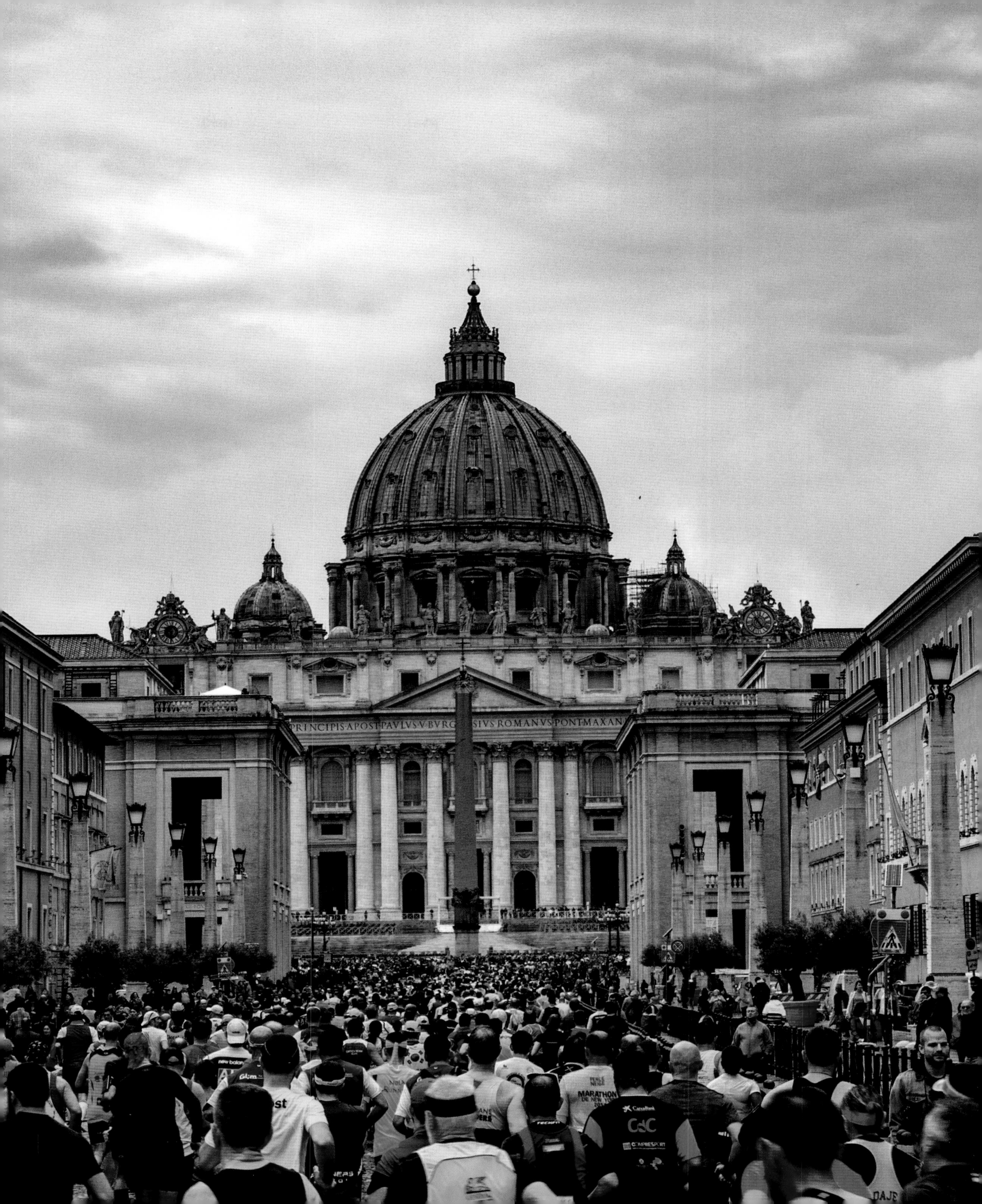
PRINCIPIS·APOST·PAVLVS·V·BVRG
SIVS·ROMANVS·PONT·MAX·AN
MARATHON
DAJE

as usual, but not before the organizers had gone to the trouble of devising no fewer than 17 different possible routes to avoid the 200,000 pilgrims who were likely to turn up for this historic occasion.

THE ROUTE

As we've seen, the Rome Marathon has typically been held in March, but in 2018 it was held in April. The start line of the event was moved in front of the Coliseum and runners travelled past St Peter's Basilica, the Trevi Fountain, Piazza Navona and the Spanish Steps and through many scenic, narrow streets in the old part of the city.

You may not wish to try to go for a personal best in this race, as you'll probably prefer to enjoy the sights and the history. The course is mostly flat but there are cobblestones to contend with and some of the route does take place on narrow streets. The course has been described by previous runners as "stunning".

The event finishes at the Domus Aurea. There is a hill near the finish line, part of which takes place in a tunnel, but there's a downhill section on the final 1km of the race that is a popular sight for runners anxious to reach the end.

The significant number of cobbled streets mentioned above can be a problem for runners. When marathon runner and author Lisa Jackson completed the race in 2013, she loved the course but was surprised by the amount of the course that took place on the cobbles. As she recalls, "Few marathons can boast a more impressive start or more interesting course – according to the race brochure it bypasses no fewer than 500 historic sights, ruins and architectural treasures. But what the brochure didn't say is that, although the chosen route was relatively flat – rather ironic in a city built on seven hills – it featured numerous lengthy stretches on cobbles.

"And," she continued, "unlike the London Marathon course of old, where the cobbles were covered in cushioning carpet, these cobbles were hard as nails. Imagine grabbing a hammer and then spending two hours hitting your feet with it . . . you get the joint-juddering picture! So thank goodness, then, for the distractions thoughtfully provided en route – numerous soul-stirring military bands, refreshment tables groaning with orange slices, bananas and biscuits, and even sugar cubes, and, of course, that endless list of Eternal City must-sees, ranging from the Trevi Fountain to the Circus Maximus, where charioteers used to stage death-defying races to entertain the Roman masses."

The Rome Marathon offers great support and there's a rumour that even the city's priests and cardinals will come out to cheer you on. On a more practical note, there are plenty of energy gels and drinks available around the course, too.

A CITY TO EXPLORE

When in Rome, as the saying begins, there's plenty to see and do. This capital of Italy is a cosmopolitan, bustling city, with around 3,000 years of influential art and culture to see. There are ancient ruins, such as the Forum and Colosseum, and the Vatican Museums, which are the home of masterpieces from Michelangelo.

The Colosseum is one of the most iconic landmarks in the world and at one time held gladiator tournaments and was regularly visited by Roman emperors. This famous structure is incredible to look at and is close to the metro station, so it's easily accessible. There's also St Peter's Square, which, despite the name, is actually circular and has some beautiful statues and figures of previous popes. While you're there, it's also worth seeing St Peter's Basilica, a celebrated religious building, which is at the far end of St Peter's Square. Another sight worth seeing is the Pantheon, a beautifully preserved ancient Roman building erected in 118 AD by Emperor Hadrian. The inside of the building features a dome with a series of stone patterns.

In Rome, there are plenty of pasta restaurants to power those marathon miles, but a quick Internet search before you leave home can prevent you from spending needless hours on your feet hunting for some elusive carbs. The same goes for breakfast – unless you're staying in a hotel with ties to the race, it's unlikely that you'll be able to get anything to eat that early on race day, so be sure to scrounge some bread rolls and butter at your meal the night before, or, better still, bring some muesli or instant porridge, along with a kettle, as not all hotels have tea-making facilities.

▽ Runners streak away from the Colosseum as they begin their 26.2 mile journey around Rome.

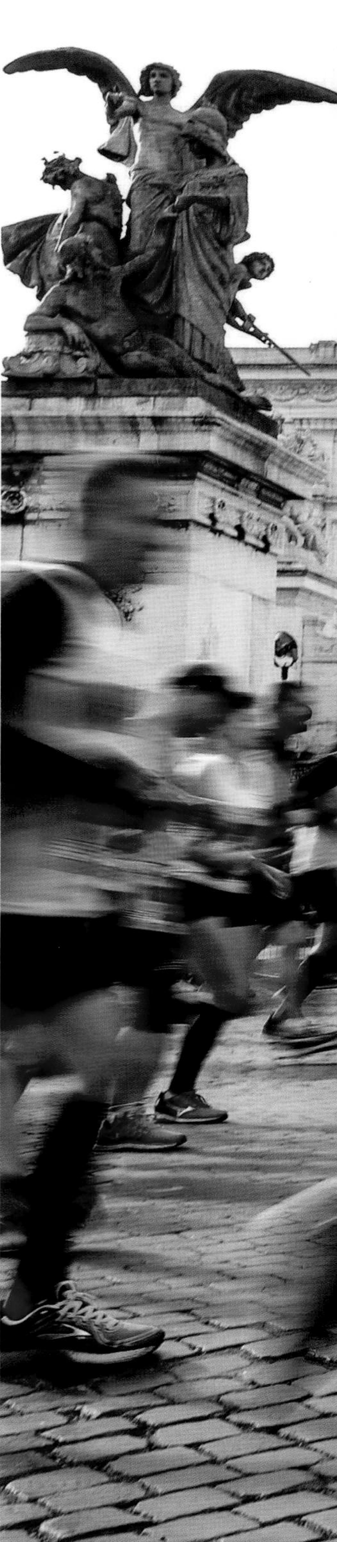

▶ It can be tempting to stop and marvel at the sights of Rome during the run, but try to resist.

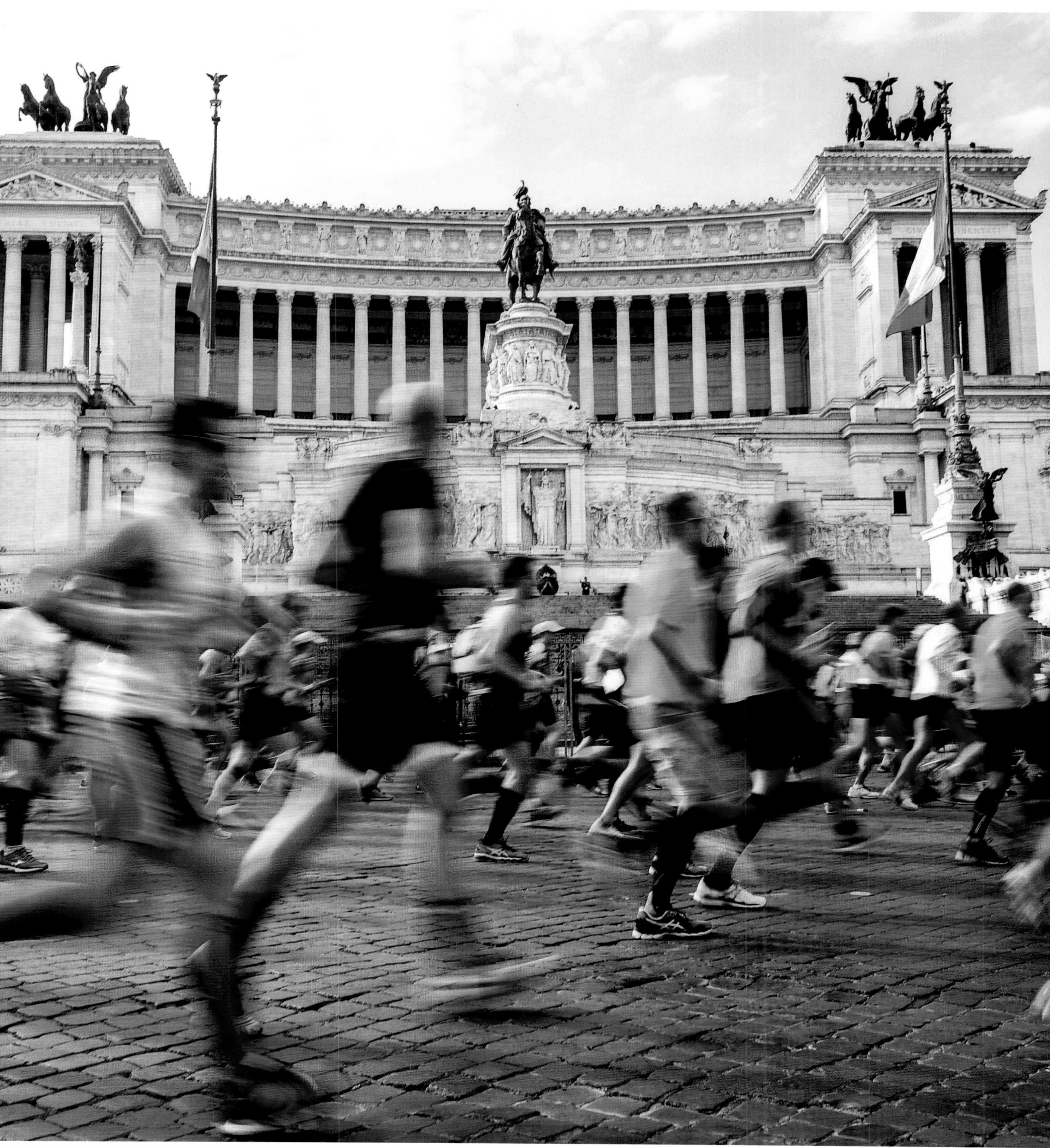

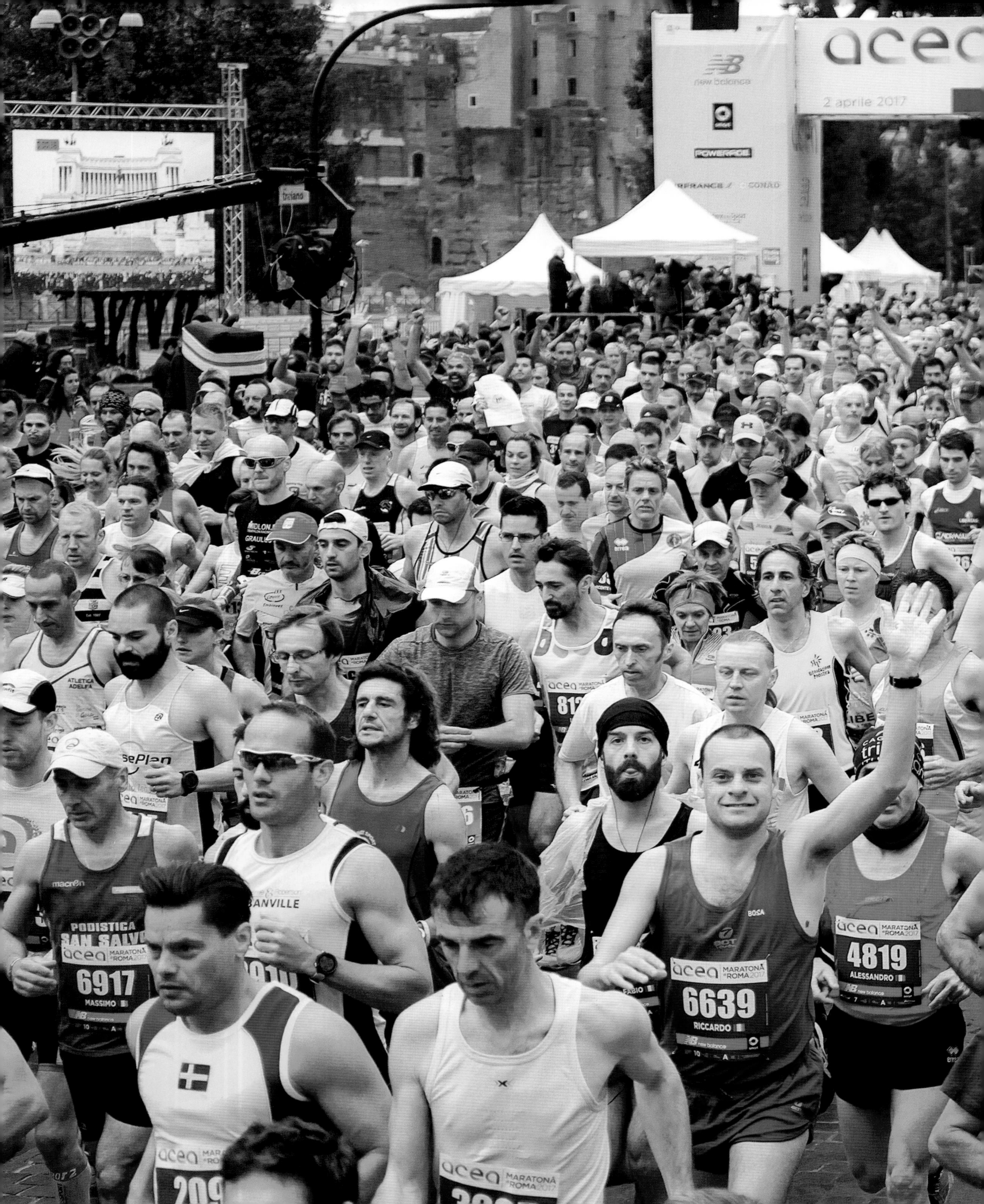

acea
new balance
2 aprile 2017
POWERADE
CONAD
traiano
ATLETICA ADELFIA
BANVILLE
PODISTICA
acea MARATONA di ROMA 2017
6917
MASSIMO
6639
RICCARDO
4819
ALESSANDRO
812
BOSA

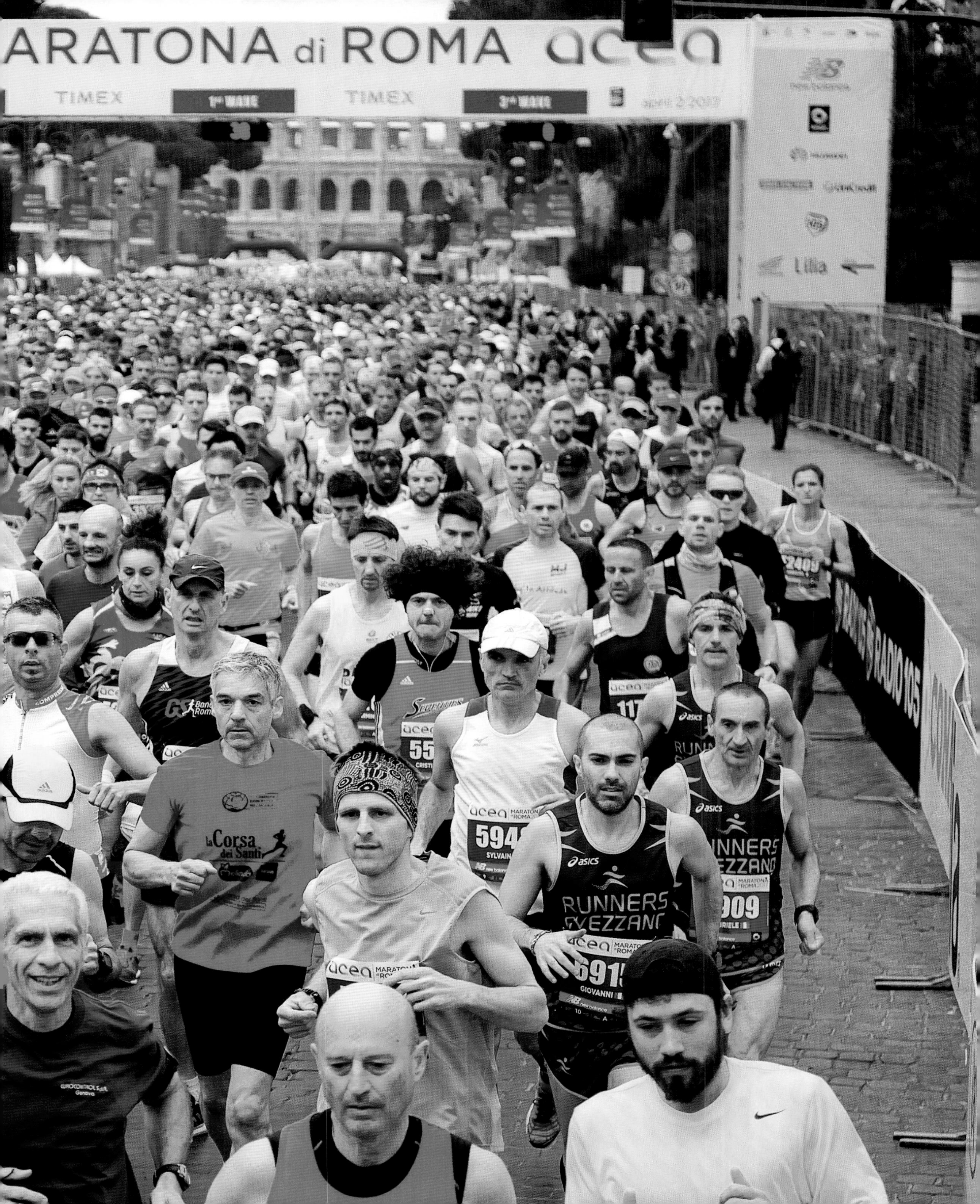

ARATONA di ROMA acea
TIMEX
TIMEX
RADIO 105

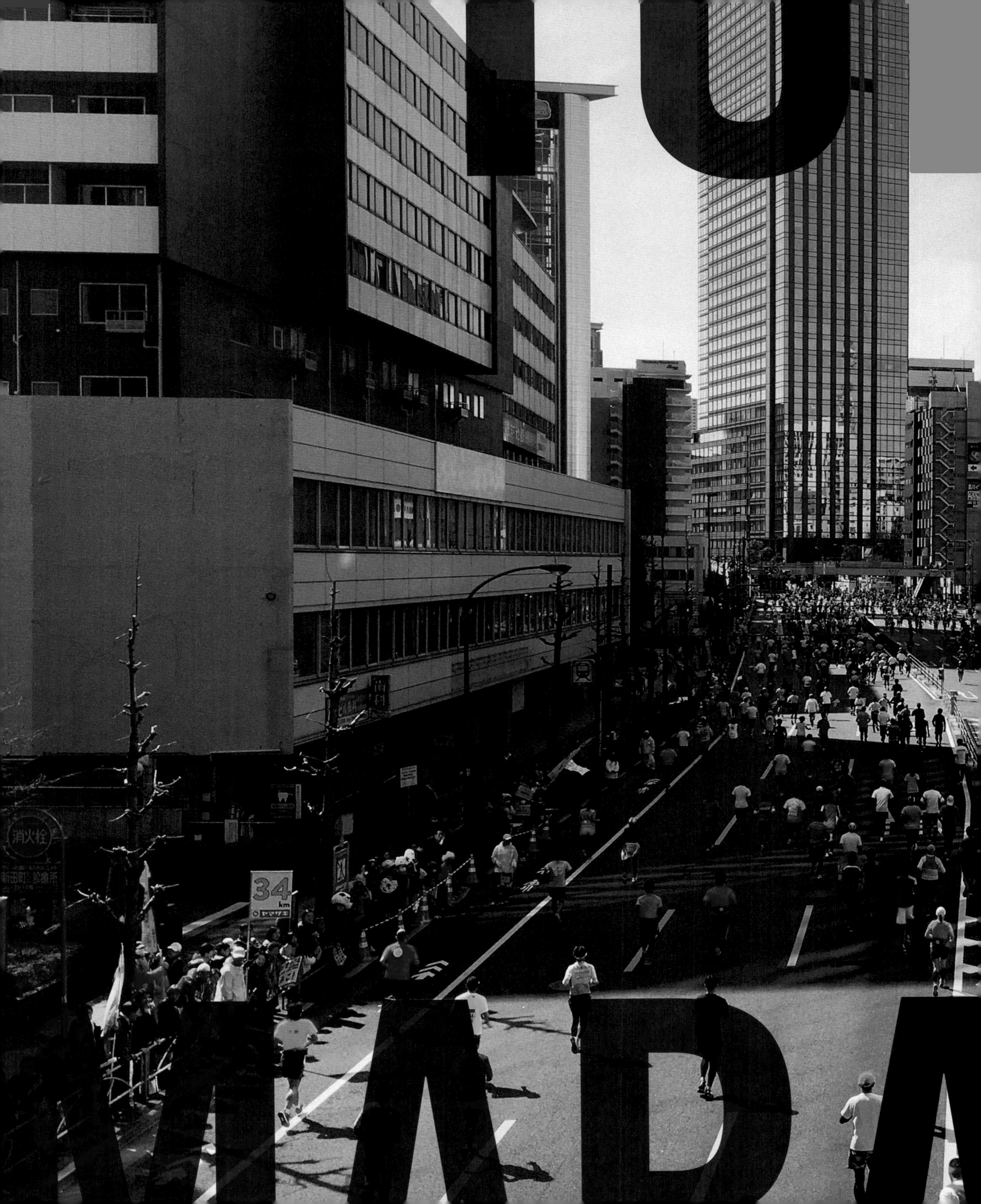

消火栓
34
km

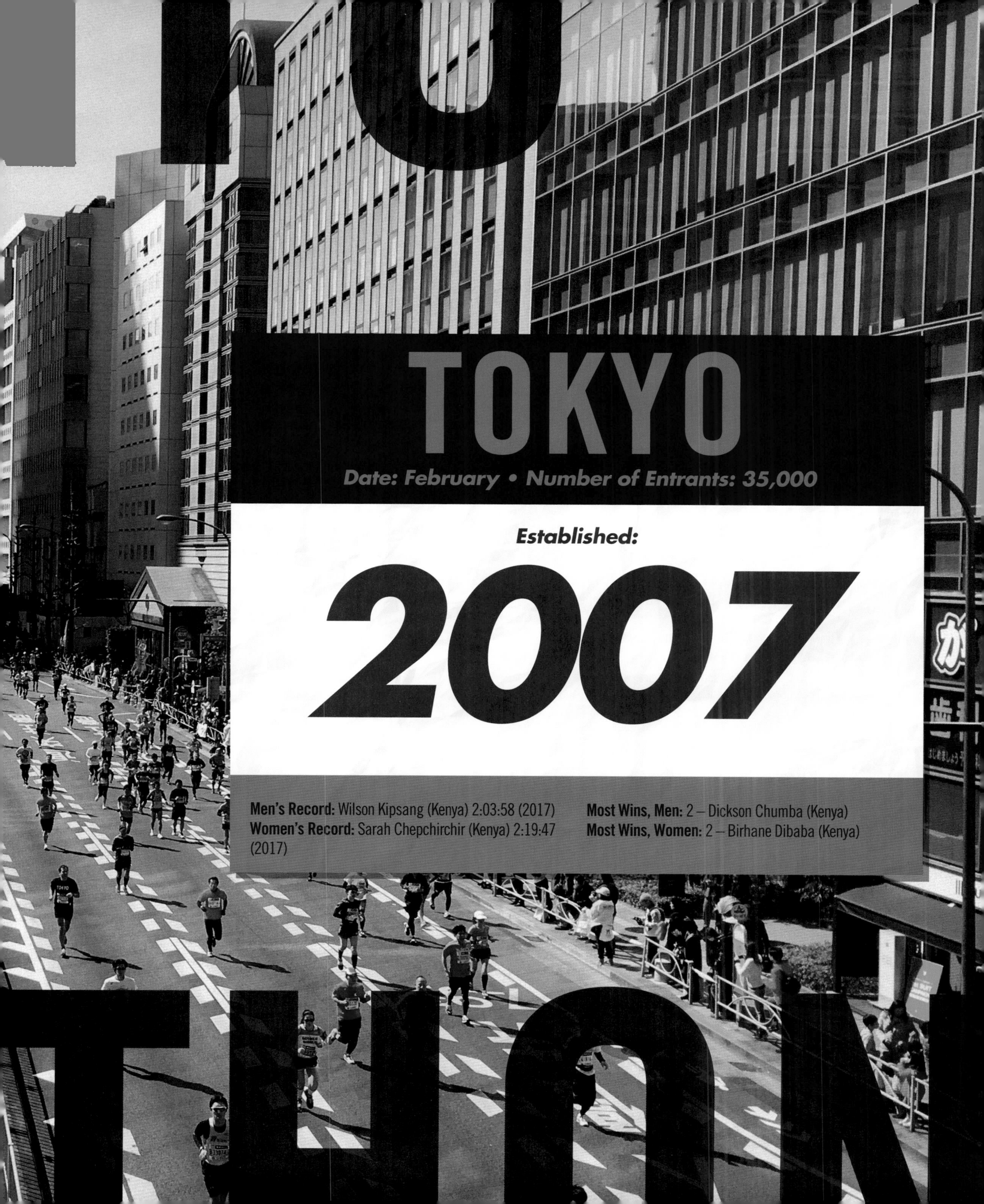

TOKYO

Date: February • Number of Entrants: 35,000

Established:

2007

Men's Record: Wilson Kipsang (Kenya) 2:03:58 (2017)
Women's Record: Sarah Chepchirchir (Kenya) 2:19:47 (2017)

Most Wins, Men: 2 – Dickson Chumba (Kenya)
Most Wins, Women: 2 – Birhane Dibaba (Kenya)

THE TOKYO MARATHON

Well organized with great crowd support, this race offers a mostly flat course through one of the world's most populous cities. Expect a lot of encouragement, along with some unusual fuelling snacks along the way.

▶ Tokyo is a heaving metropolis on any day, and that's even more apparent during the marathon.

▼ A huge crowd of athletes runs in the inaugural Tokyo, held in 2007.

The highly acclaimed Tokyo Marathon is one of the Abbott World Marathon Majors – a series of six of the largest and most renowned marathons in the world. The other five are Boston, London, Berlin, Chicago and New York.

To gain recognition from the Majors, athletes score points for their finishing place in each race with the top male and female runners at the end of each cycle receiving an equal share of the $1 million prize. The organizers of these big marathon events are all keen to advance the sport and increase the level of interest in elite racing among running enthusiasts.

Even if you aren't an athlete, and you just want a marathon experience that doesn't involve trying to win any prize money, the Tokyo Marathon, which takes place in February, has more than just prestige: it can be a great race experience for runners of all abilities. It's fun, friendly and very well organized, which may be one reason why it has become one of the largest and most popular marathons in the world – not bad for a race that began only in 2007. In fact, it's the largest race in Asia.

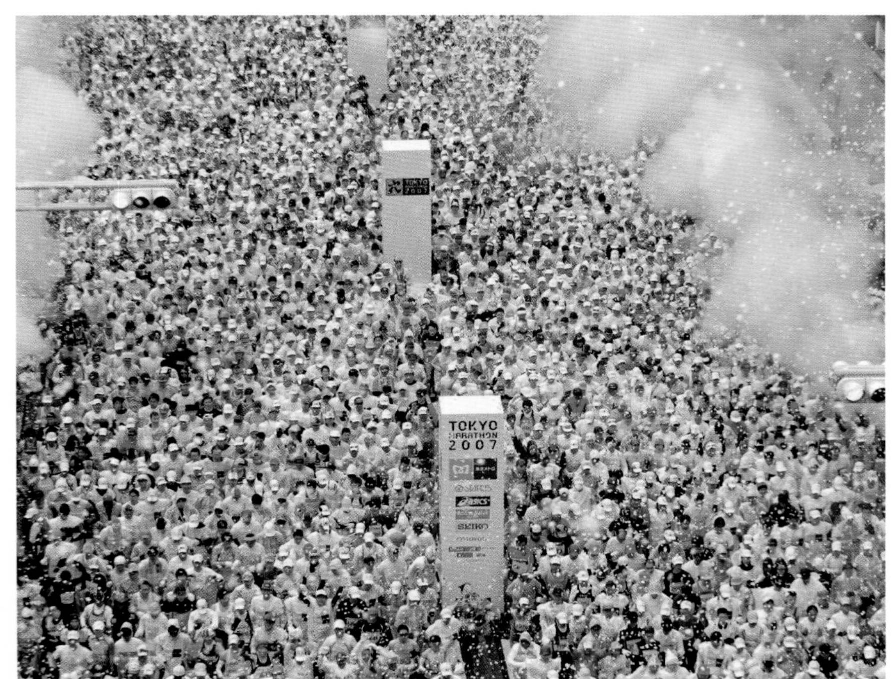

THE HISTORY

Before the launch of the Tokyo Marathon, there were just two separate ones in Japan. One was called the Tokyo International Marathon, and took place every other year on even-numbered years, while the Tokyo New York Friendship International Marathon took place on the alternate years.

Organized by the Tokyo Marathon Foundation, the event is also co-organized by the Japan Association of Athletics Federations (JAAF), the Tokyo Metropolitan Government and various media, including the Fuji Television Network, Nippon Television Corporation and the newspapers *Sankei Shimbun* and the *Tokyo Shimbun*.

Apart from the marathon, there are also individual wheelchair marathon races for men and women, a mixed 10km race for men and women and for juniors and youth, as well as separate races for visually impaired and intellectually challenged people.

RACE CAPACITY

The event has capacity for around 35,500 runners, and final selections are made on a lottery basis. There's high demand for this race, so it can be difficult to get into.

In 2010, the marathon attracted 272,134 applicants for its 32,000 places and it has continued to grow in popularity. In 2015, those who had registered to take part totalled 308,810. You might think there's little chance of getting

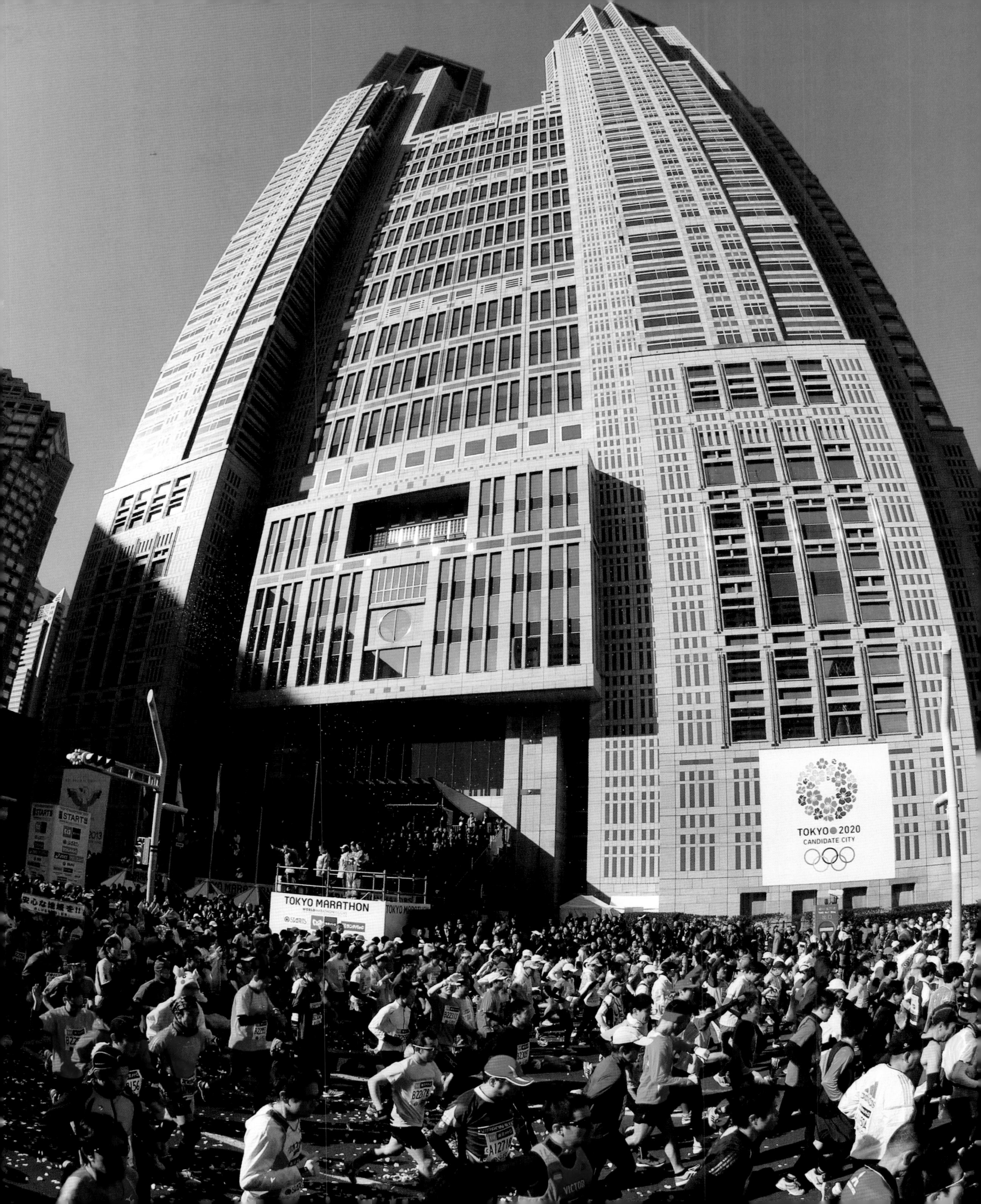

TOKYO MARATHON
TOKYO 2020
CANDIDATE CITY

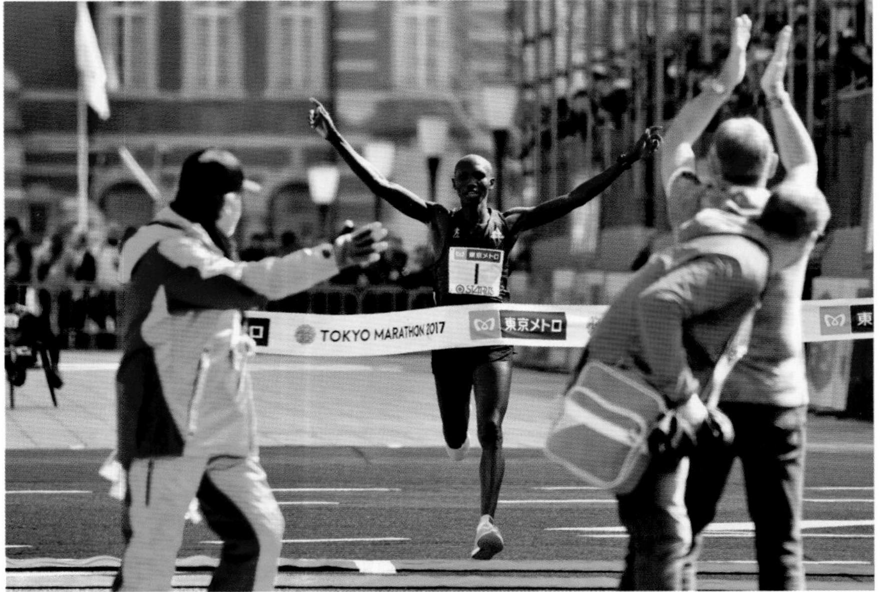

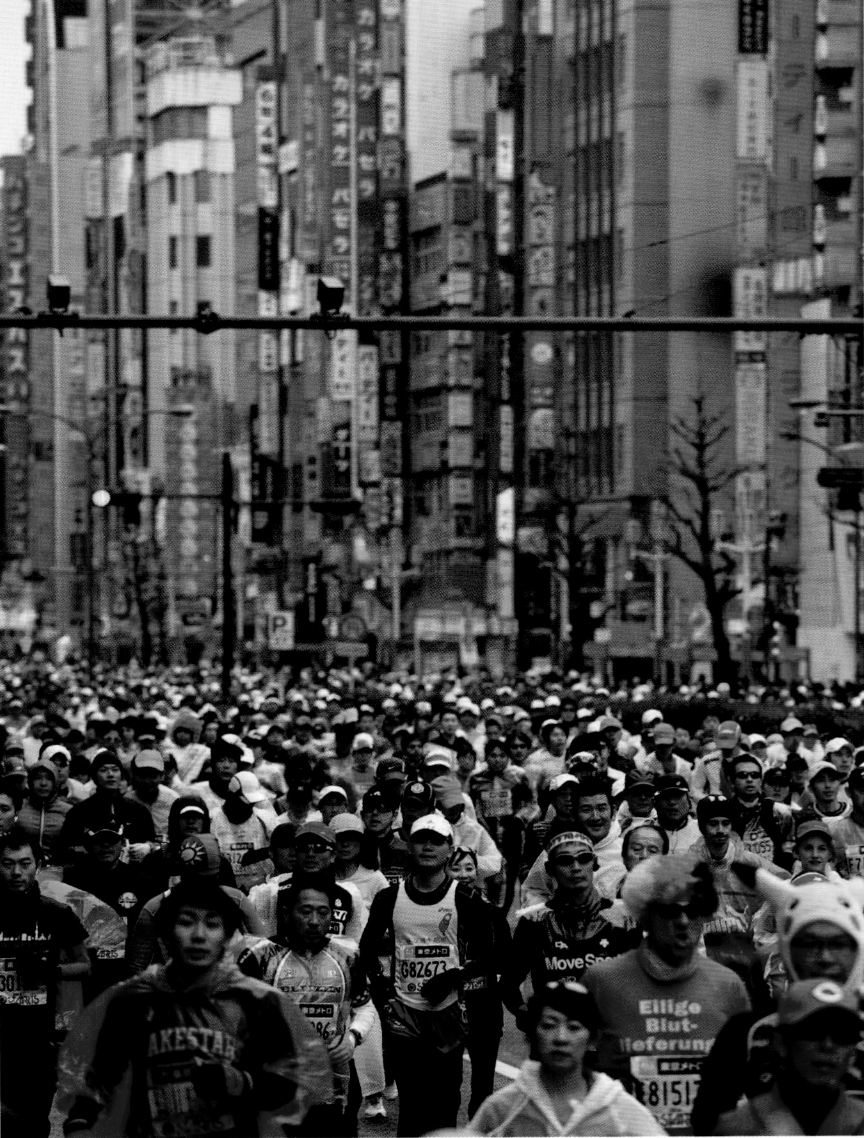

into this event, and you'd be right in saying it can be a challenge. However, if you're a fast runner registered with the JAAF, then you could register in the Elite field. The race time requirements in 2014 were 2:23 for the full marathon for men and 2:54 for women. Otherwise, as with the London Marathon, you're at the mercy of the ballot, unless you choose to go with a tour operator.

As with many other marathons, participants must collect their race number at an expo before the race, where there's an outdoor food festival at which you can fuel up on delicious Japanese cuisine.

RACE-DAY WEATHER

The weather for this race is typically around 44°F – ideal conditions for runners. Many of the previous marathons in Tokyo have been rainy. The mostly flat, urban course starts by the Tokyo Metropolitan Government HQ, a large 45-storey building, close to Shinjuku station. It then goes through the high-rise city areas, via six districts, including Iidabashi, a district of Tokyo, the Imperial Palace and the cultured city of Nihombashi, and up to the Tokyo Skytree Building. It then goes through Ginza, another district of Tokyo, which is famed for its shopping, and the Tokyo Tower, before finishing near the Mitsubishi Shoji Building. The views of the Tokyo Tower, Tokyo main station, the Tokyo Skytree, Tamioka Shrine and the Rainbow Bridge are all outstanding.

There are some short inclines in the earlier stages of the race but, other than that, it's a largely flat course with fantastic crowd support. Marathon runner Matthew Stears, who ran the race in 2017, describes the course as relatively fast and straightforward. "There were no real bottlenecks at any stage, so following the course was less challenging than other marathons I've done in the past," he says. Another bonus to doing this marathon is the markers that measure the course in kilometres. Some runners may find this motivational. "The entire course was measured in kilometres, rather than miles, which meant the distance markers seemed to come around much quicker and helped with the mental battle of the race," adds Matthew.

◤ Wilson Kipsang of Kenya crosses the finish line to claim victory in the 2017 Tokyo Marathon.

◀ Tokyo's status as a World Marathon Major makes it priority for elite athletes.

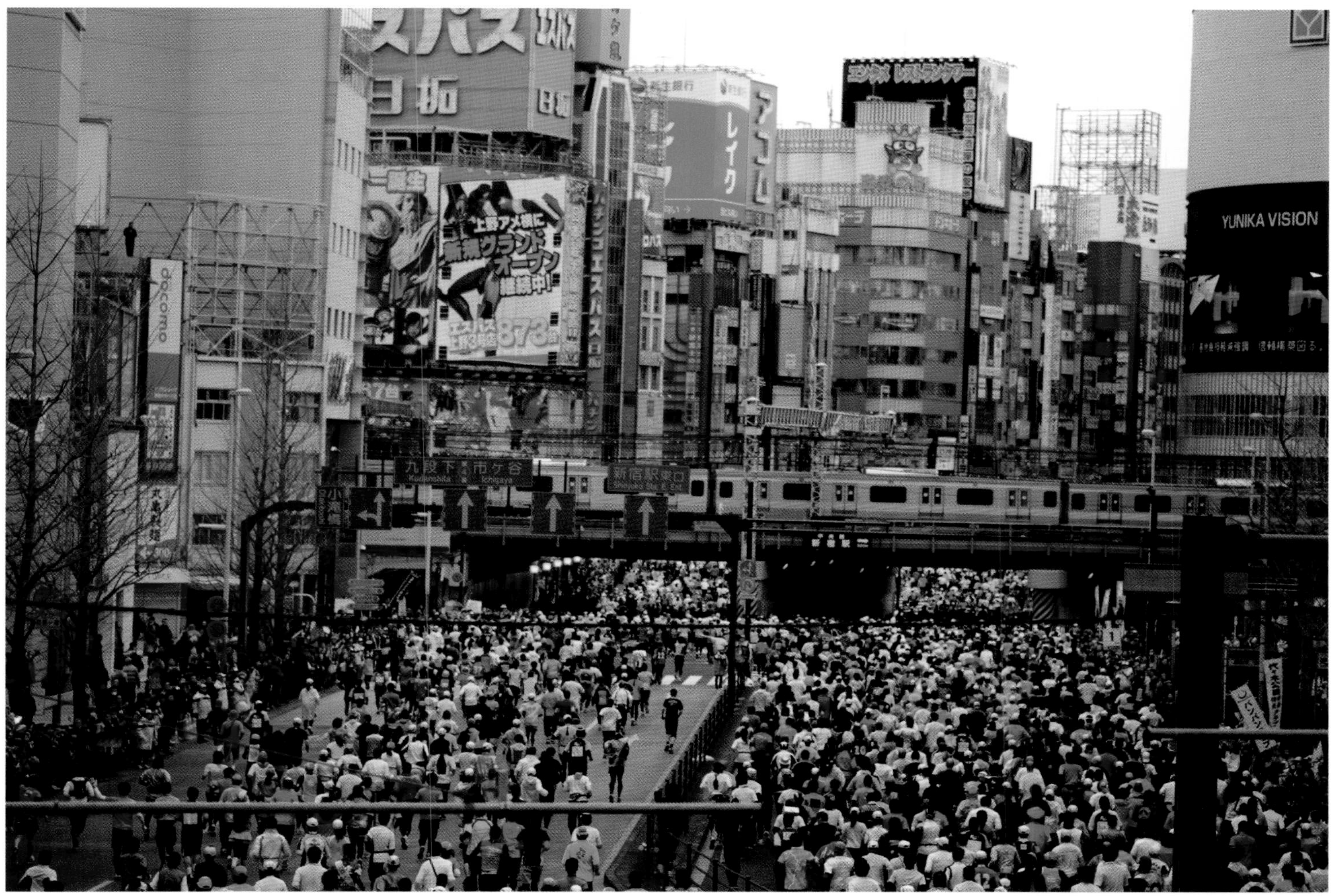

▲ With thousands of competitors and more than a million spectators, just staging the Tokyo Marathon is a major logistical feat.

There are few inclines along the way with two relatively long but gentle climbs, at about 36km and again at 41km just before the Imperial Palace area. There is then a short downhill run before runners turn the corner for a 200m flat dash to the finish line. The easiest part of the race is the first 6.4km, or four miles, which is downhill. Matthew says, "The natural temptation is to run this section way too fast relative to your target race pace, and, with the euphoria of a unique mass start, it is almost impossible to avoid the blood rush."

There are three memorable, 180-degree turns on the course (at about 15km, 20km and 36km, respectively) but they are all easily manageable without any pace lost. The course has wide roads and the asphalt surface is in noticeably perfect condition.

HELPFUL VOLUNTEERS

The race has a lot of volunteers, who help to manage the queues at the toilet stops, and many hold bags for your rubbish. The water stops are also well staffed and managed, and the volunteers, known for their huge smiles and exceptional politeness, are called Team Smile. Volunteers who can speak English wear green jackets so that overseas runners can identify them, and there are also around 1.6 million spectators.

You get to fuel up with snacks, too, as volunteers along the way hand out tomatoes, sushi and cakes. The drinks stations are miraculously free of debris with an army of volunteers on continuous clear-up duty.

Former participants report that the overall organization is exemplary at every level. This applies to the setup of the expo as well as the marathon. It's easy to understand why an event like this must be so well planned and prepared in a country where earthquakes can be a risk. The organizers take health and safety around the expo and the race very seriously, and have special procedures for earthquake alerts.

The Japanese tend to enjoy dressing in bright colours and flamboyant clothes when doing races. You won't find too many black outfits. Runners are welcome to complete this race in costume. Running

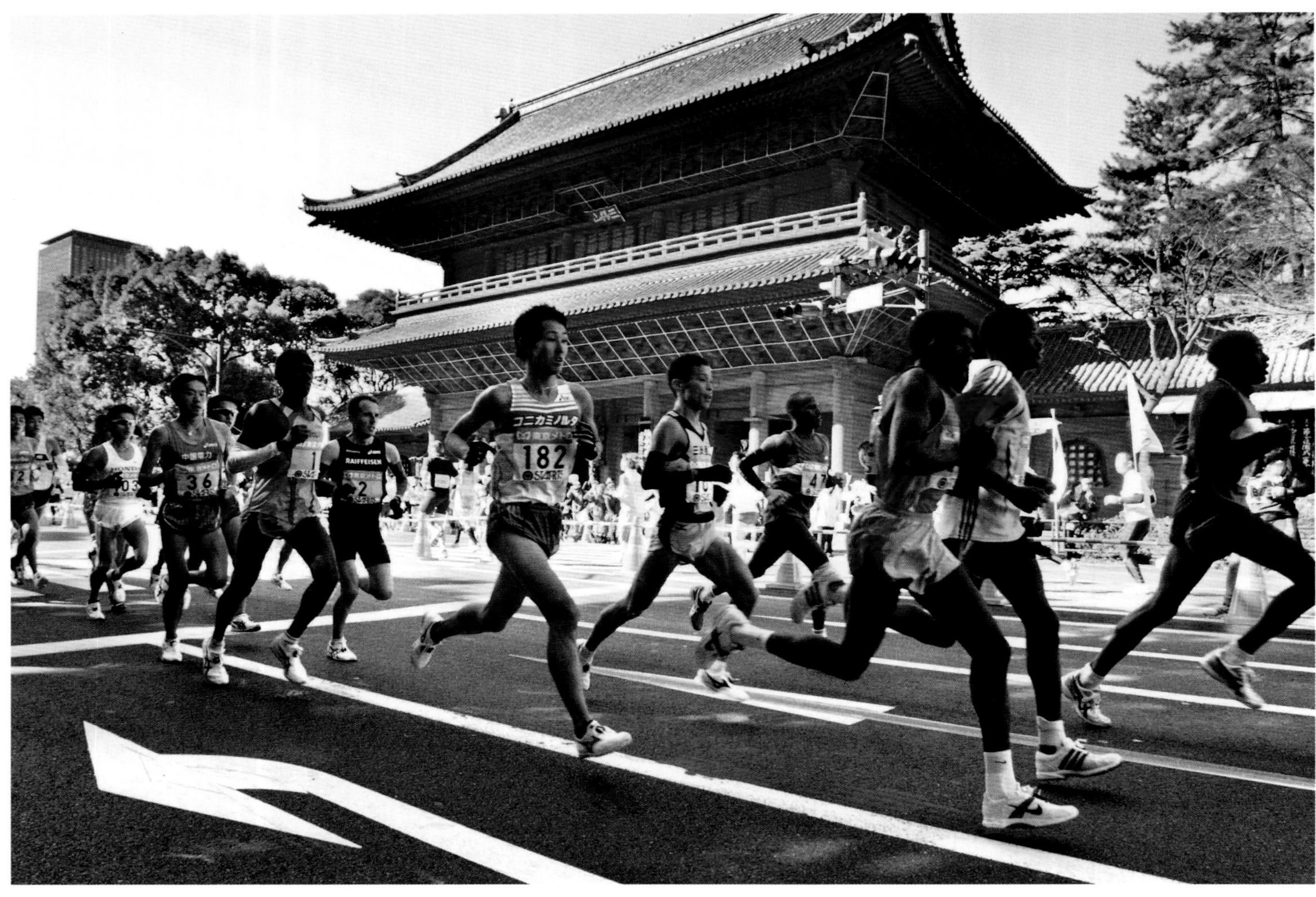

▲ The spectacular Zojyoji temple is just one of the Tokyo landmarks that runners pass on the route.

blogger Charlie Watson, who ran the marathon in 2018, says, "The costumes were amazing, and although the organizers are strict on the sizing of the outfits – meaning you won't see some of the rhino-type outfits you find at London – they went all out. It's the only other Marathon Major where I've seen so many people wearing fancy dress."

There have been some outstanding moments in the Tokyo Marathon. In 2017, Wilson Kipsang from Kenya set a course record of 2:03:58. This was notably faster than the previous record-holder, Dickson Chumba from Kenya, who finished the course in 2:05:42. Another course record was set in 2017 by the female winner Sarah Chepchirchir from Kenya, who completed the course in 2:19:47.

There is a seven-hour time limit for the marathon and a 2:10 cutoff time for the wheelchair marathon.

LOCAL CULTURE

While you're in Tokyo, you must take some time to view the local culture and explore the sights. You can go to Sensō-ji, Tokyo's most visited temple, which has a golden image of Kannon, the Buddhist goddess of mercy. You'll also want to see the Meiji-jingū, Tokyo's grandest Shinto shrine (a place of the gods and a place of worship), which was destroyed in World War II air raids and rebuilt in 1958.

Tokyo is a truly international city, while also subtly preserving its own culture. The Japanese love shopping, and there are many shopping outlets, where you can shop for everything you would expect in London, New York and Paris.

There are great bars (which are usually English-speaking) and the most immense range of International restaurants (including the usual fast-food chains, if you're in a hurry). While you're there, you must make it a personal mission to try sushi at a Japanese restaurant.

Matthew Stears made the most of his time in Tokyo. "The city is incredibly clean and litter-free," he says. "The subway system is vast and efficiently operated. All signage is in English and Japanese, making navigation relatively easy.

"I participated in the Mario Kart tour, involving riding in a go-kart, where I dressed up as my

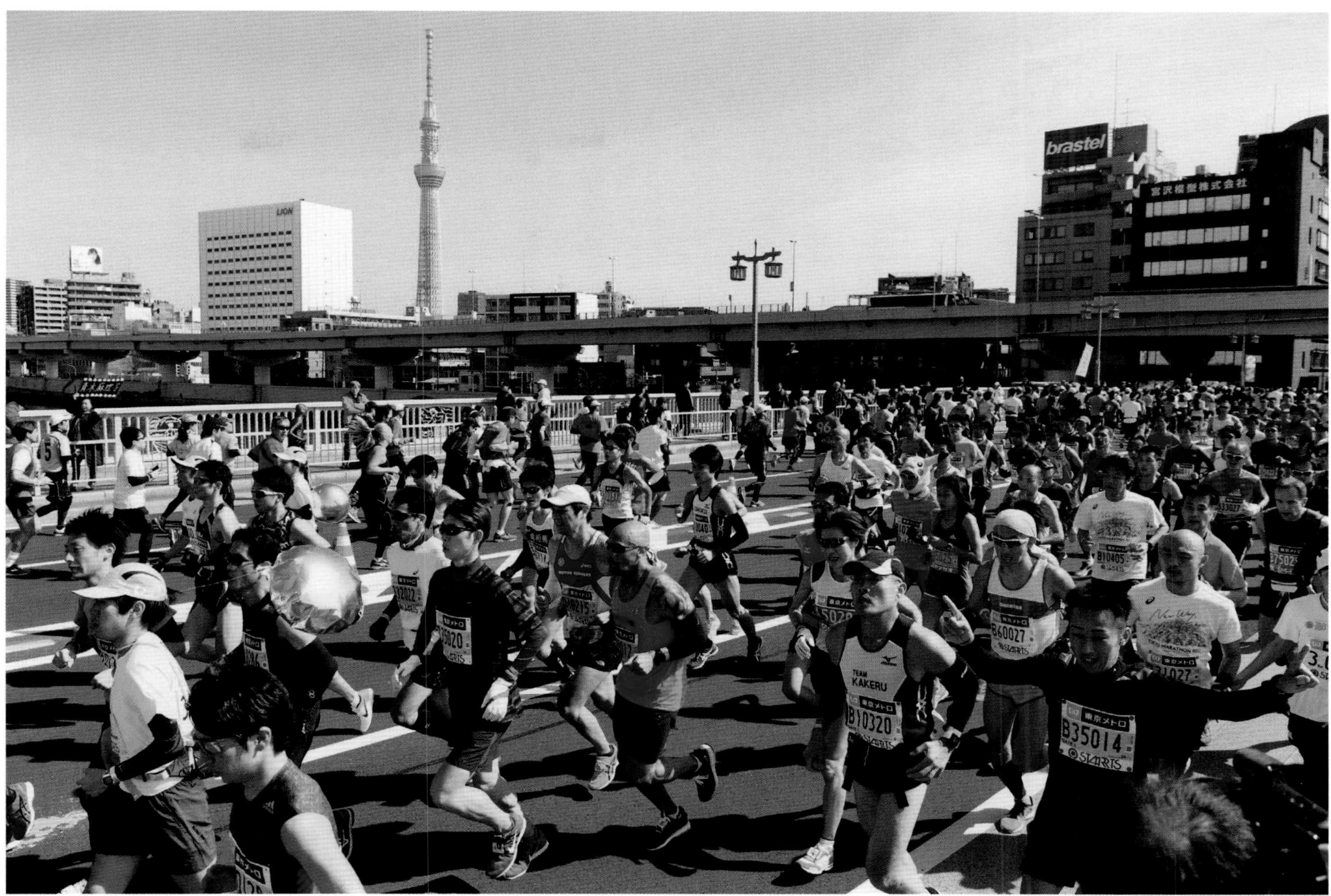

▲ Though most entrants are understandably from Japan, Tokyo attracts runners from all around the world.

favourite Mario Kart character. The professionally guided tour lasts about three hours, starting at Tokyo Bay, and tours the city. I did the night tour, which added to the magic of my time in Japan."

You can also visit Mount Fuji and the snow monkeys in Nagano, as well as experiencing the famous, very high-speed Bullet Train, which can reach 200mph.

As with other marathons in faraway territories, you're well advised to fly out at least a week before the race, to give you time to get used a different time zone and overcome jetlag. Stears says, "There is a nine-hour time difference between London and Tokyo and a twelve-hour flight. This makes for some potentially serious difficulties in sleeping and in acclimatizing sufficiently before the race – unless you arrive a week ahead of race day. This must be factored in if you want a quality running experience."

However, if you're prepared to make the long journey, it's well worth it. Stears says, "The Japanese are wonderful. The vast city of Tokyo and its populous were incredibly welcoming. The crowd support throughout the race course was simply fantastic. It felt like half the city's population was out there entertaining and cheering all the runners along and encouraging every kind of runner–spectator interaction. There seemed to be cow bells at every corner and the crowds were unique."

Watson agrees that crowd support during this race is "really great". She says, "There were people lining the streets the entire route. Most of the cheering was in Japanese of course, but it still gave me a boost to hear so many people out cheering. It also made anyone shouting in English even more special, like they were cheering just for me!"

Apart from the marathon, there's also a Tokyo Fun Friendship Run the day before the marathon. The distance is 4km and it attracts runners from all over the world, along with friends and family members of those doing the marathon the next day. If you're planning to cheer on a loved one doing the marathon, it's worth noting that the Friendship Run also earns you a wristband that you can use to gain entry to the grandstand finish line for the marathon.

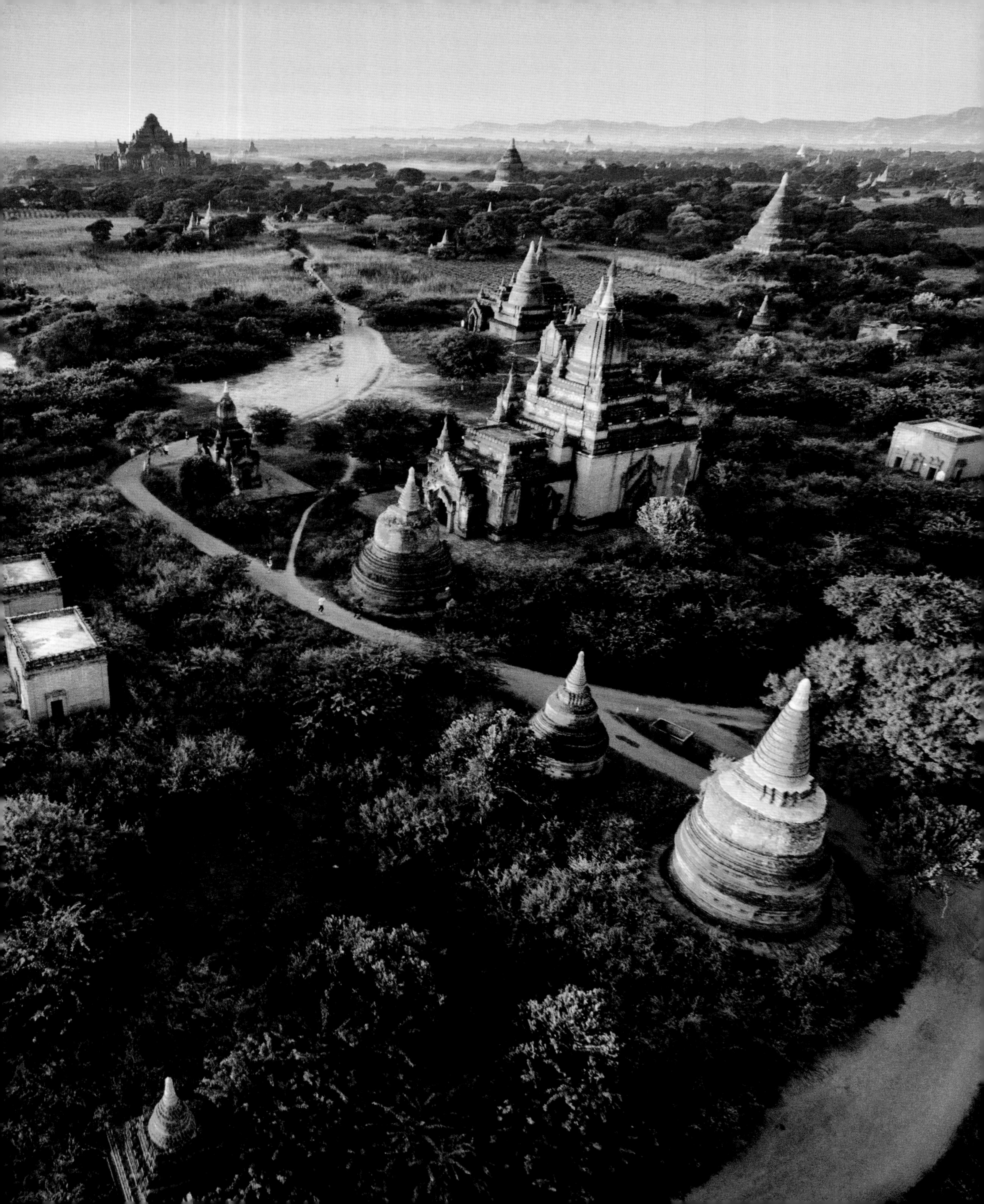

WEIRD & WONDERFUL MARATHONS

BAGAN TEMPLE MARATHON

A MYANMAR MARATHON THAT'S UNLIKE ANY OTHER

MYANMAR

Established:
2013
When: November

Tourists may have been banned from climbing the ancient temples of the Bagan plains in Myanmar, but running for 26.2 miles around them is still an option, even if the climatic conditions for distance running are challenging, to say the least. What you lose on the speed front, however, you more than gain on the scenery.

The course starts and ends at the Htilominlo Temple and also offers a half-marathon and 10km. This is one of the biggest ancient places of worship of the many to be admired during the run. In the rosy glow of the 6.15 a.m. start, its crumbly red bricks look truly spectacular. The 10km, half-marathon and marathon courses all start here, and then continue along dirt tracks with a few stretches of asphalt, through the dusty plains, dotted with thousand-year-old temples and pagodas. Runners who opt for the 10km peel off at Old Bagan to reach the finish. Half-marathoners part company with their longer-running comrades at the Dhammayazika Pagoda.

The longer-distance runners carry on towards New Bagan, running on sandy paths, passing through agricultural land. There are rice and peanut crops, and every now and then a cart loaded high with grain and pulled by oxen trundles past. Children run out to wave and smile. There's quite a festive atmosphere in the final miles, which take runners to the villages of Nyaungdo and Pwazaw and onto the homeward loop back towards the temples passed earlier.

This race is certainly not personal-best material. November is a hot and humid month in Bagan (with temperatures at around 80°F), so it's the weather that will slow you down, rather than the terrain, which is relatively flat. The course itself is semi-trail (think dirt roads and rutted paths), with occasional stretches of tarmac roads where cars and scooters zip along. The field is never very big, so you're often left with just goats and cattle for company, and temples to admire. The punishing humidity makes it difficult to run all the way, but there are frequent rest stations where runners are encouraged to do just that.

There's a five-hour cut-off point around Mile 16.5 and the overall cut-off point is seven hours.

▼ Watching the sun rise during your marathon run is a truly unforgettable sight.

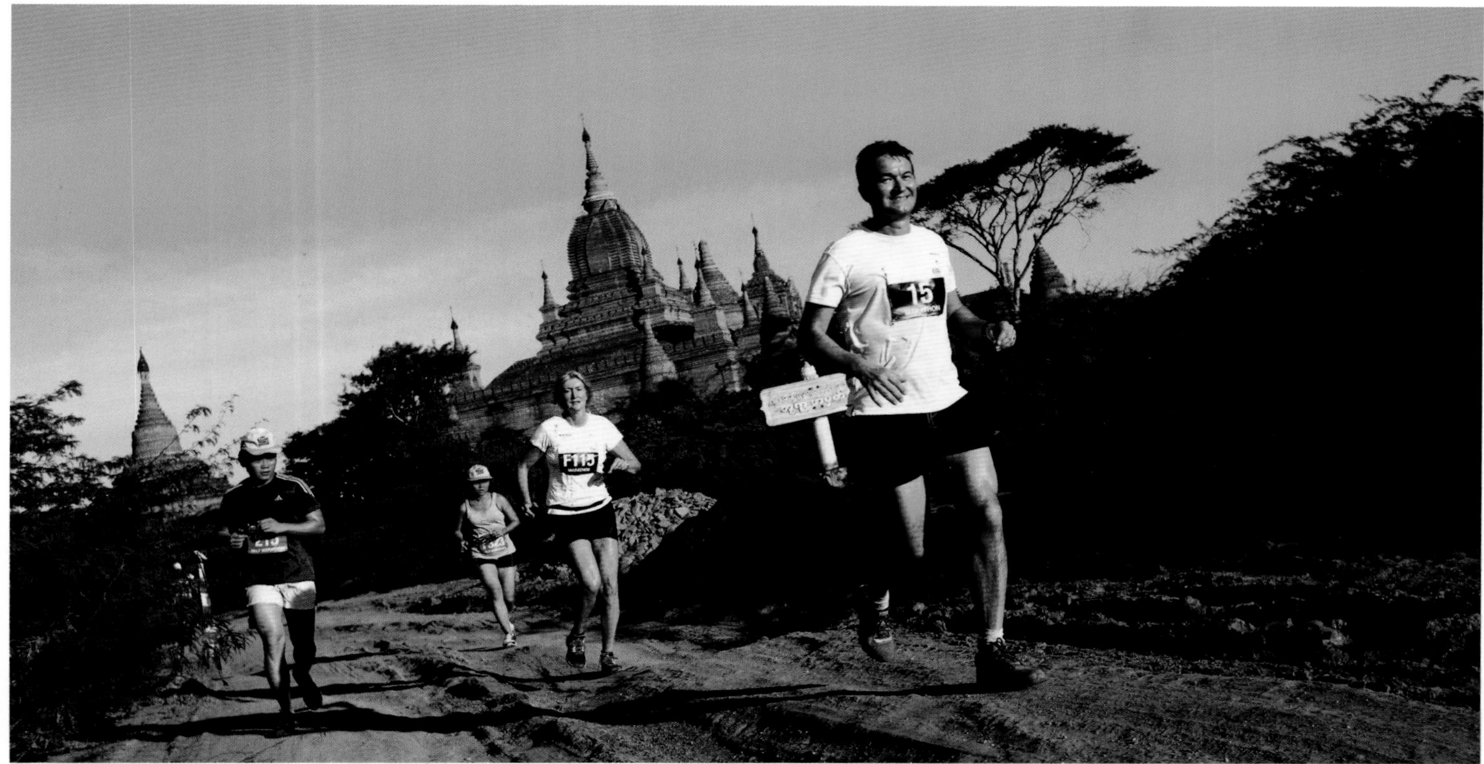

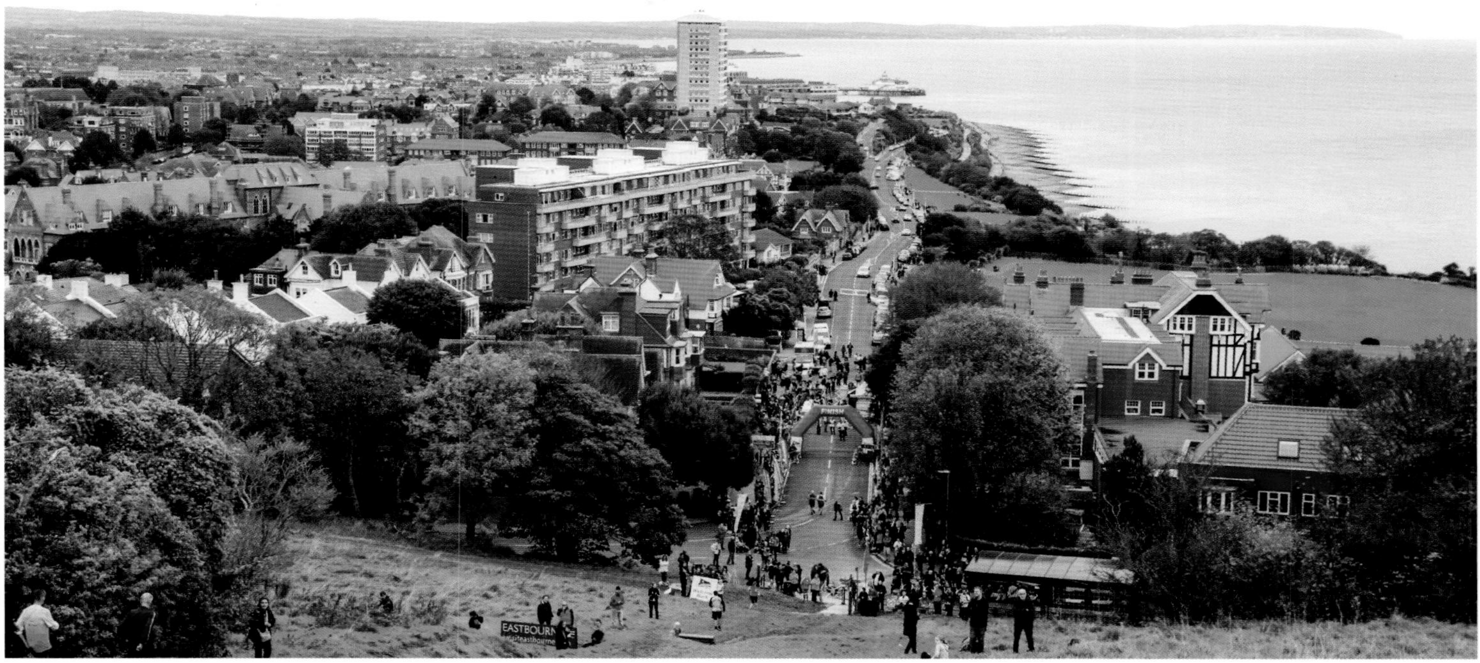

BEACHY HEAD MARATHON

GORGEOUS VIEWS APLENTY ON THIS QUINTESSENTIALLY BRITISH COURSE

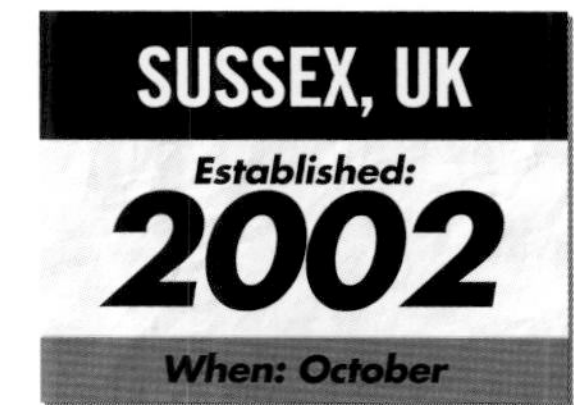

Nobody ever plummets down the final hill of the Eastbourne Beachy Head Marathon feeling disappointed or underfed. It's a huge yet difficult 26.2-mile cross-country race, but is so well supported you'll want to run it again and again. The race takes place in the stunningly pretty, coastal South Downs National Park in Sussex, and tackles the steep, grassy slopes of the Seven Sisters, a series of spectacular chalk cliffs that undulate their way to Birling Gap. This race is a never-to-be forgotten experience. Just over a mile to the east of Birling Gap is the imposing Beachy Head, the highest white-chalk sea cliff in Britain at 531 feet (162m) above the English Channel, and the spectacular spot that gives the race its name.

On race day, there's also a fiendishly difficult 10km race, a great taster for the main event. Finish times for both races bear no relation to road events of the same distance – in addition to the hills, runners must contend with steps, stiles and gates, as well as a veritable banquet along the way. The food at the refreshment points seems to be designed to slow you down: hot cross buns, sausage rolls, mugs of tea, chocolate biscuits, flapjacks.

The start and finish points are also food central, with all manner of race-fuel concessions to provide you with go-faster snacks before the race and refreshments afterwards. Ticket entry also covers a hot meal in the canteen.

There is a 6 p.m. cut-off point, and the race starts at 9 a.m., which allows you time to snack and chat, run the flatter bits and stop along the way to take photographs if the autumn weather is being kind.

Beauty spots along the way include the delightful down-land villages of Jevington, Alfriston and Litlington, all of which have some gorgeous old pubs for celebratory pints and Sunday lunches. The course also includes the historic woodland of Friston Forest, with its stately trees and leafy, twisting trails, so it takes in the full range of English countryside.

▲ Twisting trails and winding roads await keen runners at Beachy Head.

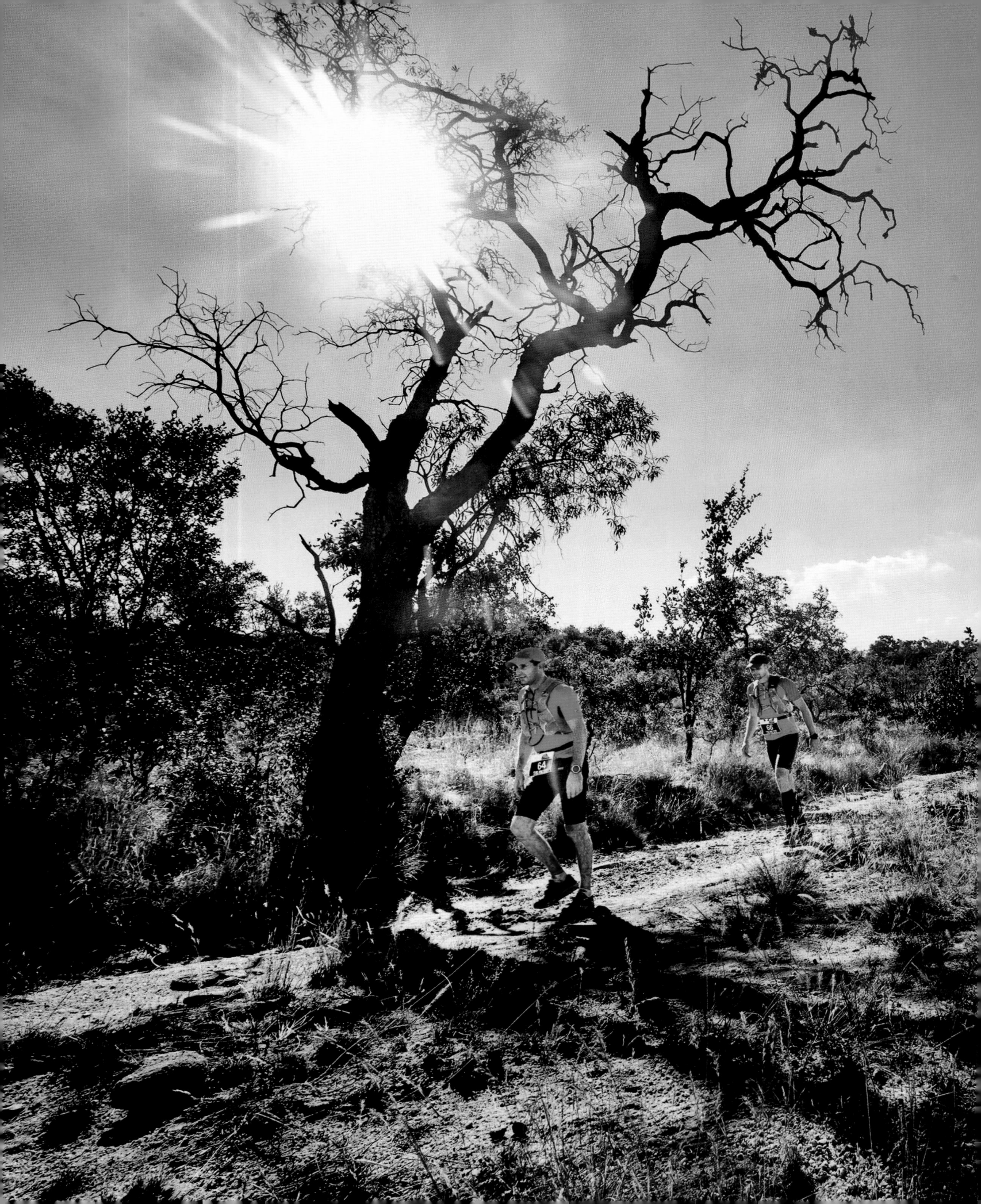
64

BIG FIVE MARATHON

MARATHON MEETS ON-FOOT SAFARI OVER THIS GRUELLING 42KM COURSE

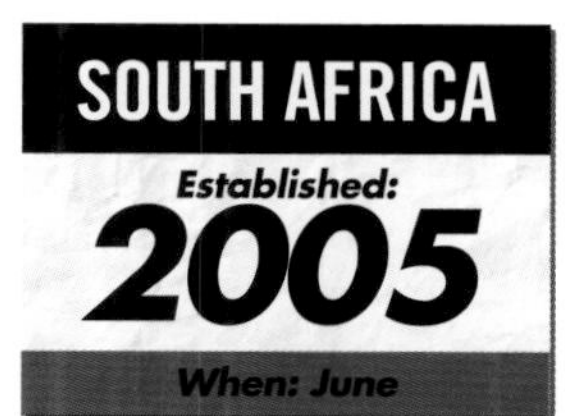

When the going gets tough, runners seek distractions. So how do elephants, rhinos and lions grab you as diversionary material? The Big Five gives its participants all of these and yet more African fauna to ease the pain of this fabulously gruelling 42km worth of the 220km Entabeni Game Reserve. This private reserve, a three-hour drive from Johannesburg, is a collection of different ecosystems, which makes for very diverse running experiences. Fortunately, the whole route is very well marshalled and there's a refreshment station (water and cola) at every 4km, so it's easy to break up the challenging course into bite-sized sections.

The terrain keeps runners on their toes – from undulating dirt tracks to a lower plateau, prior to climbing to a viewpoint before plunging into the Yellow Wood Valley, which is where the going gets tricky. The descent is punishing to the thigh muscles. After the descent, you're in lion country (not a detail course descriptions usually include) and, more punishingly, deep sand, which is tough to run through.

The lion reference explains why there must be more marshals and guides than on the average trail marathon, and why, indeed, there are three cutoff points (at 26.5km: 4 hours and 15 minutes; at 32.5km: 5 hours and 15 minutes; and at the finish line: 7 hours after start). With lions on the prowl, the race organizers can't risk allowing runners to wander around unaccompanied.

Sadly, what goes down must go up, and you must tackle the ascent, which seems to go on for miles. There's a brief respite of dirt trails, before the final 4km down a ridge, which affords spectacular views over a lake from the plateau.

The climate is kindly. South Africa enjoys dry, sunny and relatively cool temperatures (around 68 °F), so competitors are tempted to make use of the aid stations and pause to spot the wildlife, while being mindful of those cutoff points.

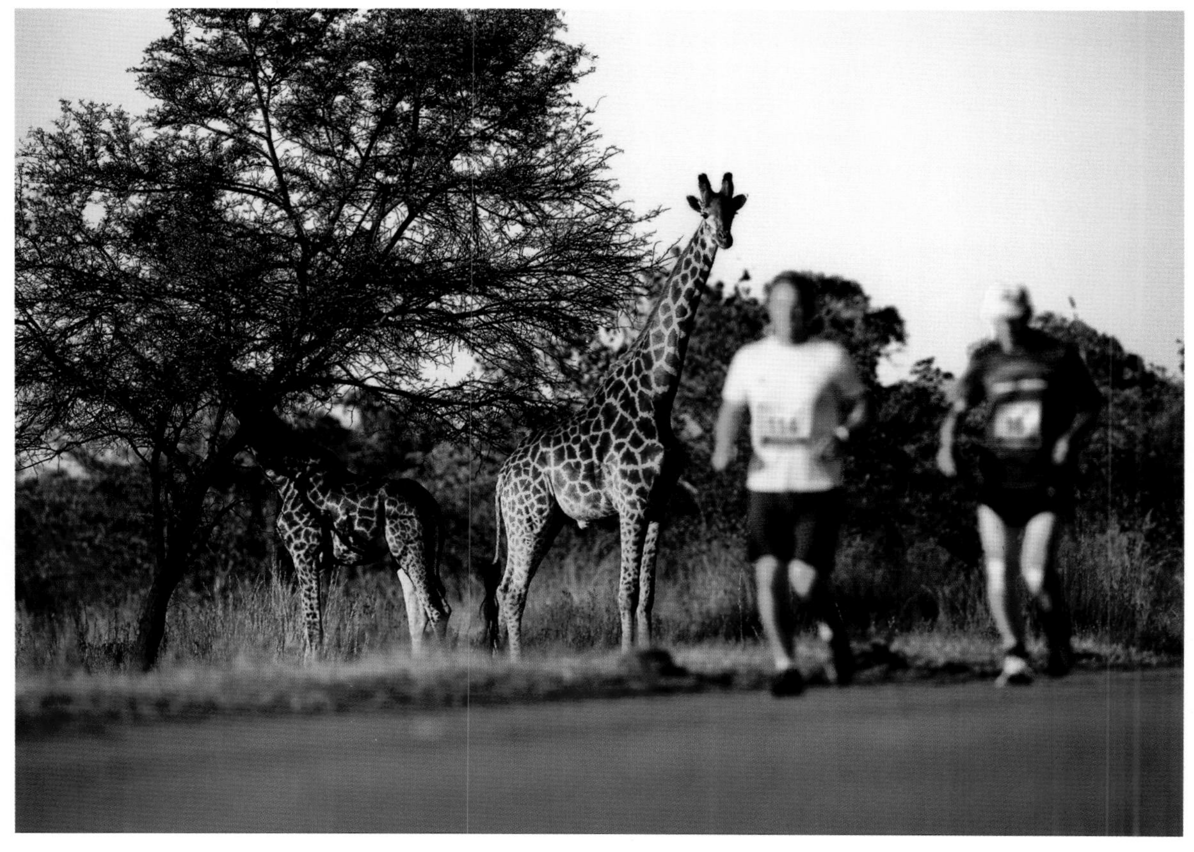

◀ The spectators for this marathon are completely unlike any other.

◀◀ The rugged terrain can make for difficult going.

AUTUMN CAKEATHON

MARATHON RUNNING AND CAKE – A MATCH MADE IN HEAVEN?

ENGLAND, UK

Established:

2015

When: October

Running for cake makes for a popular hashtag these days, which is probably why this delightful confection has gained so many followers since its inception in 2015. The ingredients are more than tempting: traffic-free, bucolic and fuelled by the sweetest of high-carb treats. The race organizers, Saxon Shore, have scheduled Cakeathons in many areas of England. This one is in Kent, contained within the lovely Jeskyns Community Woodland, an area of outstanding natural beauty, now owned by the Forestry Commission. It's a gorgeous portion of the North Downs, not far from Gravesend in Kent, full of native woodlands, community orchards, open parkland and wildflower meadows.

The route through all this beauty is on well-maintained trails, and competitors run a series of 3.28-mile (just over 5km) loops but, during this six-hour timed event, you can run as many loops as you want within the time limit. Depending on your speed and fitness. The course is undulating, so there are several gentle climbs to negotiate. Every loop finishes with a refreshment stop and groaning cake table. You don't have to run a marathon's worth of loops: you can just run one, finish, and scoff the cake. Most people, however, grab a flapjack and keep going. The six-hour time limit means that would-be ultrarunners can practise their running-and-refuelling techniques for as many miles as they can squeeze into the time. Eight laps is the official marathon distance. Anything over nine is considered (by Cakeathon standards) an ultra.

Laps are counted using a small laminated card, which you pin onto your shirt on registration. When you've completed a lap, one of the officials punches a hole in your card. You decide when you've had enough and want to sit down and have a nice cup of tea and a piece of cake.

The first Cakeathon, dreamed up to celebrate the 100th anniversary of the Women's Institute (WI), captured the bake-off zeitgeist so effectively that it has become a fixture in the running calendar. As well as an athletic challenge, it's a baking one, so there are trophies for the best cakes (categories include best brownie and best vegan contribution), which have contributed to the tempting refreshment display.

Participants (the running ones at least) receive a cake-themed finisher's medal and a goody bag, which organizers announce proudly will be unhealthy (filled with chocolates, crisps, cider). More goodies of the high-fat/sugar variety await runners at base camp. Even better news for not-over-committed marathoners is that you receive all of this even if you manage to complete only one lap. The icing on the cake, really.

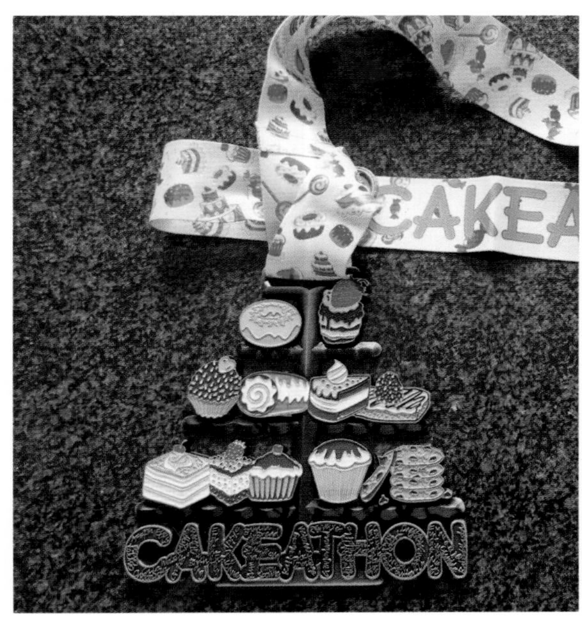

◣ The medals are perhaps the most delicious-looking of any marathon.

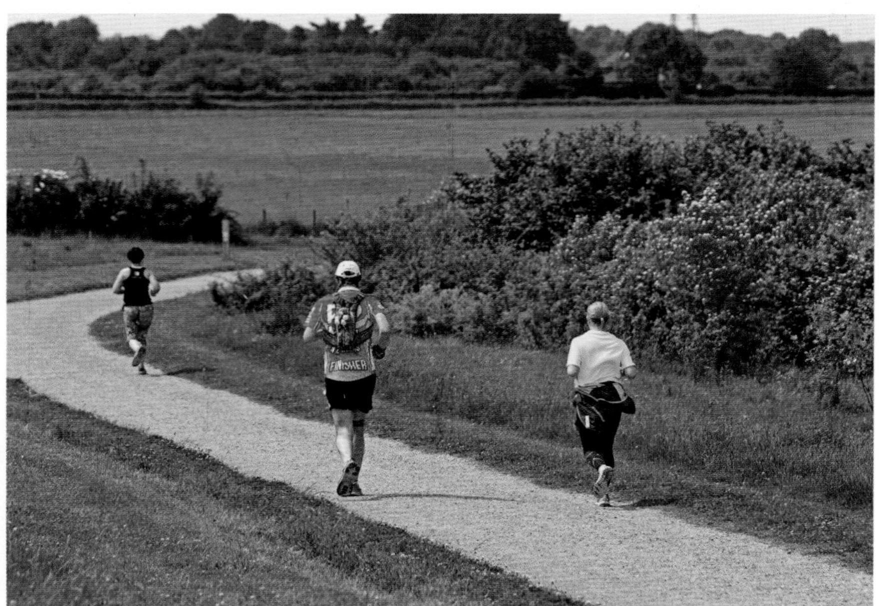

▼ The course is short, but you'll run it multiple times.

E.T. FULL MOON MARATHON

RUN INTO ALL SORTS OF ALIEN LIFE EN ROUTE

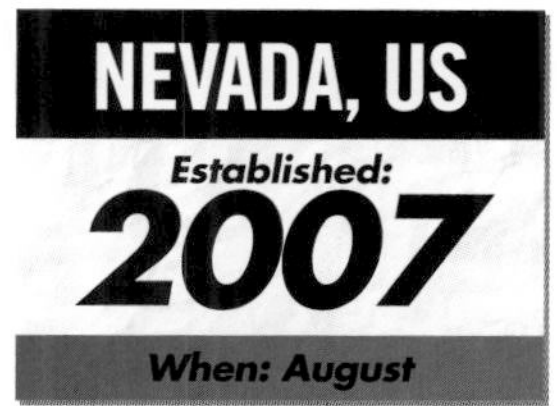

Rachel, Nevada, is a rather singular place. It's 100 miles from Las Vegas, and has about 50 inhabitants. It's famous, though, for this marathon, and more generally because of its proximity to the Nevada Highway 375, or the Extraterrestrial Highway, so called because a disproportionate number of UFO sightings have been reported on this stretch of road. The marathon start is about 20 miles outside the little hamlet of Rachel, but you run through it, then double back to the finish line back in town at the Little A'le'Inn diner on Old Mill Street, for the breakfast spread.

You'll eat breakfast after the race, because this marathon starts at midnight. It takes place on the weekend in August closest to the full moon. Head torches (or handheld flashlights) are compulsory; so too are reflective vests, and glow-bracelets are handed out, which put an even more weird and wonderful shine on this E.T. race. The organizers warn that you may run into all sorts of alien life en route, but admit it's cows and other beasts wandering the highway at that time of night. However, you should exercise caution, in any event.

The race starts at the "black mailbox", which was painted white but now doesn't even exist, but everyone knows where the start is, because marathon night is the busiest night of the year. You run along the highway, but against the traffic, on the hard shoulder. The breathtaking desert scenery and surrounding mountains add to the otherworldliness of this extraordinary event. The temperature is perfect: this area of Nevada is cooler than the mean temperature of Vegas, and the nighttime running means it's more comfortable still.

This is a very traditional event with a splendid, homely vibe. You're lucky if you can bag a place to sleep in the Little A'le'Inn – most people stay in a partner hotel in Vegas, and buses are provided to and from the event. As well as the marathon, there are 5km, 10km, half-marathon and 51km races on the same night. The longer races have a highlight called "Coyote Summit", which involves a climb of about 1.5 miles. The marathon is a Boston Qualifier, so it's certified and results are carefully graded according to age range.

There are five refreshment stops along the marathon route: runners are given isotonic drinks in various flavours by Hammer HEED. You're encouraged to carry your own water bottles to be refilled along the way from the water stations. This is an environmentally aware race, so disposable cups and bottles are frowned upon. The prizes are "something inspired by nature" and everyone is given a medal; prizes are also awarded for the best alien-themed costume. This is definitely a race you'll be phoning home about.

◣ Beginning at midnight gives this lively race a distinctly alien feel.

▼ Costumes aren't just encouraged in this marathon – they're borderline essential.

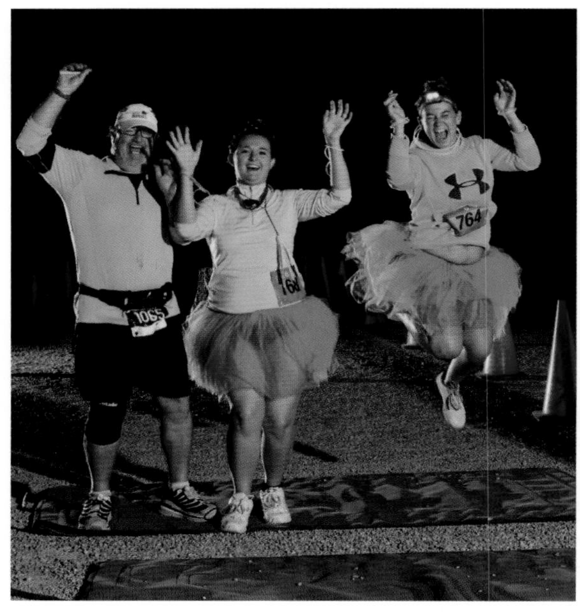

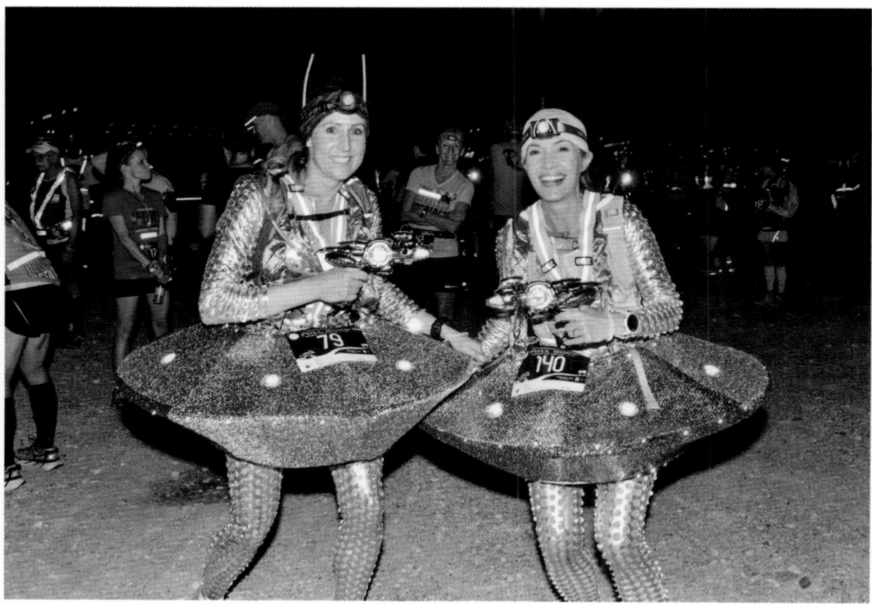

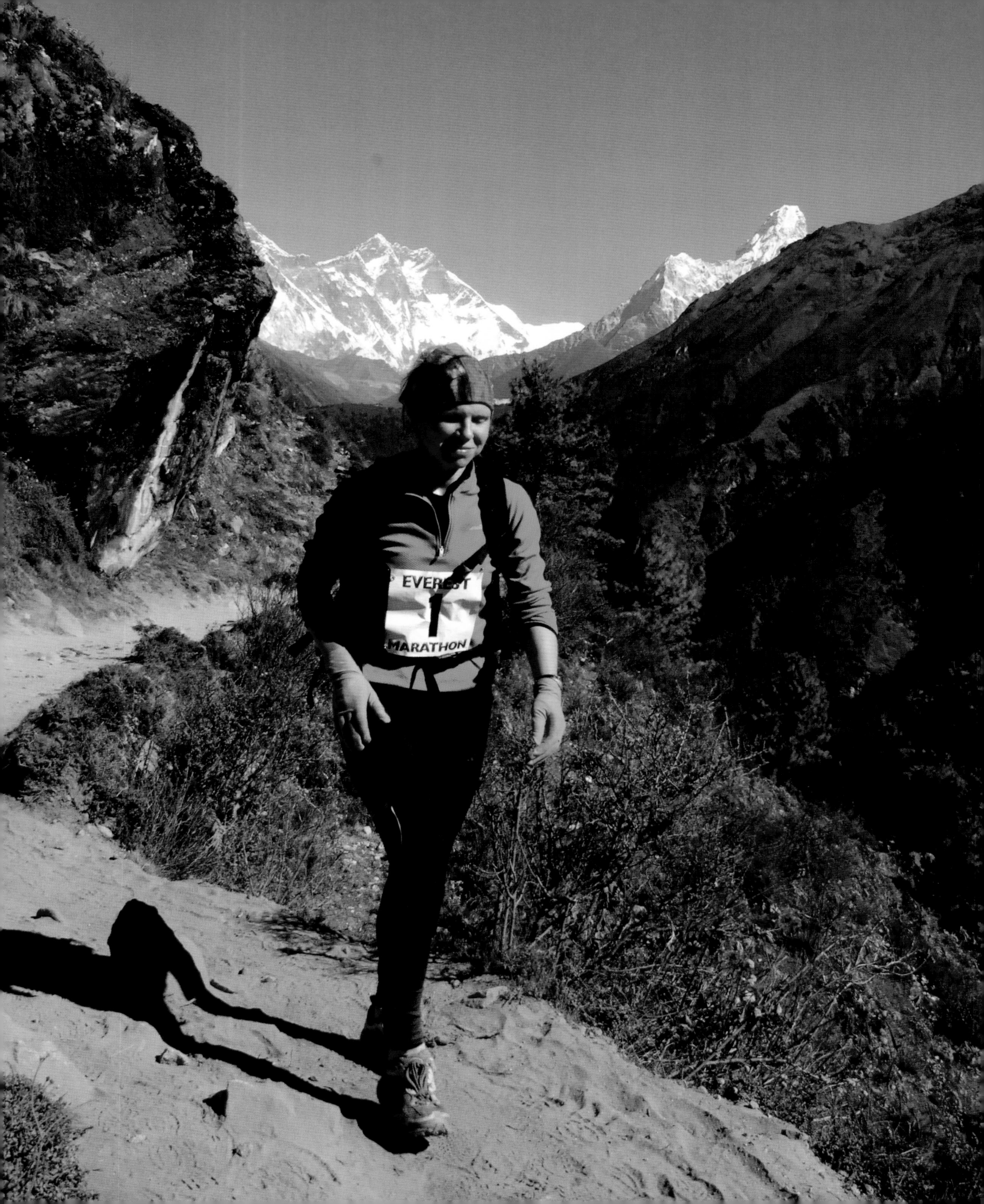
EVEREST
1
MARATHON

EVEREST MARATHON

THE HIGHEST MARATHON ON EARTH

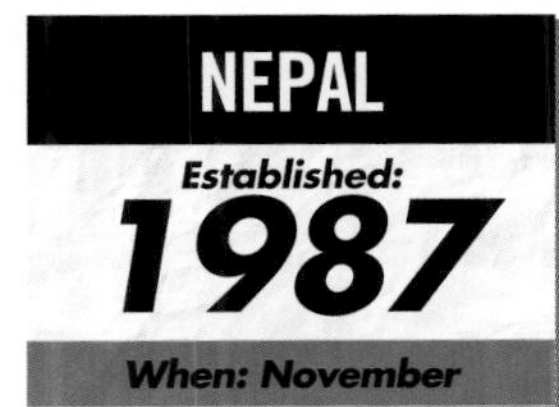

This is a marathon that selects you, rather than vice versa. The altitude, conditions, logistics and general difficulty mean that only relatively few marathoners, however seasoned they reckon they are, are up to the job.

It is, unsurprisingly, the highest marathon in the world, and it takes some preparing for. The fact that it has been staged only 17 times since its inception in 1987 (2019 marks the 18th in the series) suggests that it takes quite a lot to get it off the ground, as it were. The main barrier for most people is the fact that you're obliged to run it as part of a 24-day stay in Nepal, to allow for acclimatisation. Weekend warriors need not apply – you need to take some serious time off work for this one. During this Nepalese odyssey, runners enjoy sightseeing days in Kathmandu as well as a 15-day trek to the marathon start, while being monitored by medical staff. The trek involves ascents of two more humble mountains, Gokyo Ri (5,483m) and Kala Pattar (5,623m), both of which offer inspirational views of the big one: Everest.

Only 75 non-Nepalese runners are selected, and each must have had experience of technically challenging fell or mountain races. If you've only run road marathons, you won't make the cut.

The race starts at Gorak Shep 5,184m (17,000 feet), close to Everest Base Camp in Nepal. The finish is at the Sherpa capital town of Namche Bazaar at 3,446m (11,300 feet) and the course is a measured 42km (26.2 miles) over rough mountain trails. November 2019 marks the 18th staging of this marathon event. Although the course is basically downhill, there are two steep uphill sections. There may be snow and ice on the upper part and there is considerable exposure along much of the route.

So, the marathon course heads down Everest, winding 26.2 miles to the finish at Namche Bazaar. Although the route is mostly downhill, the elevation alone, combined with two steep uphill sections, plus snow and ice and rough terrain, make it one of the most challenging marathons around. What makes it worth it? The most breathtaking views – literally, since there's 50% less oxygen at Base Camp than at sea level – and lifelong bragging rights.

The Everest Marathon is a nonprofit event: most runners raise money both for their own favourite charities and the official race charity, the Everest Marathon Fund, which supports health and educational projects in rural Nepal.

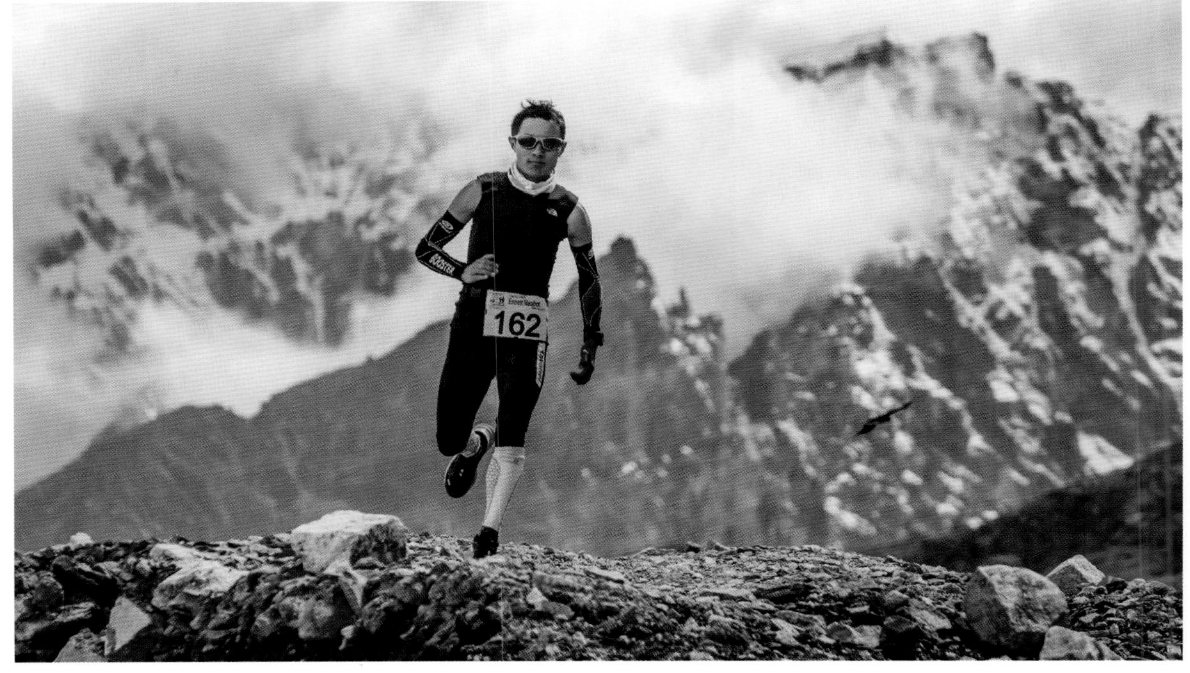

◀◀ Not every part of Everest is snow and rocks; theres a range of views to keep runners on their toes.

◀ The extreme conditions on Everest mean that this isn't a marathon for the casual runner.

JERUSALEM MARATHON

A HUGE EVENT DRAWING 30,000 PEOPLE FROM 60 DIFFERENT COUNTRIES

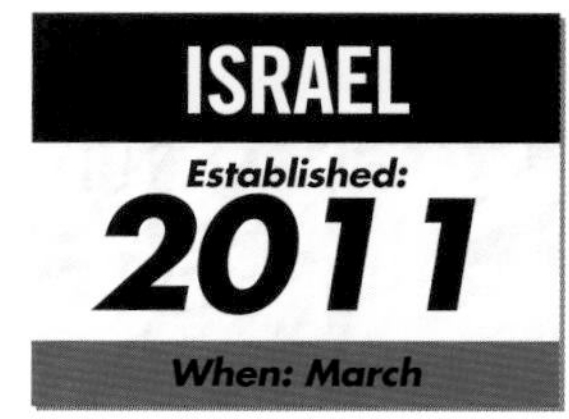

An eye-popper of a race, not just because it passes through so many holy, historic places, but because it's super-hilly. As soon as runners have hauled themselves up one long, steep incline and admired the view, there's another to consider, but the Jerusalem marathon is stunningly atmospheric.

The race is a relative newcomer on the world marathon stage (2018 marks the eighth staging of the event) but it has proved a big hit with marathon tourists, with about 30,000 people from 60 different countries lining up at the start. It's run on a Friday because of Shabbat (the Jewish Sabbath) on a Saturday. The brainchild of the city's mayor, Nir Barkat, it's generally hailed as one of the toughest urban marathons in the calendar. Barkat had run the New York City marathon to celebrate his 50th birthday (his pacers were paratroopers he'd led in the Israel Defense Forces) while planning his own city's signature race. He loves running and has worked hard to create a major race in this challenging location.

Runners gather not far from the Knesset (parliament building) at 7 a.m., and it's elbows out as a couple of thousand stream through the city and out towards Ammunition Hill, the site of one of the bloodiest battles of the Six Day War in 1967. From there the route circuits the university and snakes back into the Old City, through Jaffa Gate, passing by the Tower of David, part of a fortress built in 2 BC.

Around here, everything has cultural significance. The pack runs not far from the Via Dolorosa, Jesus's final journey according to the Bible. Then it's through the Jewish quarter, near the Western Wall and out towards Zion's Gate. The last part of the run is through the sad, beautiful Valley of the Cross and back into town for the finish on the Ben Zvi Boulevard.

The whole marathon journey is dotted with reminders of this sacred city's turbulent history and continued fragility. Security is high, but, as Nir Barkat says, it always is: "We are alert all day, every day." However, the mood is celebratory, and the views are out of this world. In the after-race festivities in the park, you're reminded, once again, just how running is a universal language and it brings diverse nationalities all together in one collective effort.

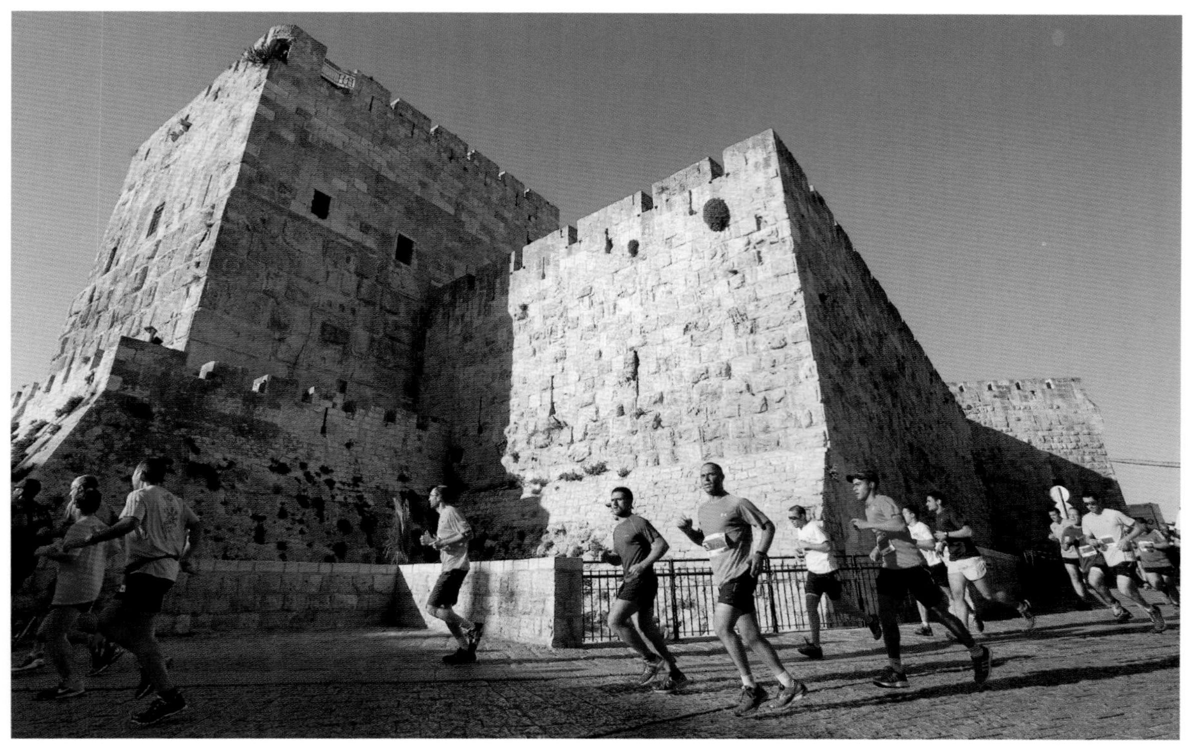

◀ The marathon route takes in many of the ancient sights dotted around Jerusalem.

▶ Though it only began in 2011, the Jerusalem Marathon is already proving a popular event.

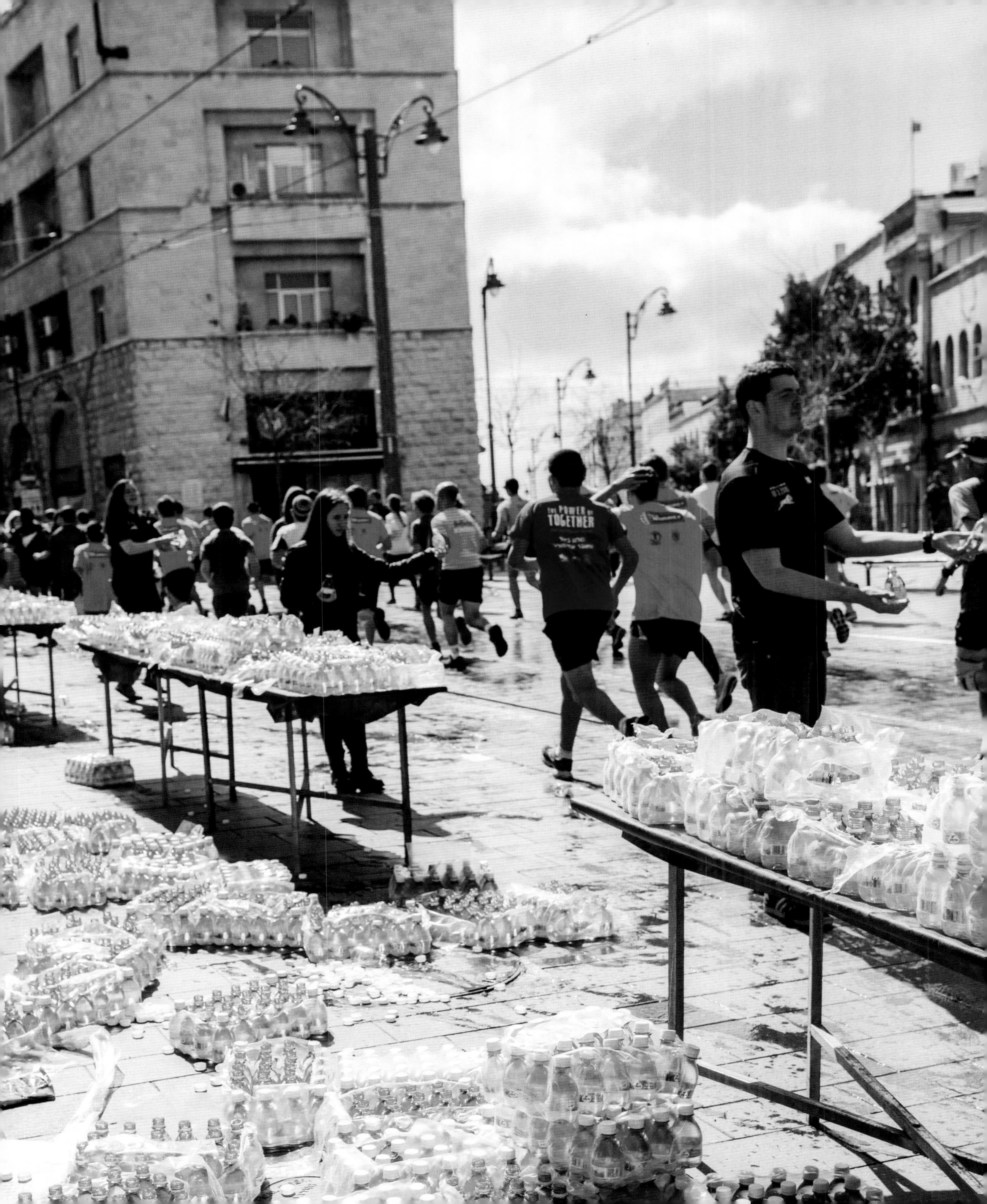
THE POWER OF
TOGETHER

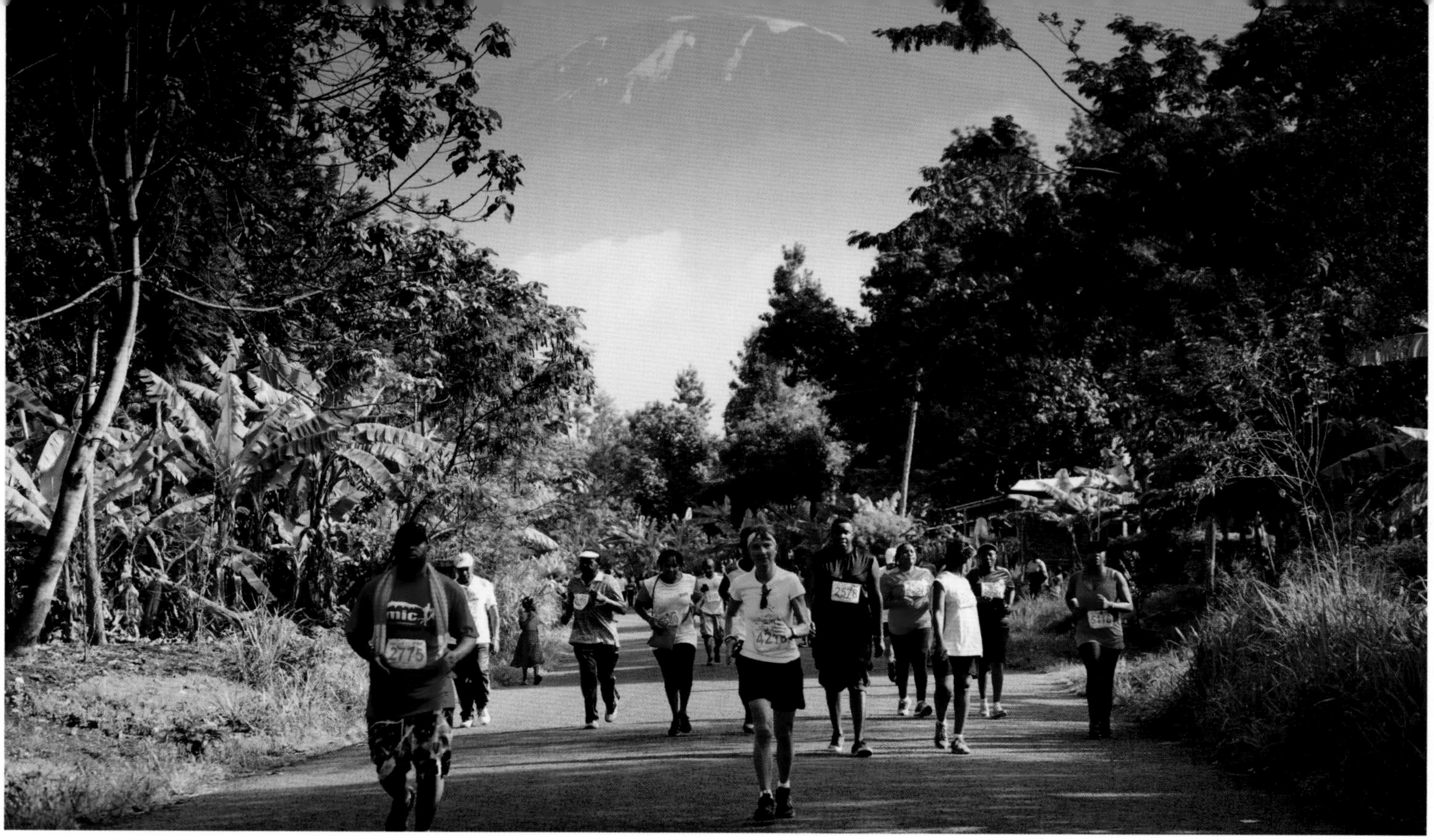

KILIMANJARO MARATHON

RACE AROUND THE ROOF OF AFRICA

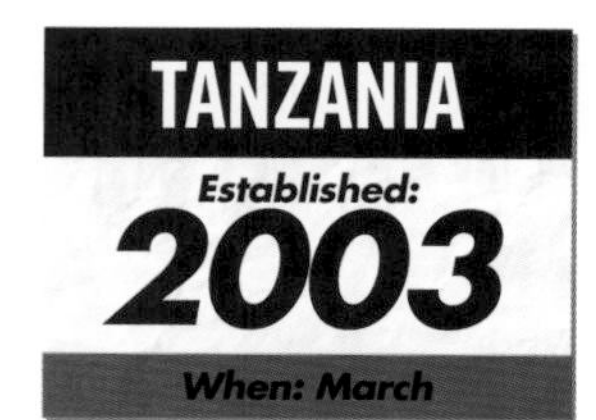

The fact that this race takes the name of Africa's tallest mountain gives it a huge amount of kudos, perhaps more than the course's modest altitude gain would suggest. The course takes runners from the sports stadium in the town of Moshi, at the base of Kilimanjaro, out on the road towards Dar es Salaam, before looping back through farmland, including coffee and banana plantations, and a few forested areas giving welcome shade. The terrain is largely tarmac road, with some dirt trail during the second half.

The countryside around here is beautifully green and lush (coffee-plantation tours are a popular attraction in Moshi), and running through the roads and having farmworkers and children cheer you on is a delightful experience. It's hot, though (hence the 6.30 a.m. start), so there are multiple water and cola stations throughout the route, in addition to well-equipped medical-aid points.

This well-organized and beautiful race was initially planned to draw in a new tourist stream to Tanzania, who would then further invest large amounts of cash into climbing the mountain, or going on safari after running the race. Today, the event is a major event in its own right and has become a landmark marathon for those who want to get some special ones under their belt. This is the largest organized annual sports event in the country, so it's a huge deal. The whole town of Moshi gets involved, and the atmosphere during the marathon festival (there's a 5k fun run, a 10k for athletes with disabilities and a half-marathon the same weekend) is terrific. One of the best things about the event is the music, as so many local bands are booked to provide entertainment.

When the event was first staged, 700 runners turned out; these days the number is nearer to 9,000, which has quite an impact on the pretty, mid-sized town of Moshi. However, because it's used to tourist interest from those wanting to climb to the "roof of Africa", Moshi is well set up for visitors, with many affordable bed-and-breakfasts (book yours well ahead). It's well worth staying on for a while after the race, because there are so many beauty spots within reach of Moshi and it seems a shame not to explore further.

▲ Serious heat and altitude make this a super challenging run.

LA MARATHON, LOS ANGELES

LOS ANGELES' MOST EXHAUSTING SIGHTSEEING TRIP

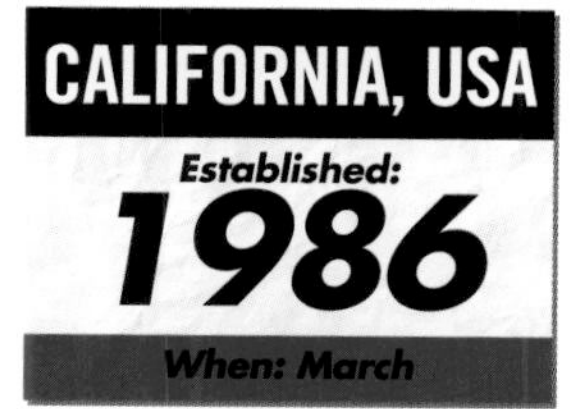

"Awesome!" is the oft-repeated verdict about this popular marathon, dubbed "Stadium to the Sea". The course and the crowd support ensure it gets the biggest thumbs-up. The race starts at the Dodger Stadium in Los Angeles, a 56,000-seat "icon of American sports history", which boasts the best basketball following in the world. In March, however, the buzz is around this colourful event, where the costumes are as glitzy as the city.

From the historic stadium, the course takes runners on the most exhausting sightseeing trip of LA ever. You can be distracted from your pain by picture-postcard LA landmarks: Hollywood Boulevard, Beverly Hills, the Walk of Fame, Sunset Strip and that Hollywood sign on Mount Lee, in the Santa Monica mountains. Who can resist stopping for a selfie with those 44-foot (13.4m) white capital letters as a backdrop?

There's a huge hullabaloo at Mile 18, known as Cheer Alley, when runners are greeted by hundreds of local cheerleaders making a lot of noise. Known as the "Pep Rally of the Year", this huge mêlée of teenaged enthusiasm comprises middle- and high-school cheerleaders from across Southern California The course is quite a testing one (so selfies may be the order of the day), as Los Angeles is a pretty hilly city. The first six miles or so are undulating, which, in the often humid conditions at this time of year, can feel like a bit of a slog. The biggest hill is at Mile 4, but at least it's over and done with early on. The last couple of miles is downhill, which comes as a massive relief.

Thankfully, organizers do a great job of creating treats along the way, and LA firefighters and police also come out to provide support. This marathon has become well known for the quality and diversity of musical interludes from start to finish: all manner of rock and indie bands, percussion ensembles and dancing disco divas create a spectacle and celebrate the city's diversity.

It attracts a big field, about 24,000 runners, so there's a certain amount of jostling at the start, finish and water stations. There are 22 aid stations along the way, all providing water and Gatorade endurance drinks, and spectators are as generous with goodies and snacks as the organizers are. The finish line is a huge party, ending as it does in Santa Monica, and there's a great spread of food for finishers to enjoy once they've walked away from the finish pens and had a stretch along the way.

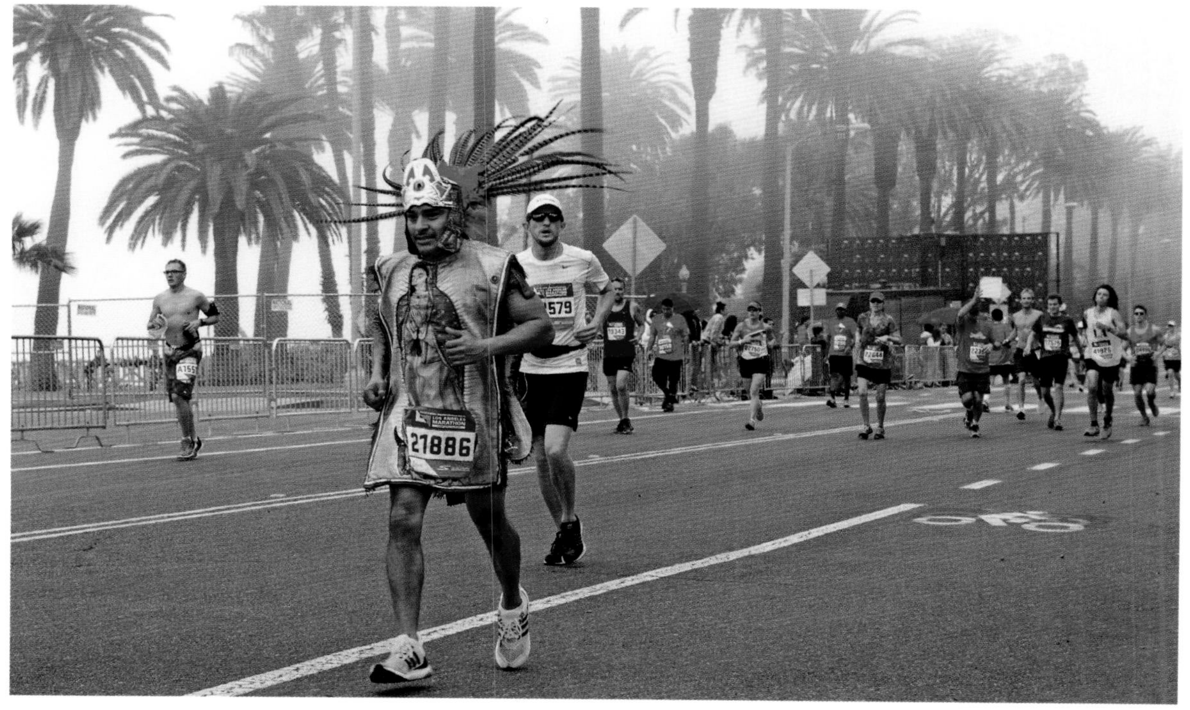

◀ LA is known for being home to some crazy characters, and that extends to the marathon too.

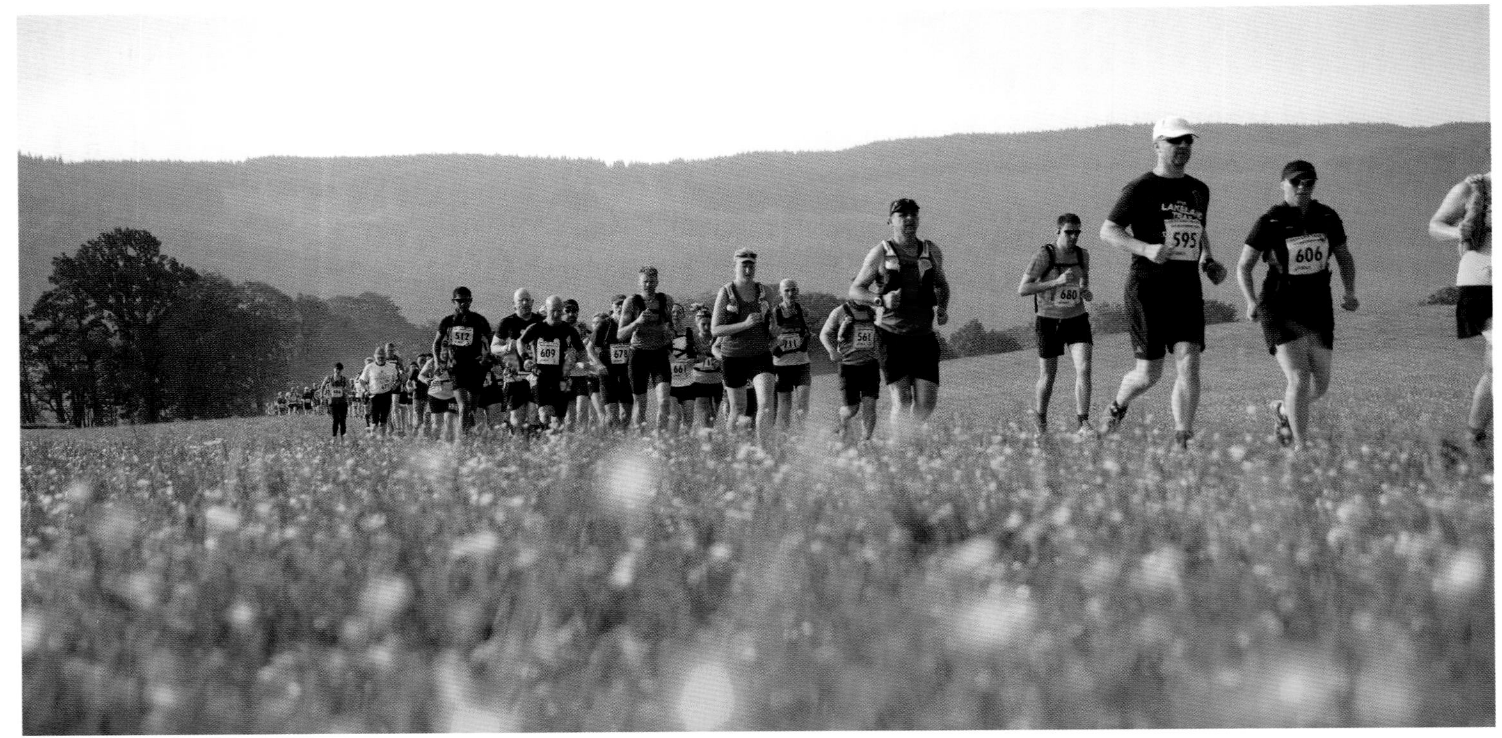

LAKELAND TRAILS MARATHON

MUCH MORE ENERGY-SAPPING THAN A ROAD MARATHON

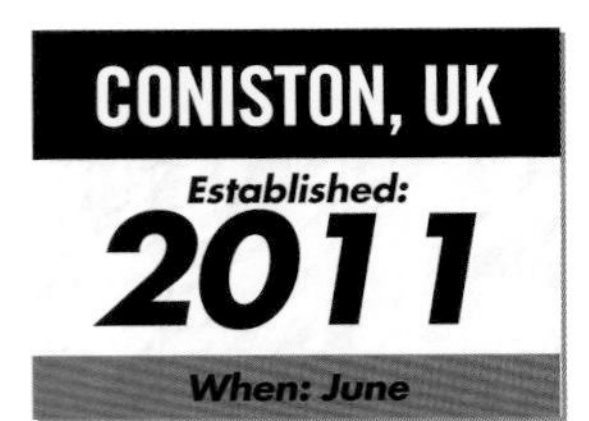

Held in one of the most scenic places in the British Isles, this tough but gorgeous trail marathon loops around the five-mile expanse of Coniston Water (scene of Donald Campbell's fateful 1967 speed record) and takes your breath away, not just because it has some tough hills to climb, but because the scenery – especially if skies are blue and those handsome peaks are reflected in the glassy waters – is astonishing.

The course around Coniston Water diverts up hill and down dale through wooded trails and grassy paths between dry-stone walls, taking in many gruelling hilly stretches, and views (thankfully not climbs) of lofty peaks of the Old Man, Swirl How, Wetherlam and Dow Crags. The terrain is a mixed bag, including trail, track, woods, fields, bog and loose scree, so is much more energy-sapping than a road marathon, but very rewarding (the temptation to stop and take photos is hard to resist).

The race starts and ends at Coniston Hall landing point, a small promontory of land that juts into the lake's glassy surface. It then climbs up the valley towards Tilberthwaite, and involves some stiff climbs before coming to a welcome refreshment point in the well-known beauty spot of Tarn Hows, where the path rolls around the mountain lake before making another climb up to Grizedale Moor. This stretch of open fell side can be punishing if there's no cloud cover, but reveals stunning panoramas across South Lakeland and towards Morecambe Bay. You can also see the start/finish area, behind you, which seems very, very far.

There are water stations and feed stations on the course, but many runners carry rucksacks to stay hydrated all the way round. The sun can be harsh at this time of year, and dehydration can be a very real problem. The trails are well signposted and there are many marshals out on the route, but the nature of the race means that there are periods when runners feel they're out on their own. However, there's little danger of becoming lost, as this is a race well known for its camaraderie.

A carnival atmosphere is guaranteed for both spectators and competitors at the start and finish, where there's live music, race commentary, food and drink. It all adds up to a really family-friendly day out.

▲ Coniston Water offers one of the most spectacular and varied landscapes which should spur weary runners on.

MAN VS HORSE MARATHON

MUCH MORE ENERGY-SAPPING THAN A ROAD MARATHON

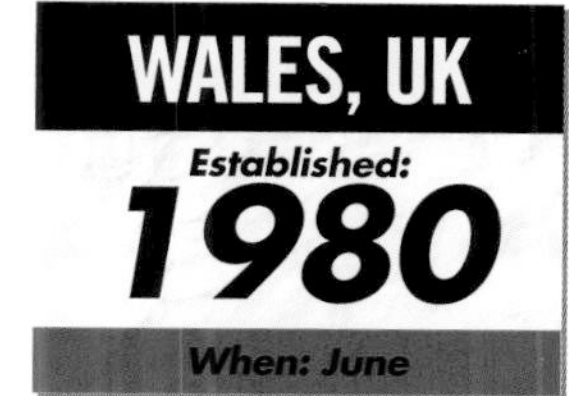

Is it a case of "four legs good, two legs bad" in this now world-famous race that pits the human elite athletes against their equine competitors? Not so in 2004, when Huw Lobb managed to cover the 22 miles of rugged Welsh terrain more quickly than the horses (his time was two hours and five minutes). Three years later, the feat was repeated, by one Florien Holtinger.

The event (not, strictly speaking, a marathon, being four miles short, but it certainly feels like the full 26.2), was founded in 1980, when the landlord of the Neuadd Arms Hotel in Llanwrtyd Wells, Powys, overheard some customers discussing the relative speed and endurance of men and horses over mountainous terrain. His idea certainly put his little town (population 850) on the tourist map, and guaranteed a bit of income before summer's high season.

In its 38-year history, the finishes have been excitingly close. The drawbacks of this kind of endurance race for horses is that they become overheated more quickly and catastrophically than humans do, which is why they must stop for a compulsory vet check.

The downside for the humans is the technical terrain – plenty of loose scree, rocks and streams, which can really slow you down. The beauty of the Welsh countryside and the unusual challenge are enough to make this race a hugely popular event, but there's also the cash prize. The runner who beats the first horse and rider cashes in: the jackpot at the time of writing stands at £2,500.

The runners set off 15 minutes ahead of the horses at 11 a.m. This is to prevent the animals spooking at all the cheering and jostling. Horses must also be checked by a vet before, after and during the race. Riders are duty-bound to call to runners they're gaining on: trampling a runner is poor form indeed! Horses aren't allowed to gallop or canter on the few tarmac stretches of the course, which gives the springier humans the edge on manmade terrain.

The whole event is very green: it's sponsored by a wholefoods company and attracts the type of hardened mountain runners who sneer at the very idea of road running, anyway. Typically, for an event in this niche, the entry limit is quite strict: only 650 runners can take part.

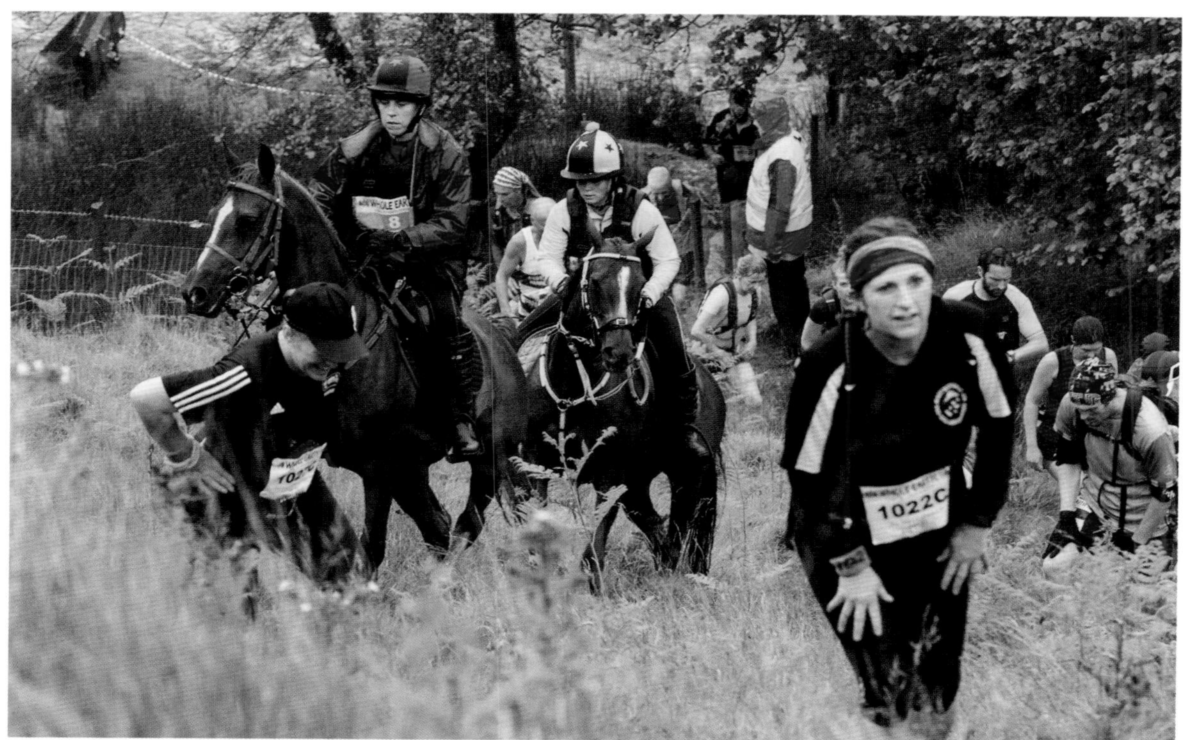

◀ Horse and human alike compete for victory in scenic Wales.

MARRAKECH MARATHON

EXPERIENCE A DIFFERENT VIEW OF MOROCCO

MARRAKECH, MA
Established:
1987
When: January

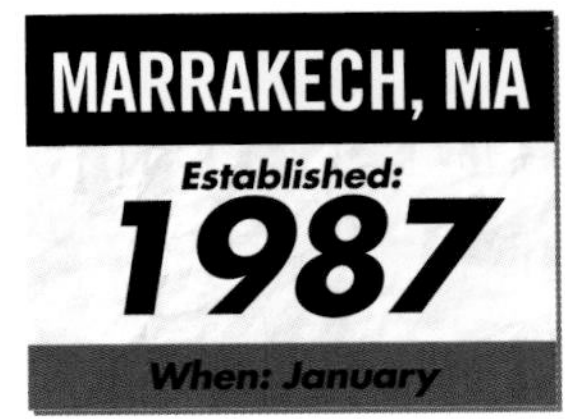

The country that breeds phenomenal endurance runners also lays on one of the world's loveliest marathons in its elegant capital city. The Marrakech Marathon charms all those who run it: the route is beautiful (camels, palm trees) and the entry fee is modest. It also doesn't cost too much to get to Marrakech, or stay there in the days before and after the race, so you can combine it with a holiday in the sun and enjoy a few treats to alleviate post-marathon soreness. It's a great, flat and fast course, and the Marrakech Marathon Village (a pleasantly simple marathon expo) is super-friendly at registration time. The 2019 Marrakech Marathon will mark the 30th staging of this much-loved and well-supported race, which comes highly recommended. The weather in January is mild, blue skies are the norm, but hydration is taken seriously: there are water stations, which are also laden with sweet orange segments, every 5k along the route.

The race starts and finishes just outside one of gates in the old city walls and, as is the norm, there aren't quite enough Portaloos (so, if you've booked into a hotel nearby, it pays to make full use of its facilities.) It's an 8 a.m. start and narrow streets mean it's hard to lose the crowds. You run past Marrakech's awesome train station, then through the historic Menera Gardens, then past the pit area for the Marrakech Grand Prix race, which is held here every year, then, to finish out the first half the race, the course runs down a road through the Old Royal Agdel Gardens and off to a short detour out of the city. Around Mile 15 the field takes the turn after Bab Al Khamis, the fifth of twelve gates in the 12km-long, rose-pink 12th-century wall that wraps around this beautiful old city.

From here, the race turns into the Palmeraie area of Marrakech, a palm oasis of several hundred thousand trees at the edge of the northern section. It's impossibly beautiful here, nearly enough to distract from the agony of these final miles. They are, sadly, slightly uphill, which seems mountainous in a state of fatigue, but it makes looking forward to that prestigious medal and warm welcome back in the old city even sweeter.

▼ The distinctive Marrakech train station is one of the major sights on the marathon route.

GARE DE MARRAKECH
محطة مراكش

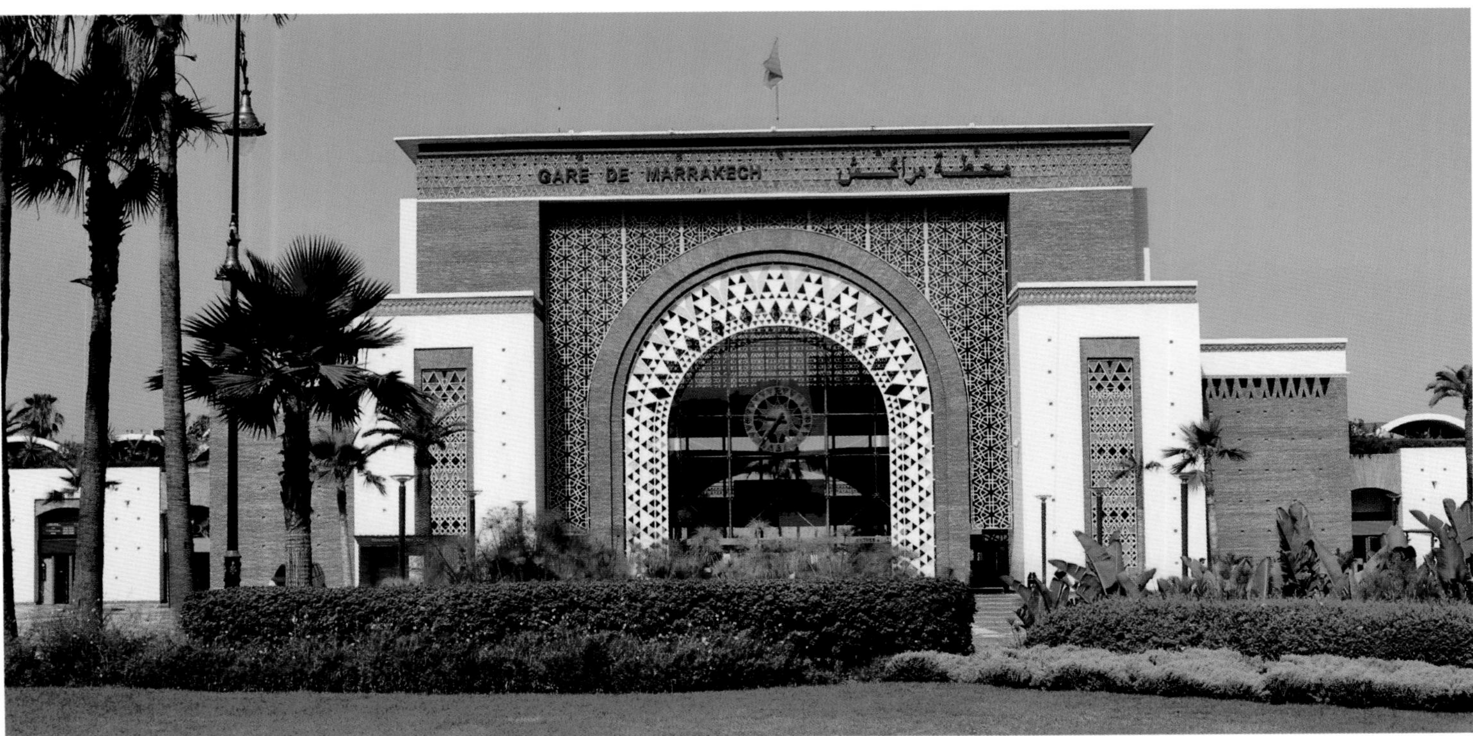

LE MARATHON DU MÉDOC

TOUR THE BEAUTIFUL WINE REGION OF BORDEAUX

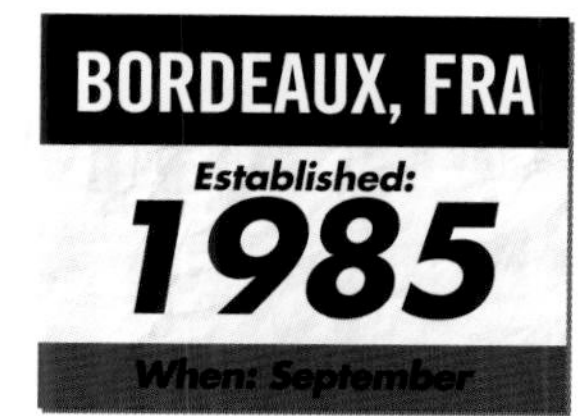

There are marathoners focused on training plans, fuelling and chip times and there are Médoc marathoners, who make their way to Bordeaux for a massive party. The latter species are the ones who have made this event, officially launched in 1985 and becoming more popular with every passing year, a highlight of the fun runner's diary. In fact, this race among the chateaux attracts 15,000 hopeful entrants, of whom only 8,500 win a place.

The Marathon du Médoc is a one-loop tour of the beautiful wine region of Bordeaux, taking in 50 chateaux. Along the way there are about 50 opportunities to eat, drink and be very, very merry. As well as the 22 wine-quaffing points, there are degustation stalls starring the very best of French fine food: cured meats, cheeses, seafood and, most welcome of all, ice creams and lollies.

The race's USP is "Health, Sport, Conviviality, Fun". As a result, runners approach the race with the belief that wine and oysters are good for you; even while taking part in an extreme endurance test in often high temperatures, you make friends and support your fellow bon viveurs as you run, and you run for the craic.

On the health front, although you may be unlucky enough to witness projectile vomiting after an ill-advised Brie-and-red-wine snack at Mile 16, this marathon is supremely well prepared for medical emergencies. The organizers say they take safety very seriously, and have more medical personnel on hand than any other marathon. In fact, the Medical Congress and the Sports Medical Symposium that take place the day before the race showcase the various field studies that have been inspired by this particular assault on the human body: more than 1,000 cardiac, blood-pressure and electrocardiograph studies have been performed on competitors to date.

The day before the race, participants have the chance to party and dance in a Médoc chateau, and, when the race is over (there's a cut-off point of six and a half hours), there's another big party, as well as a goody bag containing wine, food, a T-shirt and a medal. The day after, while nursing their hangovers, everyone, including supporters and volunteers, has the opportunity to join the Recovery Walk through the Margaux wine region, a time to really appreciate these bucolic surroundings and stretch aching legs.

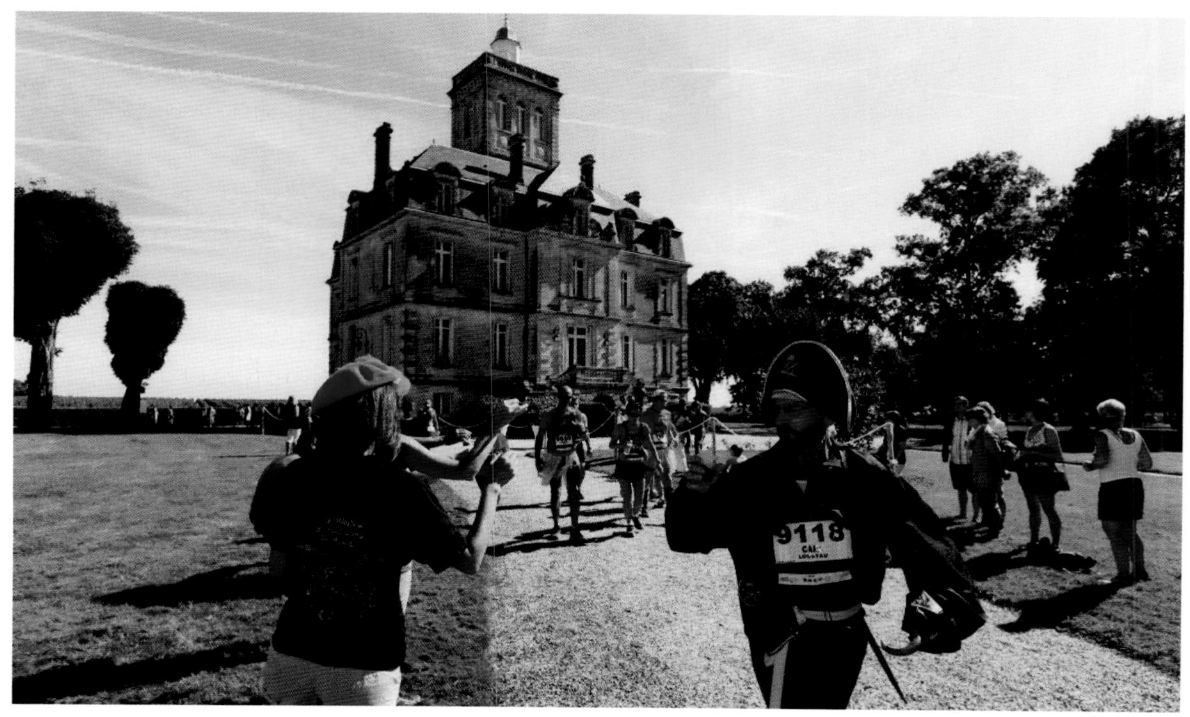

◀ Pirates, wine and beautiful scenery. What's not to like?

MIDNIGHT SUN MARATHON

THE TROMSØ BRIDGE LOOMS TWICE IN THIS NORTHERLY RACE

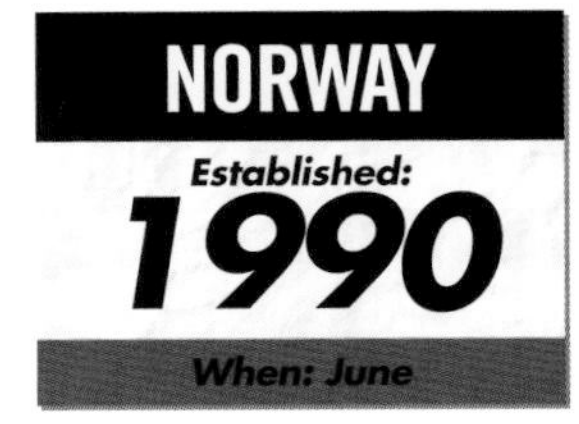

Tromsø is a small island town surrounded by a fjord, in the Arctic reaches of Norway. Its Midnight Sun marathon is the northernmost marathon certified by the Association of International Marathons. The whole town gets involved in this world-famous race, although the field is, of necessity, quite a small one – about 900 runners take part.

When all goes well, weatherwise, you really do see the sun in the middle of the night, as during the summer months you can experience up to 24 hours of sunlight this far above the Arctic Circle, as the sun doesn't set for about nine weeks. To give runners a chance to make the most of this extraordinary experience, the marathon starts at 8.30 p.m., so it's a challenge to get your sleep/fuelling strategy right.

The marathon course starts and finishes in the city centre, and stays mostly near the water, so runners can admire the snow-capped mountains in the distance, without having to climb them. That said, there is quite a steep climb near the beginning, when the high Tromsø Bridge looms into view – and runners must toil up that twice.

The bridge connects the Tromsøya island with the mainland, and runners must cope with the winds that often batter it; but running downhill off it is a delight, as the scenery is spectacularly beautiful and crowds gather in the midnight sunshine to cheer on the runners. Off the island, the pack starts to spread out and pick up the pace around Tromsdalen, although, with architectural diversions such as the Arctic Cathedral and the Polaria aquarium and natural ones such as rocky shores and snowy mountains to arrest the eye, it's easy to lose track of what the satnav is telling you. What many runners remember from this race (apart from the all-night daylight) is the sharp, clean air – a feast for the lungs as well as for the eyes.

There's that bridge to be crossed again before runners re-enter Tromsø for the final, flattish miles. At this stage, it feels as if the whole population of the town is out supporting the runners, giving them food and encouragement. This being Norway, everyone has perfect English and the huge Lycra-clad invasion of the small town is taken in very good part. The bars are all open and awaiting their new, sweating, endorphin-soaked friends. The whole event is also beautifully organized, so visitors feel very well looked after. As one happy finisher reported when asked her about this race, "If there's one race that brings on those lucky-to-be-alive feelings, it's the Midnight Sun Marathon!"

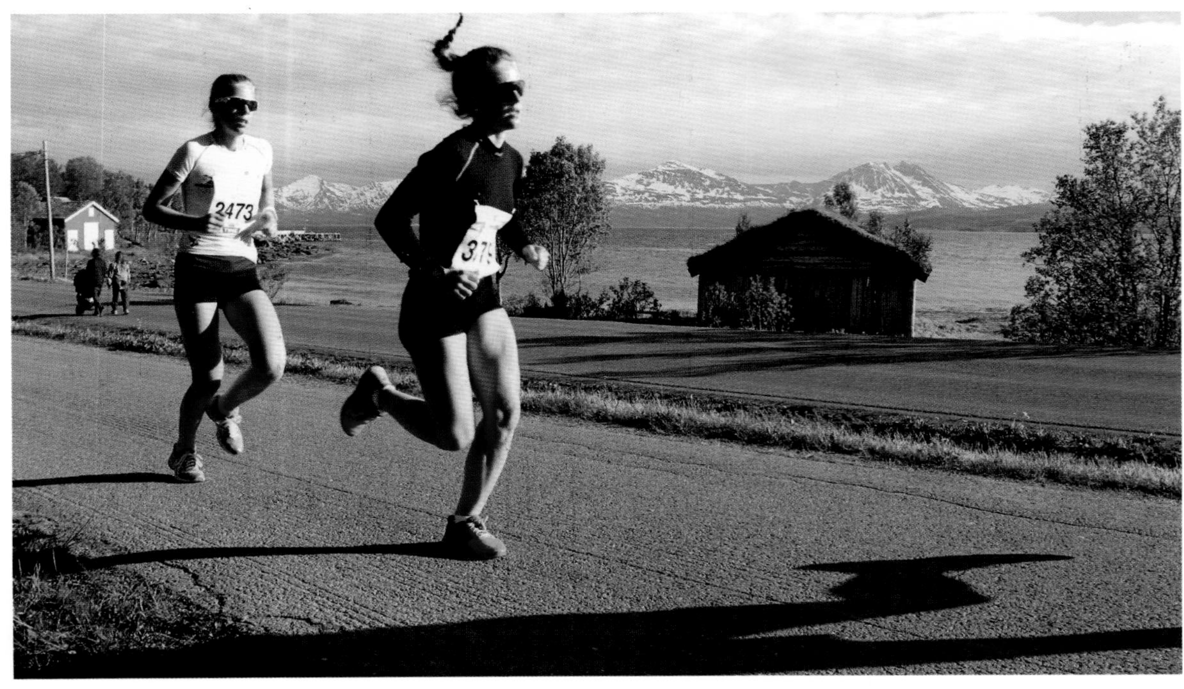

◀ Visibility is never an issue when running during the summer in Tromsø.

NORTH POLE MARATHON

DO YOU HAVE WHAT IT TAKES TO RUN A MARATHON IN ARCTIC CONDITIONS?

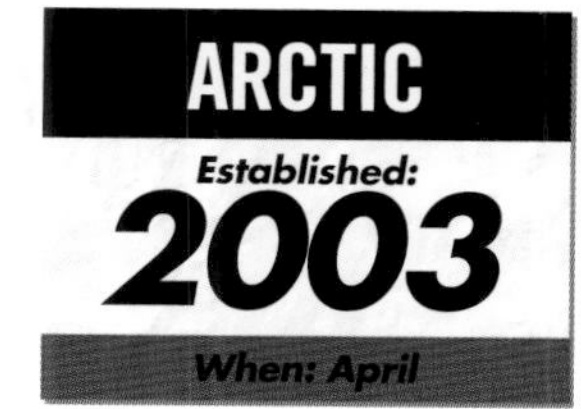

The strapline for this one is 'The world's coolest marathon', and it had to be, really, as this race takes place right at the top of the world – at the Geographic North Pole. It is quite an exclusive adventure – not least because it'll cost you about €15,000 for the whole experience, including flights and accommodation).

The race director is Richard Donovan, the first person to run a marathon at both the North and South Poles. He ran it first in 2002, when he was testing the waters – literally, as the race is run on ice floes, with 6–12ft (2–4m) of ice separating you from 12,000ft (3,658m) of Arctic Ocean. Since then, he has guided hundreds of adventurers on his frozen route and warns them before the start (probably quite unnecessarily), that this is most definitely not personal-best material. Running on this terrain is immensely energy-sapping, worse than deep sand, and then there's the fact that the winds are strong and icy, and the body is using up so much energy to keep warm. It's not all that flat, either, because the ice is whipped into slopes and hillocks, which runners must crest. This is clearly a race offering an experience of a lifetime.

Runners arrange their flights to Longyearbyen, on Spitsbergen Island off the coast of Norway, from where the North Pole Marathon organizers take over, chartering specialist aircraft to deliver them to their icy start. However, nothing can be guaranteed about the timings, as this is one of the most difficult places to fly to in the world, and delays of up to one week can scupper the start date. The organizers stress that this is a once-in-a-lifetime experience, so runners should allow themselves a couple of weeks' holiday at the Norwegian stage to allow for weather events, aircraft checks and bureaucratic issues.

The race is run from a drifting North Pole camp called Barneo, which floats about the North Pole between 89°N and 90°N. The route's a circular one, usually of about 4.2km, which must be completed 10 times (runners must stay within binoculars' view of base camp, just in case of polar-bear interest, although Donovan hadn't experienced this up to the time of writing). Leads (breaks in the ice) and safety criteria determine the maximum length of the circuit, but the finish is a triumphant one – at the ceremonial Pole, where all the lines of longitude symbolically meet.

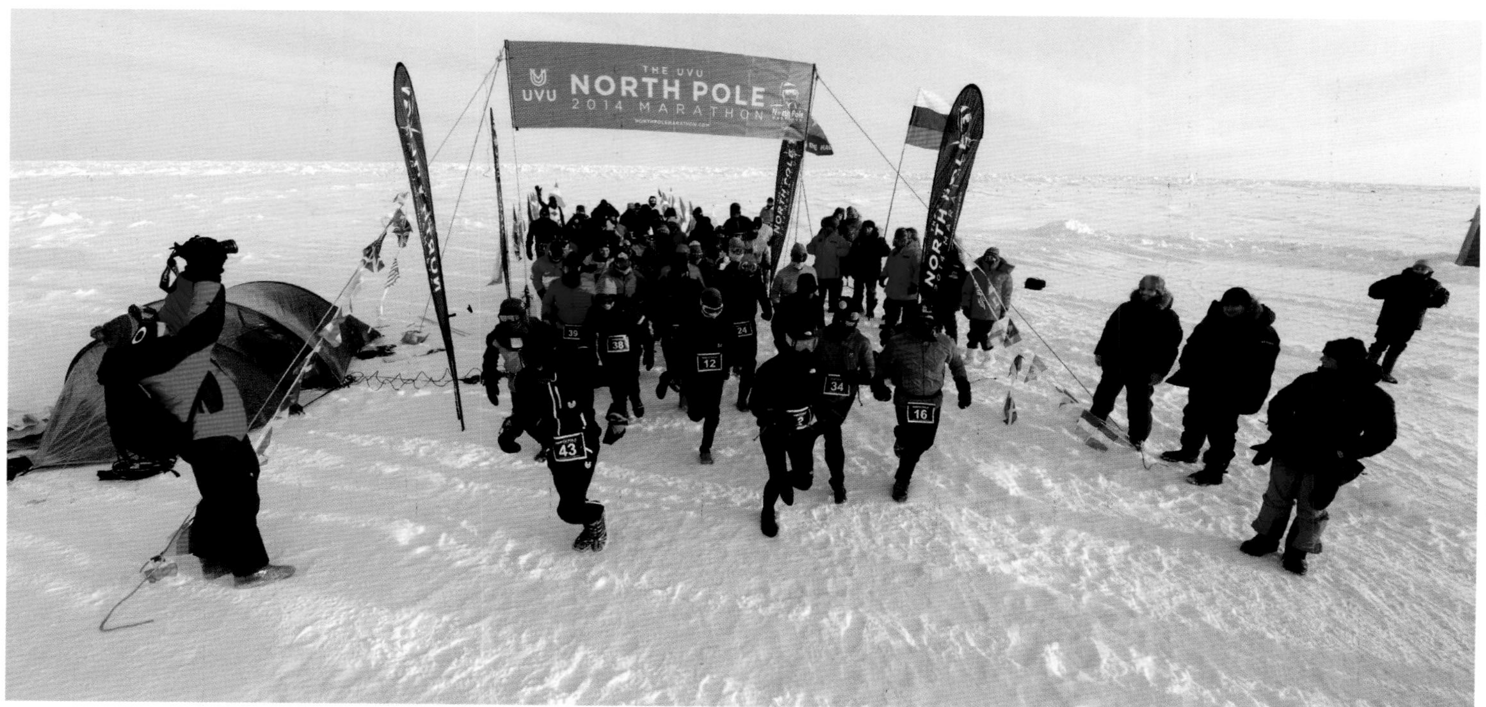

▼ Even aside from the freezing temperatures, running on snow and ice makes the North Pole Marathon hugely challenging.

PETRA DESERT MARATHON

A RACE RICH IN HISTORY, CULTURE AND SCENIC NATURE

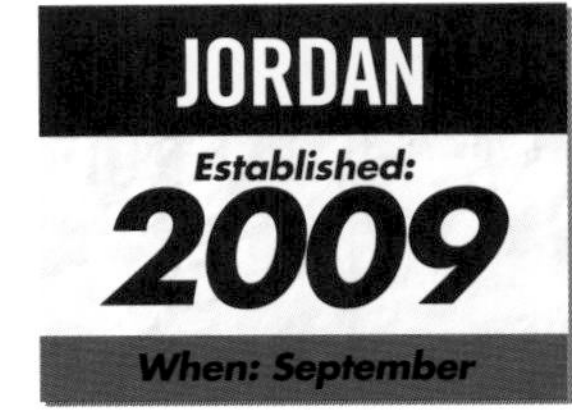

You fly to Amman to get to the start of this famously gruelling desert race, which kicks off from the ancient city of Petra and snakes its way into the otherworldly Jordanian desert, where runners must climb through the heat on punishing, pebbly paths to reach their goal. The race village is a long way from the nearest airport, so most participants invest in accommodation and transfer packages from marathon tourism companies.

The race starts at 6.30 a.m. in the Street of Facades. Petra is best known for the hundreds of ornate, classical-style façades carved into its red sandstone cliffs, the grandest of which mark the tombs of the Nabatean kings. As the sunrise washes the city's ancient monuments a rosy pink, the excitement mounts. The runners jog past ancient tombs, caves and monasteries.

After a mile or so, runners leave the Petra Archaeological Park boundaries and approach the desert on a tarmac road. Once the pack leaves the smooth road and takes the Siq, or gorge path, through the dramatic landscape, the fun begins: the path twists and turns between cliffs and sometimes becomes narrow and oppressive, as the walls loom 150m above you before opening out into the sunshine again.

It is the weirdest landscape to be running through, and of course the heat can become intense, so there are frequent water stations. Once past the 18-mile mark, full marathon runners find themselves back at Ammarine village and the route goes uphill to a mountain ridge for three miles or so, but the strenuous efforts are rewarded with an astonishing view over most of the marathon route, the mountains covering Petra. On a clear day, you can see to Israel. On this mountain ridge the surface becomes gravel for the next two miles.

The final two miles are steep downhill running on paved roads towards the finish line. Hundreds of volunteers turn out to look after the runners and the atmosphere in this ancient city is wonderful. Once the effort is over, a trip to a Dead Sea spa resort would seem an excellent idea, although many other runners undoubtedly have the same intention.

▼ Heat and uneven terrain are worth bearing for the spectacular sight of Petra.

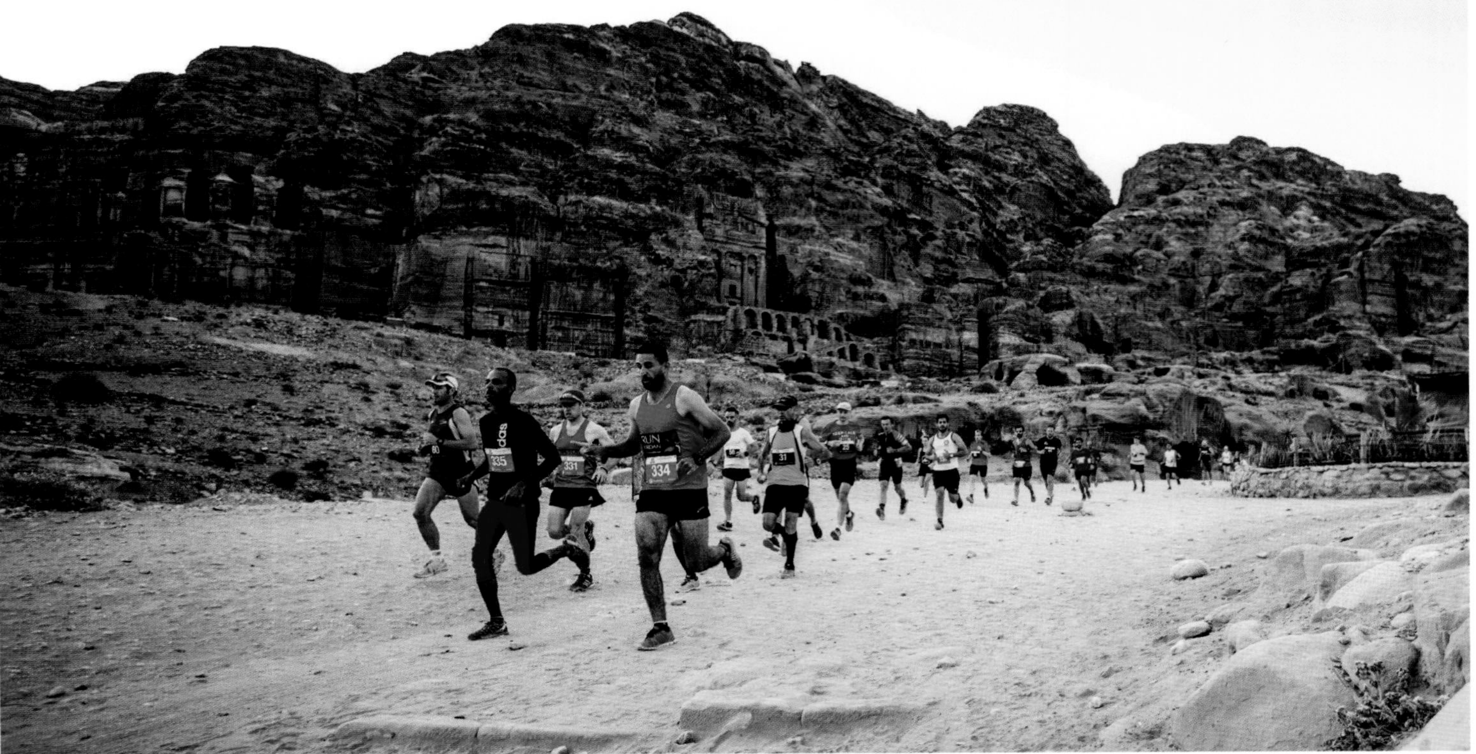

PIKES PEAK ASCENT & MARATHON

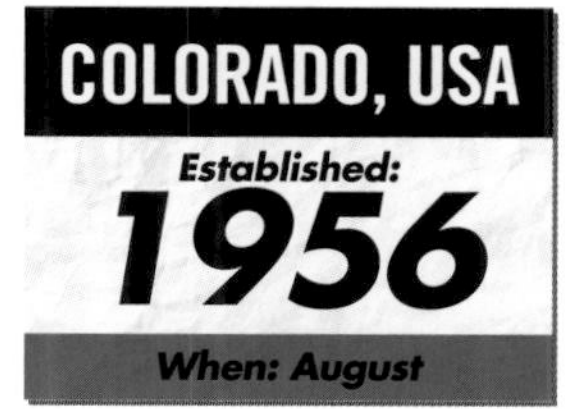

THE DEFINITION OF A BUCKET-LIST MARATHON

A venerable marathon, Pikes Peak is the USA's third oldest (behind the kingpin Boston and the recently reinstated Yonkers). Pikes Peak had its debut in 1956, and was, according to legend, originally a challenge between smokers and nonsmokers, presumably to test lung capacity. Thirteen runners, including three smokers, accepted the challenge. Monte Wolford, then 28, a vegetarian bodybuilder of a nonsmoker, won the race in 5 hours, 39 minutes. The smokers were disqualified because none of them finished the race, although one legged it up to the top very quickly – then insisted on having a smoke at the summit.

Few smokers have a go these days. Runners start fully carb-loaded in front of the town hall in Manitou Springs (elevation 6,300ft/1,920m) and race up to the summit of the hulking Pikes Peak (14,115ft/4,302m), the highest summit of the southern Front Range of the Rocky Mountains. That, of course, is half the challenge. The second half, and many people say it's the worst, is the quad- and hip-shredding descent. It's a terrible, wonderful, physical and mental challenge. The ascent can take as long as, or longer than, a full road marathon, and it pays to have trained at high altitude before you attempt it. The descent is, unsurprisingly, a lot quicker, depending on how much courage runners can muster to let themselves go fully on the steep bits. It's winding, though, so you can come across a few upland bits during the descent.

The race begins in front of the City Hall in Manitou Springs, and ends in the city, having taken its route on the Barr trail in Pike National Forest (rather than the famous Pikes Peak Highway). Once the pack has run through the city streets to get to the trail, the terrain is gravel, rocks and dirt and there are plenty of narrow, winding stretches to further slow you down.

The weather above treeline is unpredictable, and lightning is a major issue. Temperatures can vary by as much as 50°F between Manitou Springs and the upper parts of the mountain, where runners can find themselves ankle deep in snow. Storms can come out of nowhere, so competitors are advised to bring adequate mountain clothing for any eventuality. Organizers advise that, if lightning strikes, the best strategy is "for a group to spread out and crouch down with your feet planted on anything that will insulate you from the ground (jacket, fanny pack etc.). Try not to be the tallest object in the vicinity!" In short, this may be a bucket-list marathon, but, if the weather decides to kick off, ascending that Rocky Mountain high in Colorado will have to be left to another day.

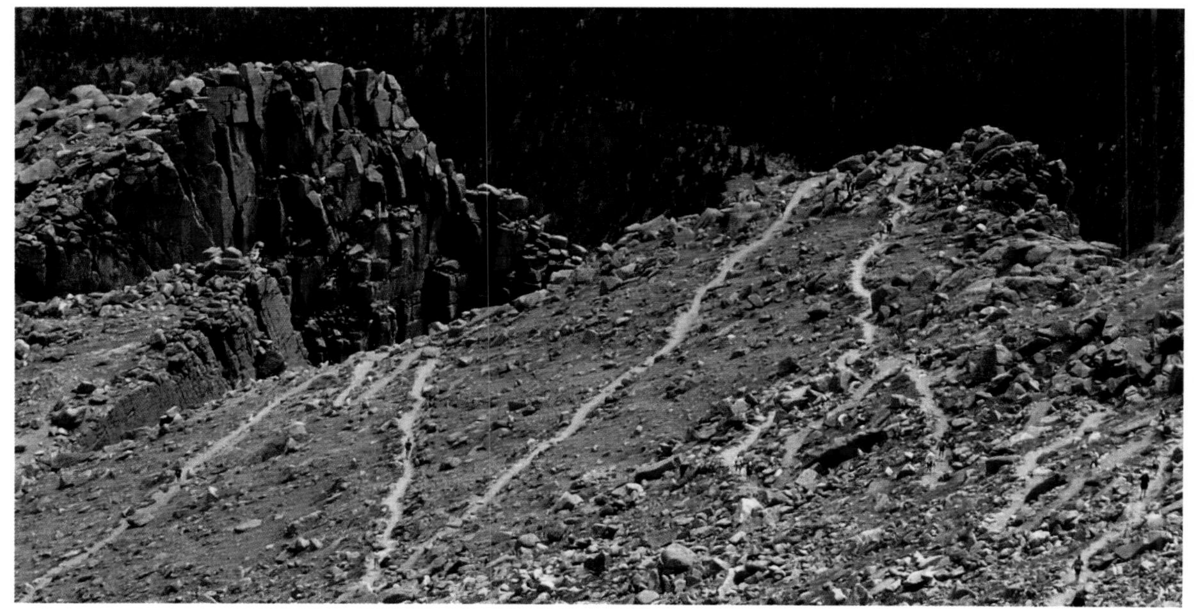

◀ The event at Pikes Peak has been running consistently for more than 50 years.

PURBECK MARATHON

A TOUGH CLIMB AWAITS ON THE SOUTH COAST OF ENGLAND

JURASSIC COAST
Established:
2012
When: September

A multi-award-winner and a favourite with tough runners not too fixated on times, this 27-mile race certainly gives you more (it's longer than standard). There's also 3,000ft (914m) of climb. That's a lot of work for the glutes and calves, so it's just as well there's a natural (seaside) ice bath for screaming tendons at the finish. The marathon is the main event in the annual Purbeck Running Festival, a community event and a not-for-profit race: all proceeds go to charity. The clifftop region of Dorset it hugs is incredibly beautiful, fascinating because of its unique Jurassic geology (you're running on dinosaur bones here) and it affords some inspirational views it would be a shame to race past.

The course starts and ends in the seaside town of Swanage. Over the first few miles, the trail is narrow and tricky but it widens out soon for those who find the cliff edge discomfortingly close. With the advent of National Trust and military land, the frequent gates and styles pop up to vary the pace. The run takes a course from the Downs overlooking the beach, then heads towards Durlston Country Park and the Jurassic coast path, before going through the villages of Worth Matravers and Kingston. From Swyre Head it passes Heaven's Gate and along the ridge towards Tyneham Cap. From here, it leaves the coast path and runs through the deserted village of Tyneham. Many runners make a note here to come back and explore this extraordinary place, requisitioned by the army in 1943 and deserted ever since. It's still military land, but walkers can wander through its ruins in wonder.

From Tyneham, it's up and up to Corfe Castle, into the village square and back along the Ridgeway, and three miles of near-continuous hills, to Swanage for medals and goody bags (they've contained cider and local beer in the past) and a well-earned dip in the icy sea.

It seems like the whole local community gets involved in this race, and, judging from the generous goody bag in previous years, many of the local producers (Dorset Cereals, Purbeck Ice Cream) put their weight behind it, too. Reviewers cannot praise highly enough the marshalling, support and encouragement they received on this testing run.

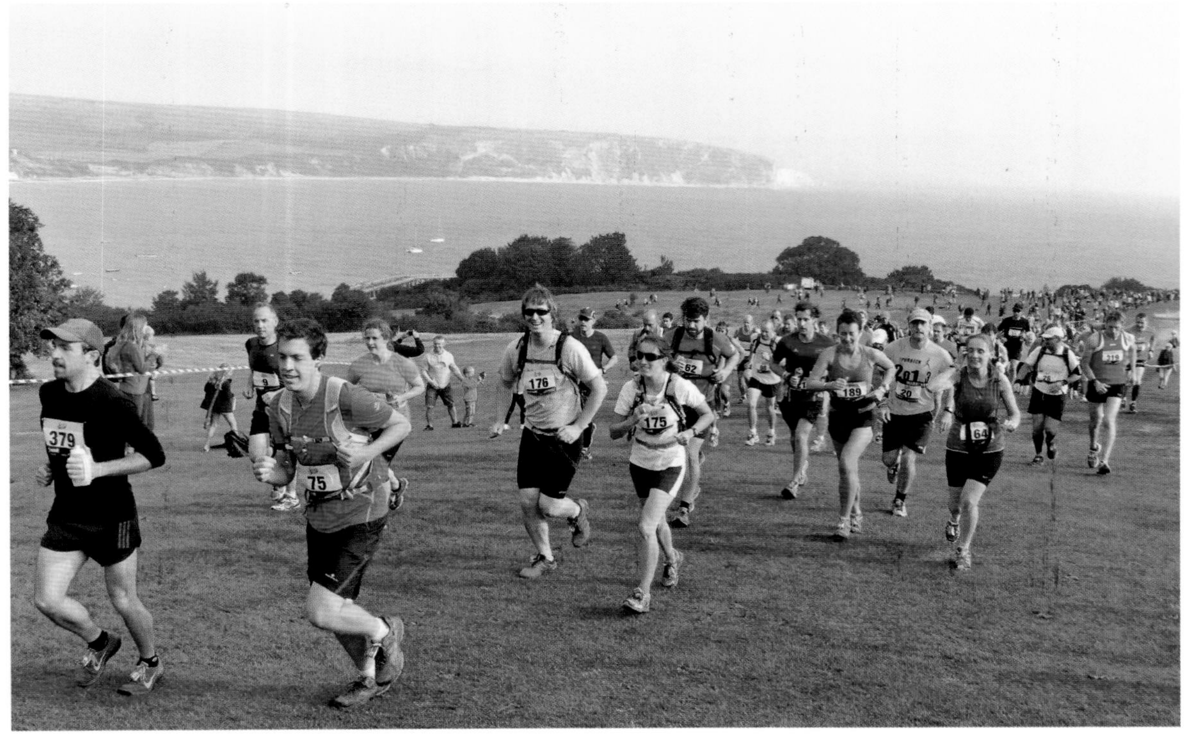

◀ A deserted village and a Jurassic coast greet runners who make it to Dorset.

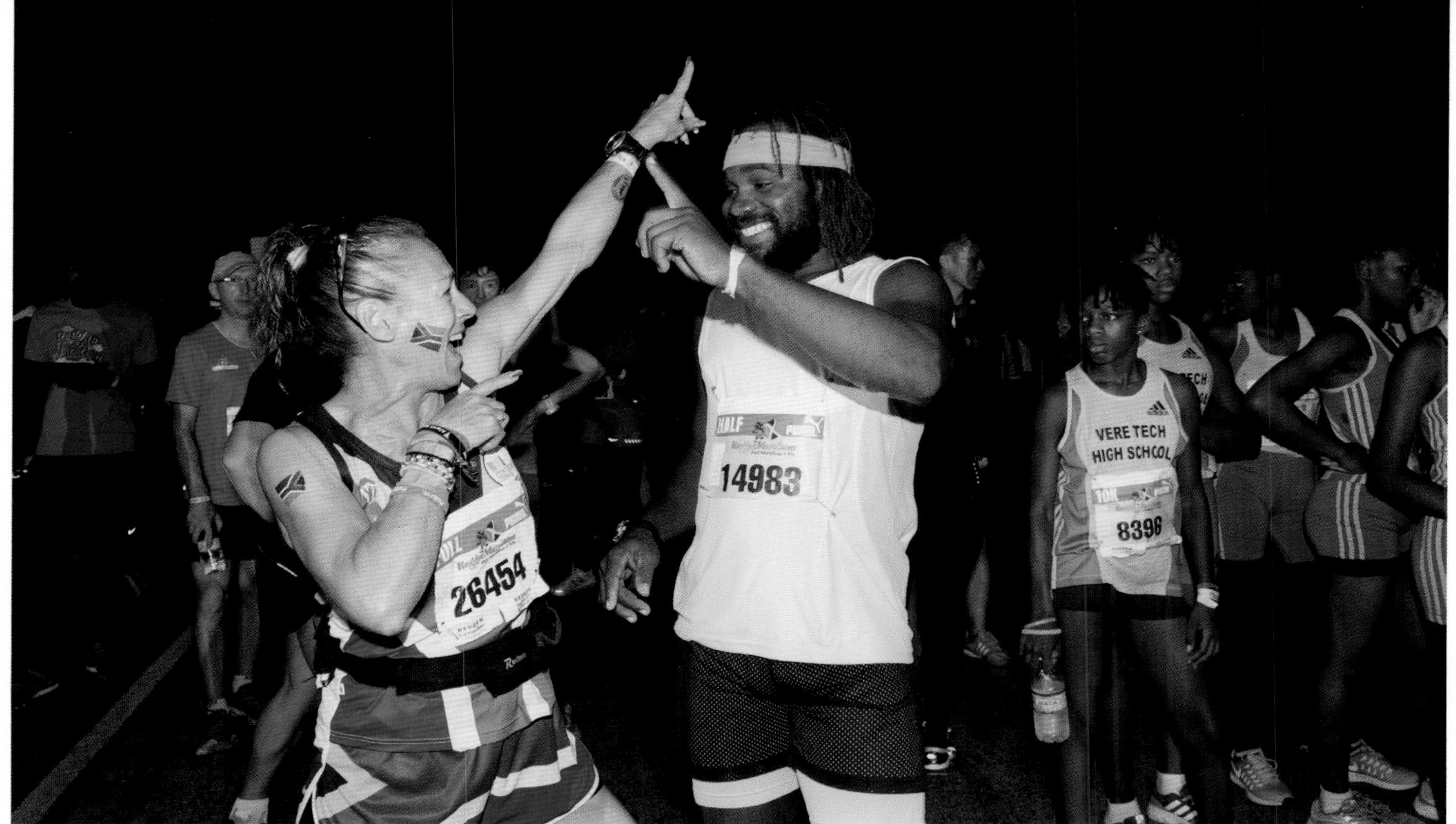

REGGAE MARATHON

ENJOY THE CARNIVAL VIBES OF JAMAICA'S MARATHON

NEGRIL, JAMAICA
Established:
1995
When: December

Expect carnival, spectacle and a whole lot of music during this totally tropical marathon. It's the one race where you'd expect your super-hydrating and mineral-replenishing coconut water to be very fresh, and so it is: the coconut sellers are out chopping the fruits for runners from dawn until dusk. The whole festival takes place in the resort town of Negril, whose seven miles of white-sand beaches have made it the holidaymakers' paradise for decades.

The party starts way before the main event. The Reggae Marathon organizers state they host the "world's best pasta party" the night before, a claim that promises much, but in this case the superlative is justified. As well as the much-vaunted Rasta Pasta, there are many different types and styles of the carb loader's favourite, and it's all free to runners signed up to the event. Live reggae music and plenty of bonhomie means it's hard to leave the party to prepare for the early start, but runners promise themselves more fun – with beer and rum cocktails to boot – the following evening.

About 2,300 runners from all over the Caribbean and the rest of the world line up for this relatively flat race, which goes from Negril town and heads north towards Green Island. Most of the route is in residential areas, but you catch glimpses of the sea (and often wish you were in it). The race starts early (5.15 a.m.) to avoid the worst of the strong sun, although the temperature at night in Jamaica is very warm. Everyone queues for the bag drop in pitch-dark. The route is, mercifully, mostly flat, and lined with hotels, supporters and volunteers providing locally made Hi-Lyte water pouches, Gatorade and gels. The support is good-natured and noisy, and there's an awful lot of reggae to help you keep a bouncy cadence.

It's the finish line that really makes the race special, though. Instead of the usual crossing the line, wandering about, then heading back to shower, you are thrown into a beach party for 3,000 runners and their supporters. With a medal around your neck, you receive a freshly cut coconut, and an ice-cold Red Stripe – which you can drink while cooling your overheated body in the clear Caribbean waters.

▲ The music and atmosphere surrounding the Reggae Marathon are perhaps the world's liveliest.

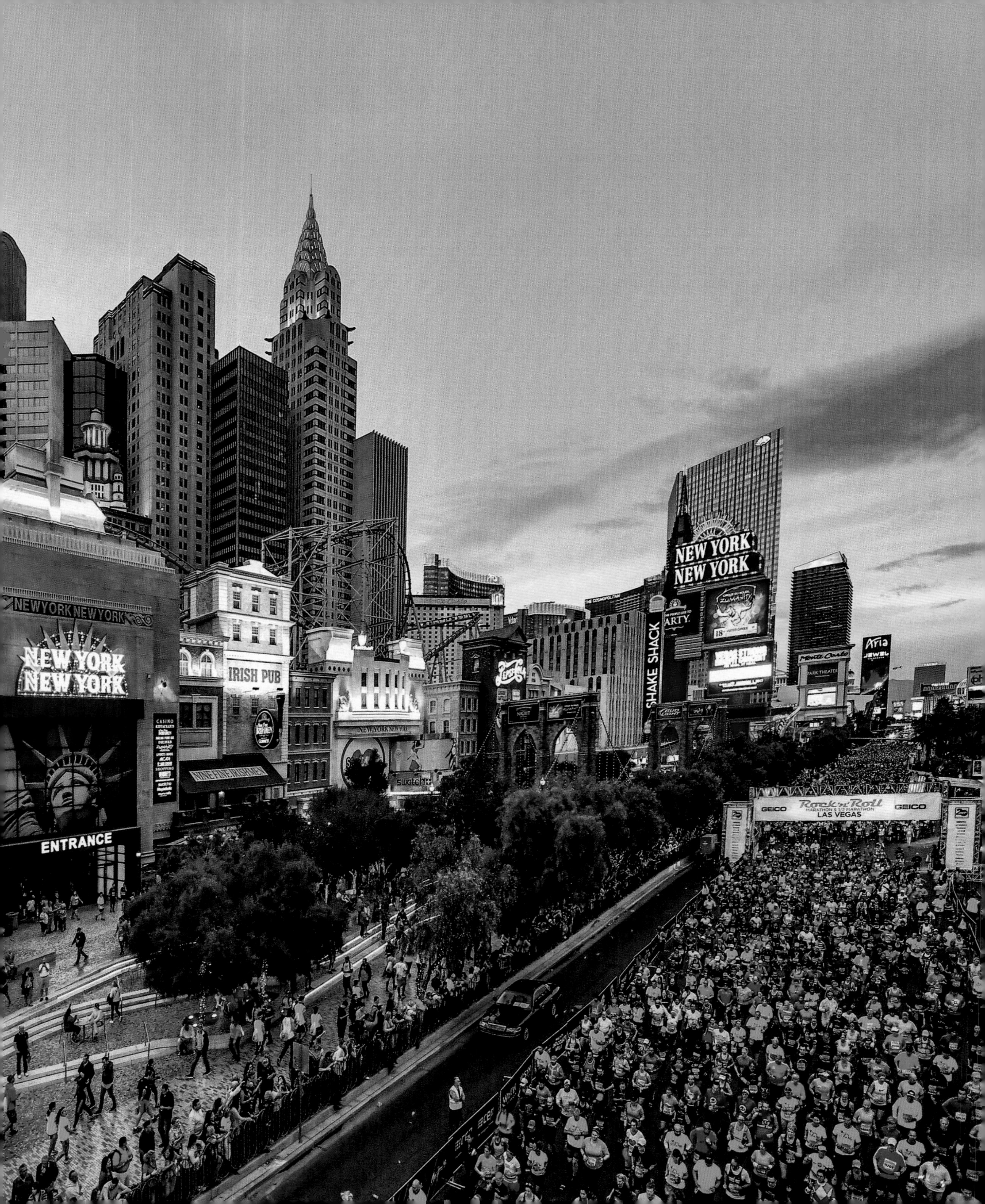
NEW YORK NEW YORK
NEWYORK NEWYORK
NEW YORK NEW YORK
ENTRANCE
IRISH PUB
SHAKE SHACK
GEICO
Rock 'n' Roll
MARATHON & 1/2 MARATHON
LAS VEGAS
GEICO
Aria
JEWEL
swatch

ROCK 'N' ROLL LAS VEGAS MARATHON

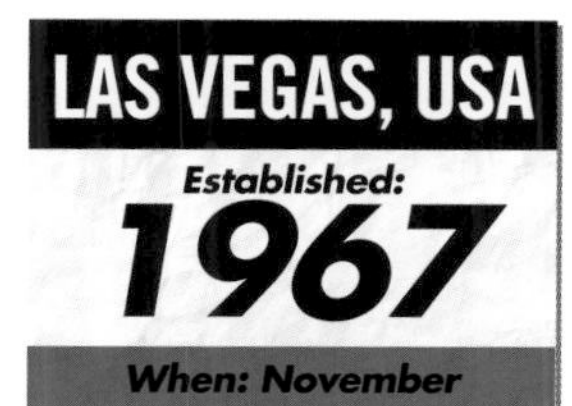

AN EXPLOSION OF LIGHT, COLOUR, SPECTACLE AND NOISE

Nightlife is everything in Nevada's sparkly town, so the late-afternoon start is cool for runners (you start balmy and appreciate the slight chill of the desert night). Then there's the neon-lit finish, which everyone raves about. Everyone seems to have good stories to tell about this well-supported race, especially the fancy-dress contingent (the fastest-ever running Elvis impersonator completed this marathon in 2:38).

Runners are also given the honour of streaming along the world-famous Strip unimpeded by traffic: marathon day and New Year's Eve are the only times in the year that this happens. The whole route is supported by enthusiastic crowds and bathed in light, so you really feel that you're part of something special.

The start line is near McCarran International Airport, and there are fireworks on the starting gun. The many corrals of runners take off and run past the uplifting "Welcome to fabulous Las Vegas" sign and past the many casinos that line the Strip, then the unbelievably opulent hotels and kitsch interpretations of world landmarks as the race opens out and streams along the city's lesser known street, where the live rock-'n'-roll bands, which are race series' unique selling point, keep runners' spirits up.

The finish line is an explosion of light, colour, spectacle and noise, finishing as it does in front of the spectacular Mirage volcano. If you're running with your affianced and don't mind adding three minutes to your time, you can squeeze in a quick Run-Thru Wedding ceremony to boot.

The marathon has a time limit of five hours, so, despite the fun element, you need to be confident you can finish in this timeframe.

This is high-end marathon tourism. The three-day event (to take in a 5km, a 10km or a half-marathon option) includes a hugely popular Marathon Expo and the city lures many visitors – attempting to have a low-key day before the big race – into too much sightseeing. The sunset start time can also play havoc with nervous stomachs (and there is always so much food around in Vegas), but, fortunately, the start is well provided for in the Portaloo department.

With aid stations at every couple of miles and live music almost every mile, not to mention all the well-wishers handing out sweeties, runners feel well catered for. The course is relatively flat, although tired runners feel the sloping routes around the World Market Center. The medal is always a blingy one (this *is* Vegas) and should be worn with much pride throughout the rest of your stay in Sin City; you may even be bought a beer from admiring fans. After the race, you can freshen up and then hit the town for a perfect post-race night out!

◀ The marathon begins with a truly stunning Nevada sunset.

▼ Runners must try not to get distracted by the bright lights of the big city in this night run.

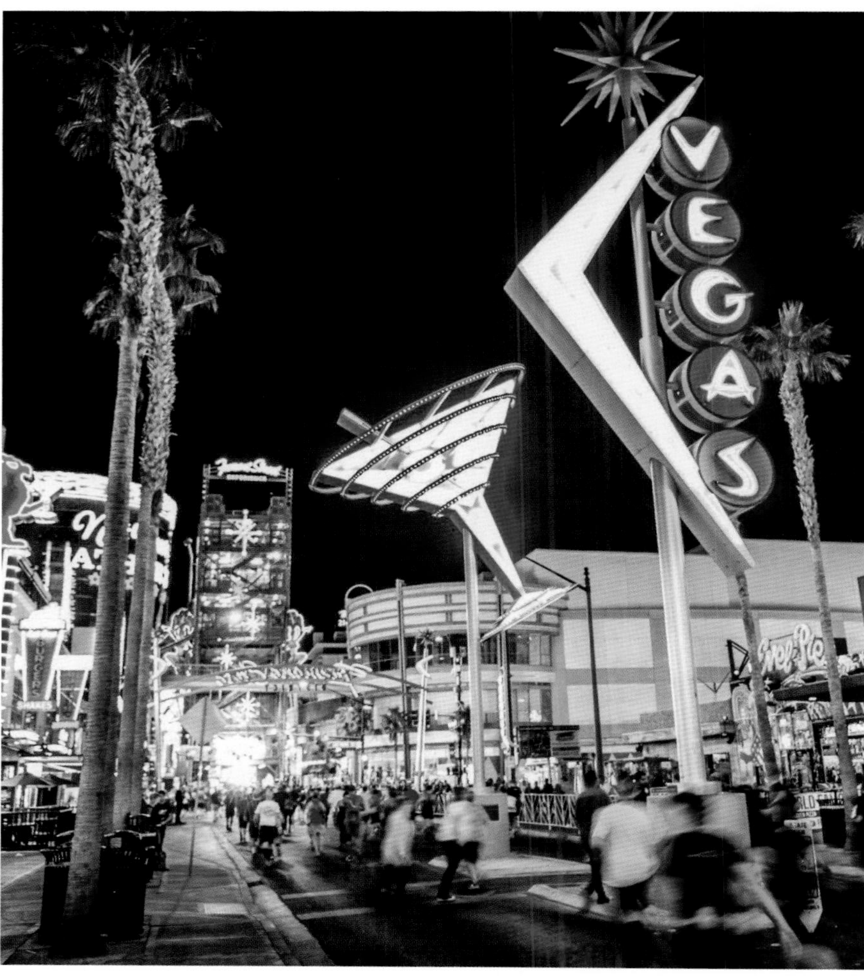

ROCK 'N' ROLL LIVERPOOL MARATHON

EXPERIENCE GREAT MUSIC AND SOME BEAUTIFUL LIVERPOOL VISTAS

LIVERPOOL, UK
Established:
2015
When: May

From the friendly city that gave the world the Beatles comes this rocking, almost-four-year-old newcomer to the UK's packed marathon calendar. It has been quickly taken to the hearts of personal-best seekers, probably because it has the full weight of the hugely successful US Rock 'n' Roll series behind it. Grey Merseyside skies may count against in the glamour stakes (its Stateside sisters have more guaranteed sunshine), but it can't be faulted on bonhomie.

Banging tunes resound along the course, and most particularly at the start and finish festivities, which put everyone in the party mood. The course route has been carefully plotted to take in the city's most appealing sights: Albert Dock, Goodison Park (Everton FC), Anfield (Liverpool FC), Penny Lane, and a wonderful reward (once you've scaled one of the series of hills that occur around the middle part of the race) of a beautiful vista of the Liverpool skyline. The last few miles take you along the River Mersey, which often means a brisk breeze off the water, but the home run is always a test on super-tired legs.

There are 11 hydration stations on the marathon, some of which have sports drinks and SIS gels; it's also very well provided with Portaloos and first aid (nine around the course). The race also has a very large pacing team, from sub-3:15 to sub-5:30.

Finishers receive a typically blingy rock-'n'-roll medal (a recent example included a spinning element in honour of the city's waterfront Ferris wheel – the Big Wheel of Liverpool) and a bright, technical T-shirt, as well as a much-appreciated free beer.

The after party takes place at the world-famous Cavern Club, but, even if you opt not to spend extra on that, the musical line up is taken very seriously. Participants are given advance information about the big-name headline act (usually a successful home-grown band) and all the live acts stationed around the course. And, as you'd expect, when you loop around Penny Lane you invariably catch the strains of the Beatles song of the same name.

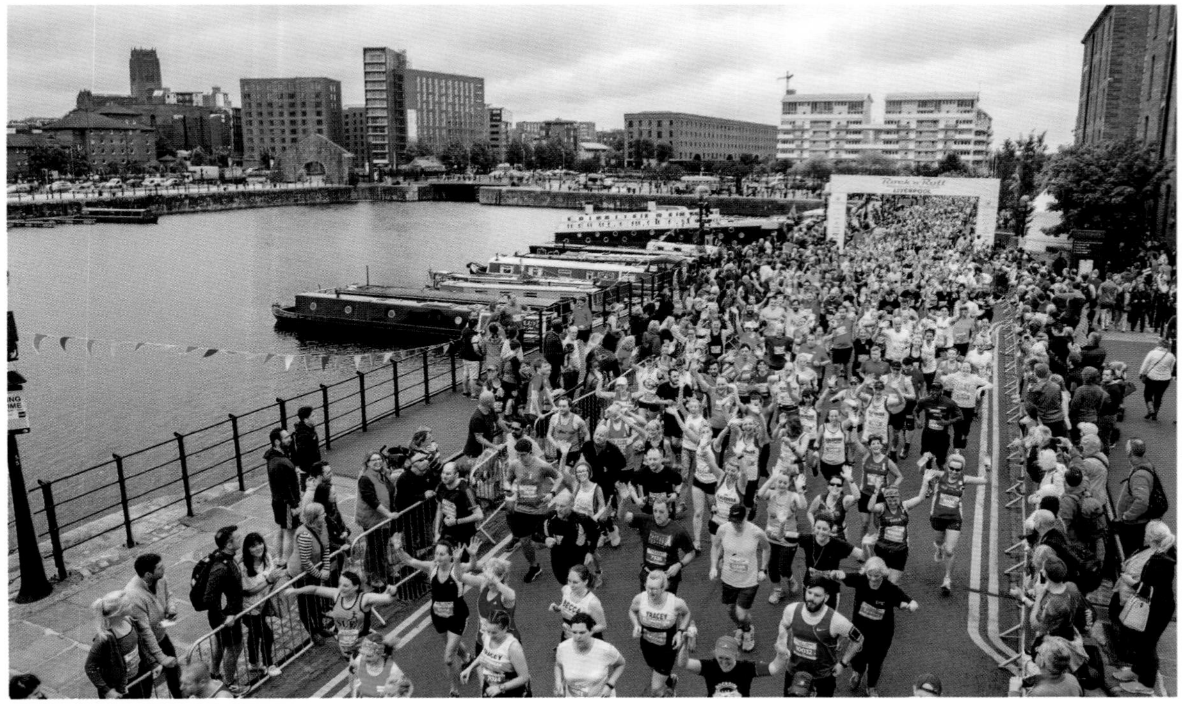

◀ The party starts in Liverpool the minute the first runners arrive.

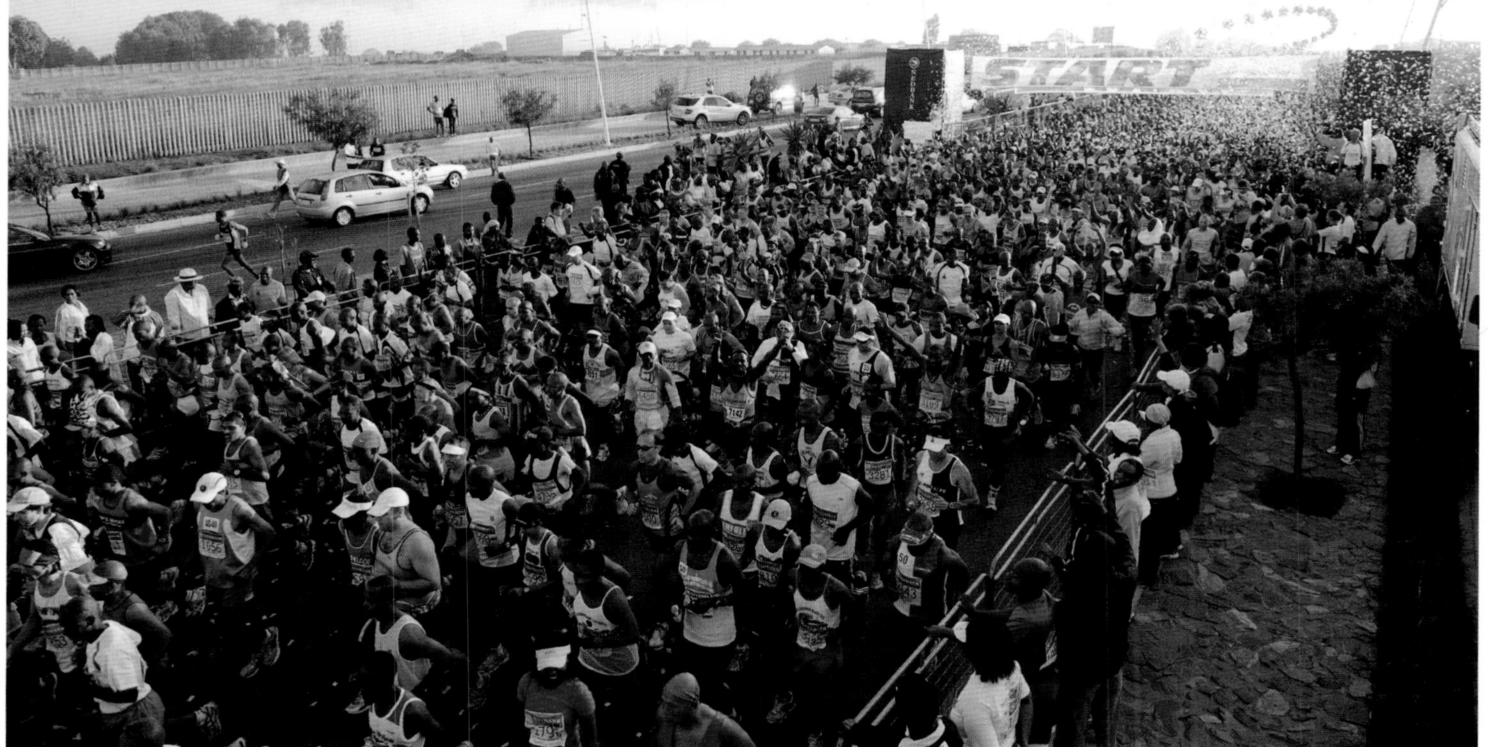

SOWETO MARATHON

A POPULAR MARATHON WITH A COURSE STEEPED IN HISTORY

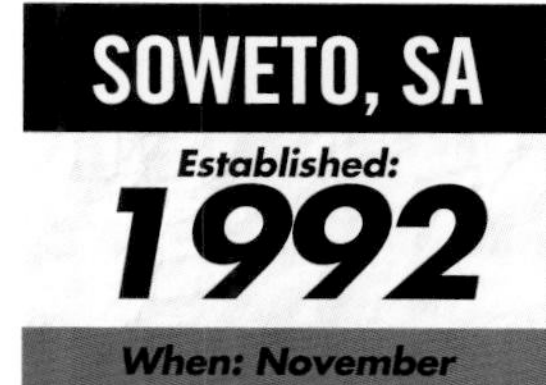

Starting and finishing in the world-famous "Soccer City", the FNB stadium in the suburb of Nasrec, the Soweto Marathon – dubbed "The People's Marathon" – takes you on you a noisy and inspiring South African history lesson and honours the characters who believed in the power of its people.

Runners pass eight significant heritage sites on the marathon route, including: the largest hospital in the world (3,400 beds), called the Chris Hani Baragwanath Hospital; Walter Sisulu Square (the birthplace of the 1955 Freedom Charter for a non-racial South Africa); Regina Mundi Catholic Church, which became famous for its role in the anti-apartheid struggle and where Archbishop Emeritus Desmond Tutu presided over the Truth and Reconciliation Commission hearings; and Vilakazi Street, not so far from the end of the race, where Nelson Mandela and Archbishop Tutu both lived – so the only street in the world to have had two Nobel Peace Prize-winners as residents. There's a long hill at around this point, where runners pass Uncle Tom's Community Hall and the Hector Pieterson Museum and memorial, which commemorates the 1976 student uprising.

With the first few miles of the race being of a largely downhill nature, it's easy to be a bit complacent. Don't be. This race saves its worst until last. The halfway mark heralds the point at which the marathon starts climbing, so you should leave plenty of energy in your tank for the latter half of the race. There are water points every three kilometres, which makes it easier to pace yourself in the heat, but this is a very hard race.

Where the 10k race joins the marathon for the spectacular, noisy finish, the route takes another climb, past the Morris Isaacson School, where the 1976 student march began. The June 16th Memorial Acre, opened in 2015, is the open-air memorial that tells the story of the Soweto youth's brave stand against the apartheid state. The climb continues for another kilometre past the Jabulani Police Station and behind the Shopping Mall. The final stretch down Koma Road provides an easy run-in to Soccer City and one huge, happy party.

The support from the people of Soweto is phenomenal. Many reviewers report that this is the friendliest marathon they've ever taken part in. The streets are lined by the community, cheering, chanting and encouraging runners throughout the challenging course, in the spirit of togetherness that forged modern South Africa.

▲ Motivational locals cheer the runners on through their historical tour of Soweto.

SPACE COAST MARATHON

FLORIDA'S OLDEST MARATHON IS OUT OF THIS WORLD

CAPE CANAVERAL
Established: 1972
When: November

A must for all space nerds, this space race has collectable medals that are out of this world. The name given to the 2018 event was Project Mercury, NASA's first human space-flight programme, 1958–63. With this amount of care taken over the memorabilia, and any number of astronaut models and other space-related paraphernalia to pose with at the expo, it's no wonder people keep coming back. Oh, and the fact that organizers encourage repeat performances so that runners can be part of their Hall of Fame Challenge.

This is Florida's oldest marathon, and it starts in the Cocoa Beach area (where the bizarre sitcom *I Dream of Jeannie*, about a man and his alien girlfriend, was famously set in the 1960s). Cocoa Beach is a charming place to hang out the day before the big race, as there are some wonderful independent cafés and vintage shops to rummage in.

The countdown to the start is a prerecorded launch audio from years past, so runners take off to the roar of solid-rocket-fuel boosters, an unforgettable experience!

The course comprises two out-and-back courses, each a half-marathon in distance, with the Cocoa Village start/finish area right in the centre. Much of the run follows a route alongside the Indian River, providing endless beautiful views along the shore, as well as clear, cool breezes aplenty. The first few miles take a winding pattern, past Indian Trail, before heading southbound on Rockledge Drive, with a turnaround at Mile 20 to take a route southbound to the finish line at Riverfront Park.

It's picture-perfect in places. The sun rising over Indian River is a beautiful sight and the crowd support is stellar. There are plentifully stocked hydration stations staffed by volunteers dressed in all sorts of costumes, be they of Doctor Who, Buzz Lightyear or characters from *Star Wars*. It's something else, being handed a water bottle by Princess Leia.

The last few miles are flat, fast and scenic, and, as temperatures rise, public-spirited homeowners bring out their spray hoses, ready to cool off overheated runners with some cool mist. At the end, there's plenty of pizza and beer and more space-age fancy dress than you can shake a lightsaber or sonic screwdriver at.

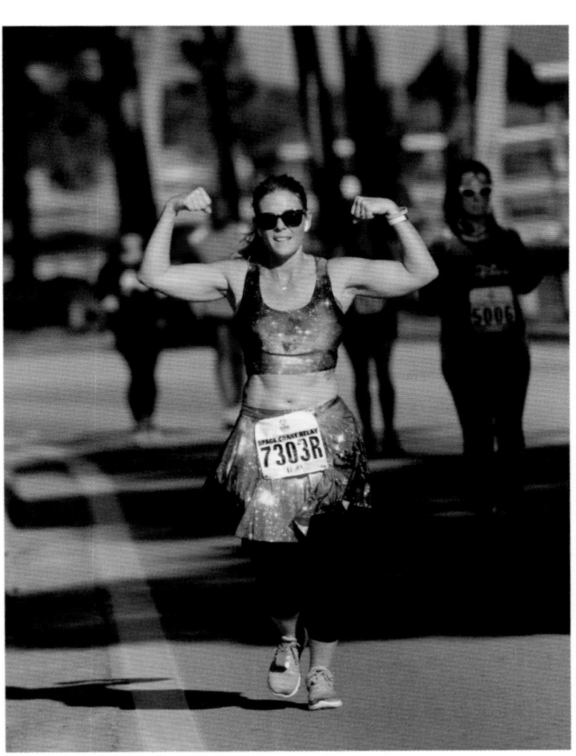

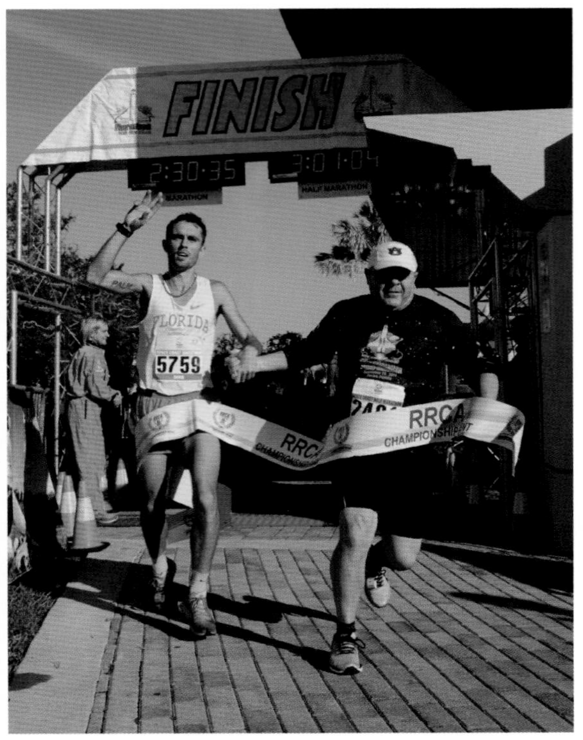

◀ Runners finish where they began, but with beer and pizza waiting for them this time.

◀◀ The galaxy needn't be so far, far away in this race.

▶ The course may be flat but the temperatures are enough to make this race a challenge.

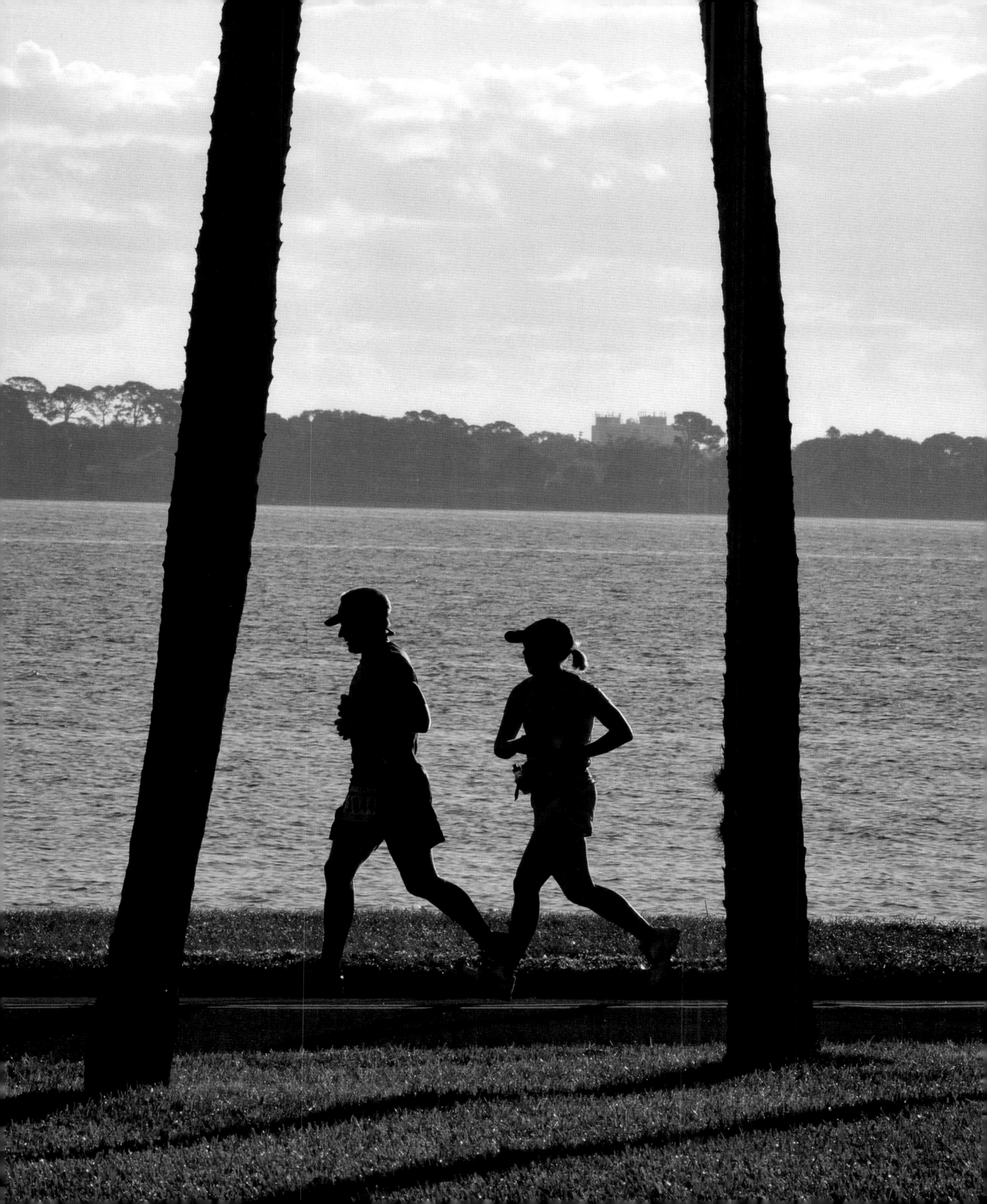

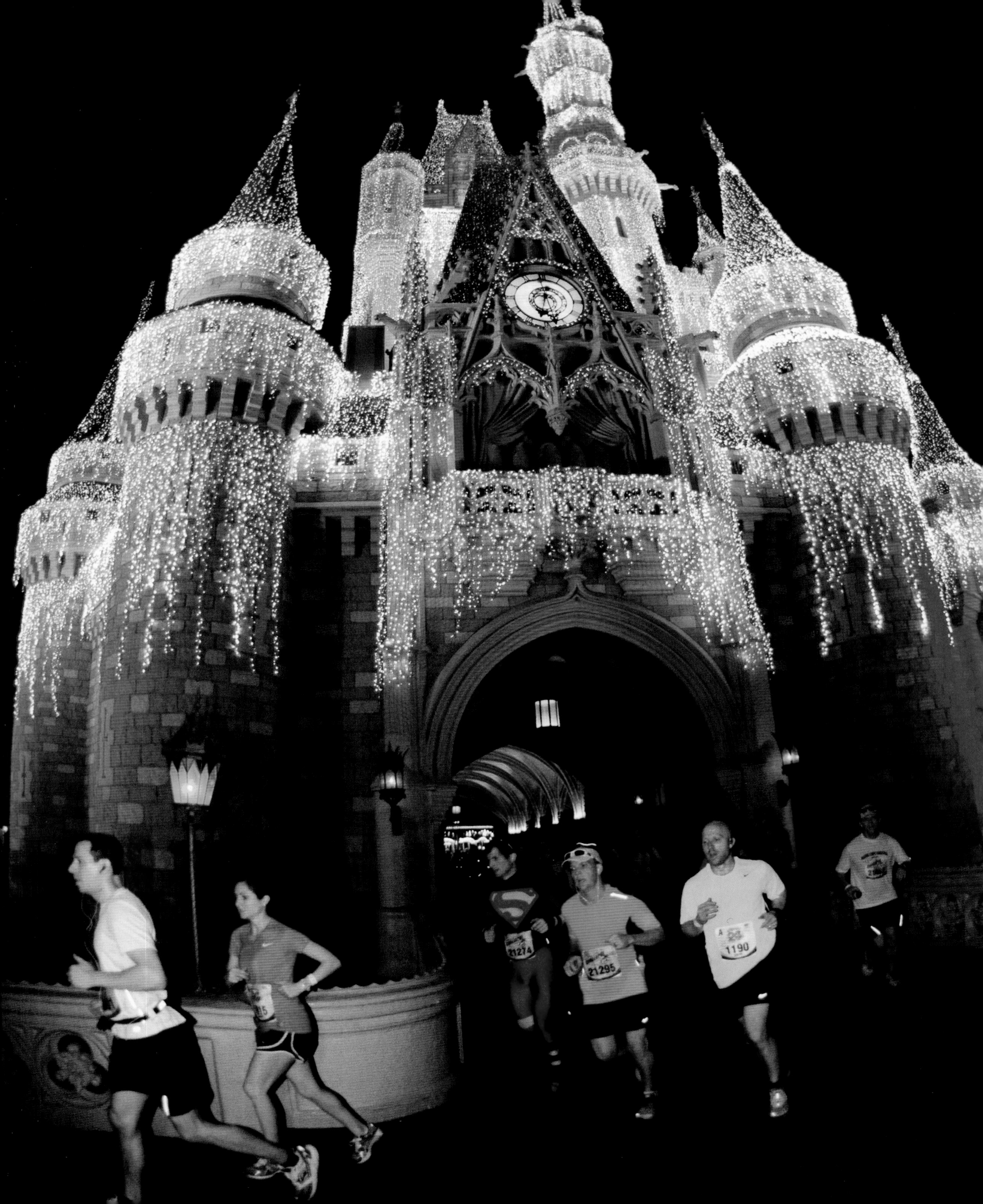
21274
21295
1190

WALT DISNEY MARATHON

A TRULY MAGICAL MARATHON EXPERIENCE

FLORIDA, USA
Established:
1994
When: January

As with all things Disney, you're required to "totally" leave any cynicism behind when you sign up to be "part of the runDisney Family". It's a dizzying, merchandising-heavy, high-octane experience, and, for those reasons, the marathon festival here is beloved by its many thousands of fans.

The humidity of the Florida climate necessitates a 6 a.m. start, which is why many runners opt to stay in the resort, and why, indeed, many incorporate their star-spangled race into a full Disney family holiday. There's certainly plenty to amuse friends and family spectators while their loved ones run.

The race takes you through four Walt Disney World theme parks, as well as the ESPN Wide World of Sports Complex. The crowds are massive – this is a hugely popular race and runners wait for ages in many corrals before the start.

The first six miles go north onto World Drive for the early-morning run to and through the Magic Kingdom, all lit up and twinkly. Then it's through the tropical landscapes, past the Shades of Green, Grand Floridian and Polynesian Village resorts, before going through some less-than-lovely areas to another lovely bit in the scenic Animal Kingdom park, where there are all sorts of domesticated animals just waiting for photo opportunities. In fact, there are temptations to stop and selfie everywhere, as Disney characters are all out in force and you don't often get the chance for a mid-race chat with Cinderella.

The paths that take runners through the ESPN Wide World of Sports Zone twist and turn and seem never ending, but, just when runners are reaching a dark night of the soul, there's a stimulating dash past Disney's Hollywood Studios at about Mile 22, then the last few miles take a serene course, past the Crescent Lake resort area into Epcot, and the last mile through World Showcase, to the finish line. The Disney Finisher medals are always a delight and it's great to pose with your hard-won honour with a beaming cartoon character. There are various race challenges for the chance to win extra prizes.

◀◀ Runners can finally live their childhood dreams of being a prince or princess as they run through the Magic Kingdom.

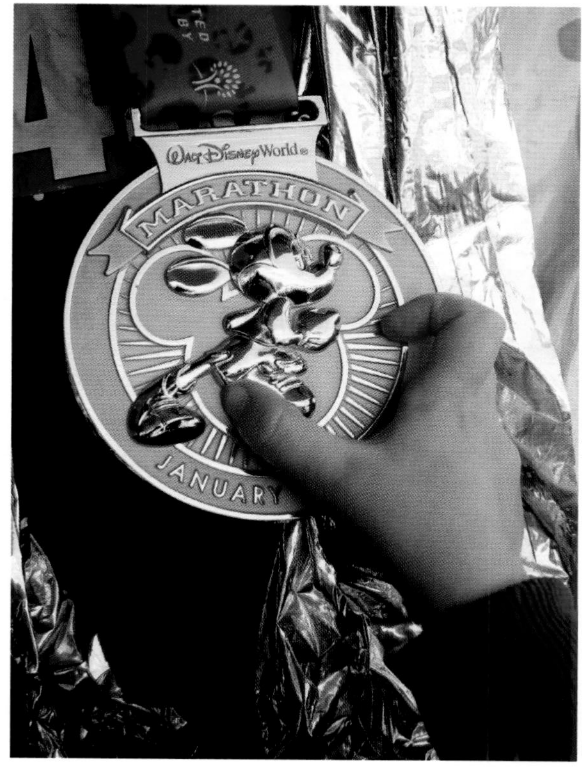

◀ It's no surprise that the Walt Disney marathon offers one of the flashier and most-prized medals.

▼ Mickey, Minnie and other beloved Disney characters celebrate with runners who make it to the finish line.

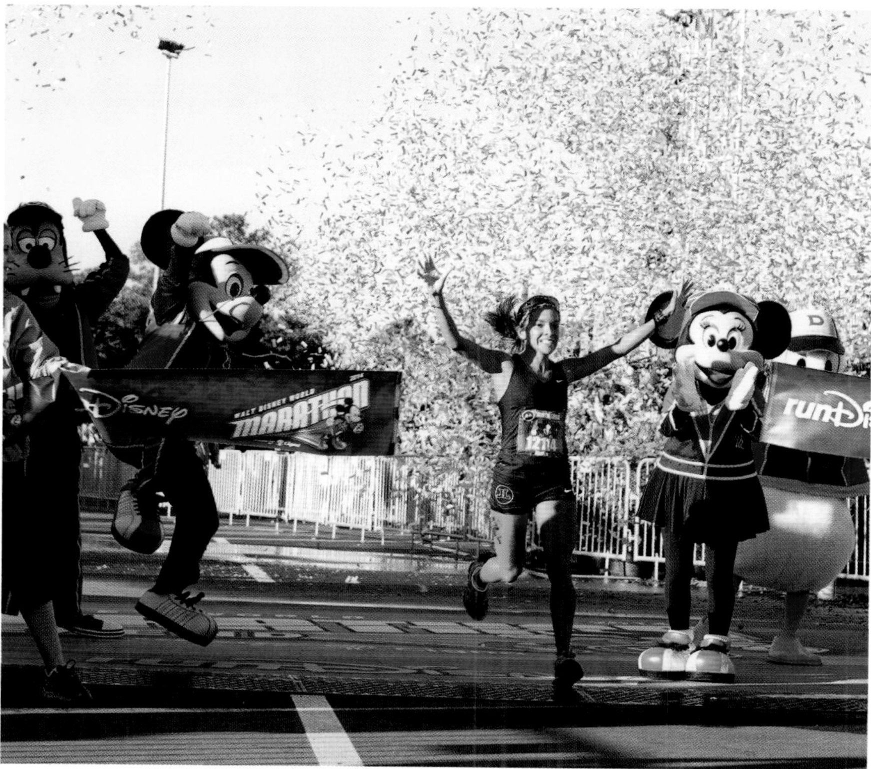

WINDERMERE MARATHON

A FAMOUSLY HARD RUN THAT FEATURES SOME EPIC VISTAS

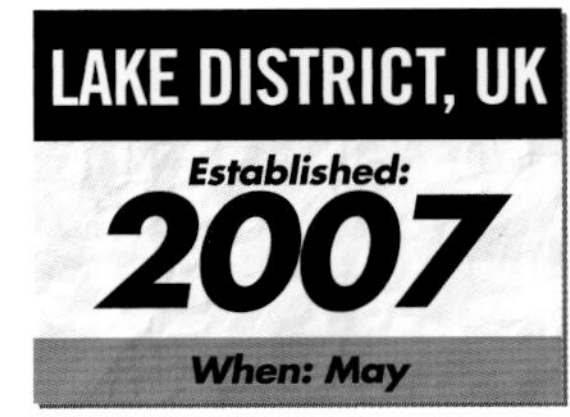

Vying with its Coniston neighbour for the "UK's most scenic" title, Windermere is held up by most Lake District aficionados as the winner in the beauty stakes because it is run entirely within a UNESCO World Heritage Site. The finisher medal is special, too, because it's engraved with a detail from the route, whose hilly course will no doubt be engraved on your memory into the bargain.

This Lakeland race starts and finishes on the manicured lawns of pretty Brathay Hall, a gorgeous 360-acre estate that overlooks the northern shore of Windermere, the Lake District's biggest expanse of water, with a backdrop of the fells. The route passes through some of the region's treasures, including the pretty villages of Hawkshead, which used to belong to Furness Abbey until the twelfth century, and Newby Bridge, another winsome settlement that takes its name from the picturesque five-arch bridge over the River Leven.

It's a famously hard run, which is why it's chosen as the course that some thrill seekers repeat tenfold – for the Brathay 10in10 Challenge. They run the marathon for 10 days on the trot in an endurance event that has been described as one of the toughest ever. Just running around it once, however, means you must dig deep.

The hills come thick and fast, but the biggest is at Mile 7, which many runners find they need to walk from halfway (where the bagpipers are, encouraging people to try even harder, perhaps to escape their drone). The course goes into extreme undulation mode at Mile 14 and, from here, every uphill is matched by a downhill and, at the summit of the hill at Mile 18, the views are spectacular. The entry into Bowness is a hilarious moment, as all the tourists in the little town seem to be partying and taking photos.

There's a cruel beast of a hill at Mile 21, which has an ice-cream van at the top. It's quite a tradition for the 10in10 runners to celebrate their 256th mile with a cornet on their lap of honour. There is a huge amount of support at this point, and a couple more feed stations. The last mile is etched on most runners' memories, because the second half is uphill – a massive struggle as you grimace at the medal wearers on their way down from the finish.

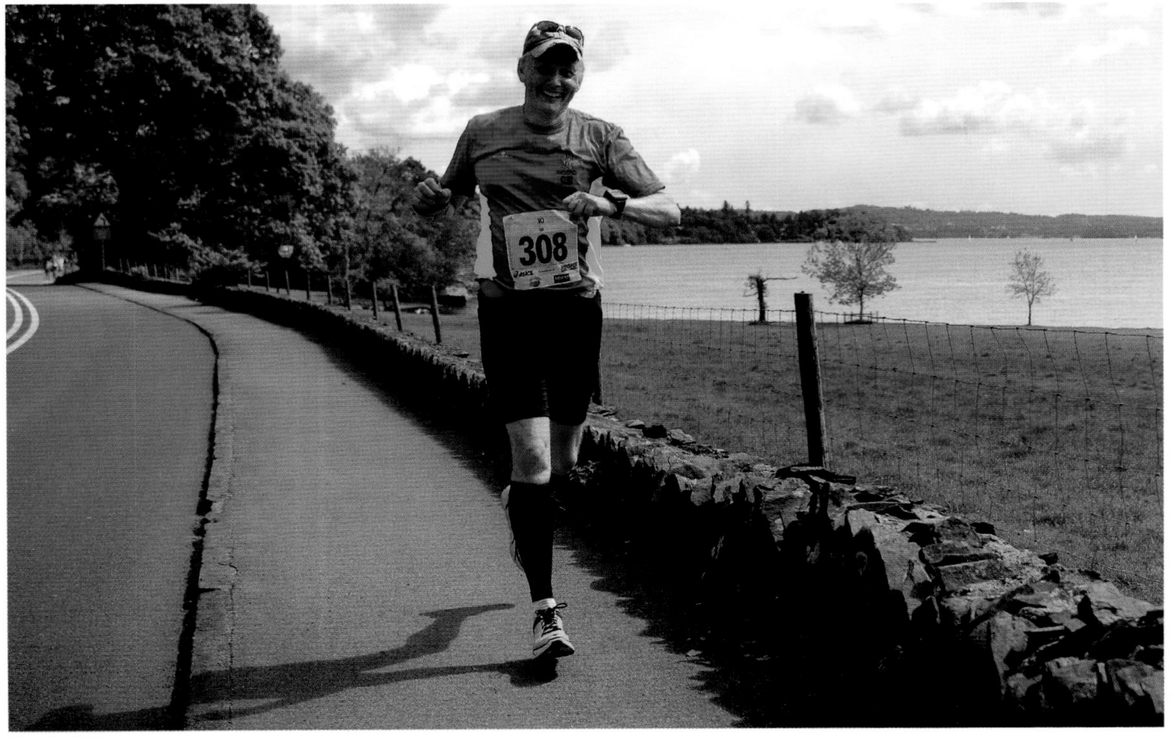

◀ You can't help but smile through the exhaustion in a setting as stunning as Windermere.

▶ The winding countryside roads lead runners down a more narrow route than most marathon veterans are used to.

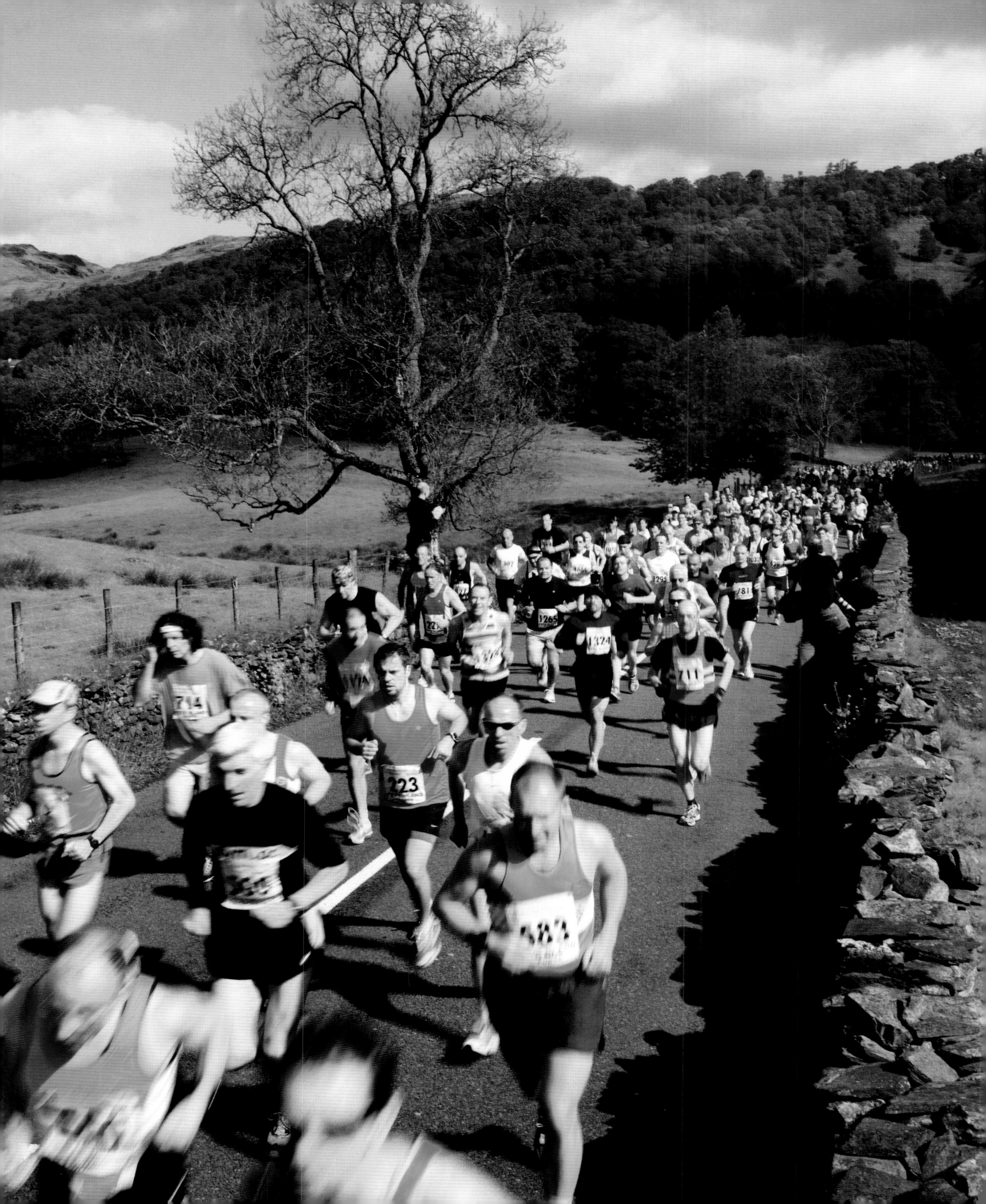
714
223
1265
1324

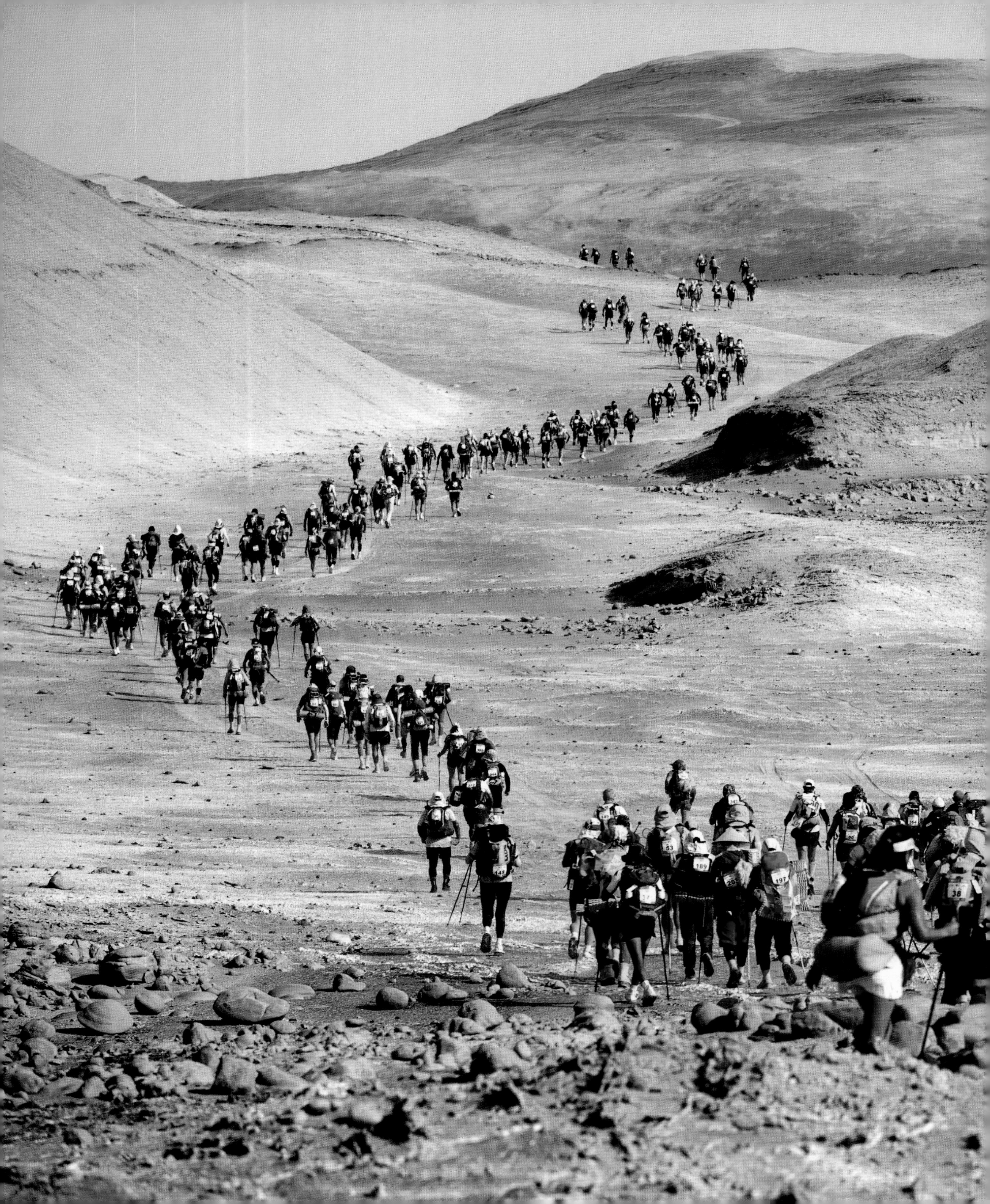

ULTRA-MARATHONS

THE NEXT STEP: ULTRAMARATHONS

If you've got the urge to become a distance runner, then beyond completing a marathon you may have your sights set on an ultramarathon. Any distance over 26.2 miles is considered an ultra, and there's a huge variety of challenges on offer.

So you don't have to make a drastic jump from a marathon to 100 miles or a similarly extreme distance. You can run a 50km ultramarathon (31.25 miles), which is only five miles more than a marathon, and still be able to say you've completed an ultra. Or you can challenge yourself to go even further. This chapter rounds up several of the best ultras that take place worldwide. Read on to discover the ultimate tests in marathon running.

If you've had a great experience training for and completing a marathon, or you've completed several marathons and want to challenge yourself further by taking your running to the next level, you may fancy tackling an ultramarathon. An ultramarathon is any distance over a marathon, which means anything over 26.2 miles. There are shorter options to choose from, so you don't have to make the drastic jump from being marathon-fit to running 50 or 100 miles unless you want to. It's worth doing your research and looking around at the options available. It may be advisable to consider starting with a shorter distance of around 50km (31.25 miles) to see how your body holds up over an even longer distance than a marathon.

But make no mistake: if you got to the finish line of a marathon recently, and felt that you could have continued a bit longer, then you could certainly tackle an ultra, and you're probably capable of more than you think. Ultrarunners often say that having a positive mindset is a huge part of being able to complete such a long distance. If you believe you can do it, and you're willing to put in the training, then there's no reason why you can't give it a go.

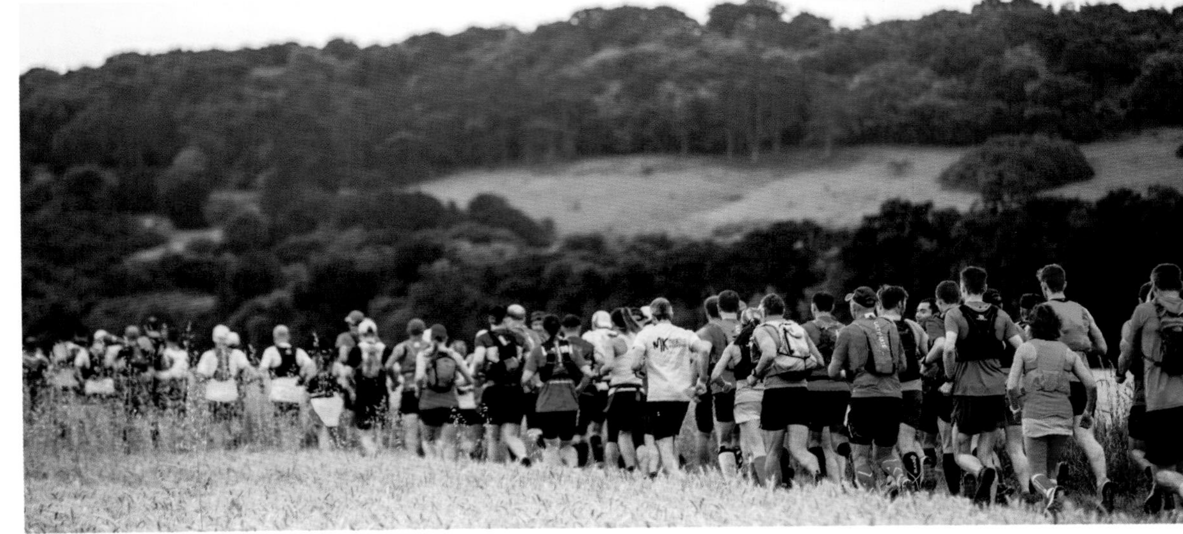

▶ More and more runners are being drawn to try ultras around the world.

▶▶ The views of the Grand to Grand Ultra are enough to tempt any marathon runner to tackle the longer route.

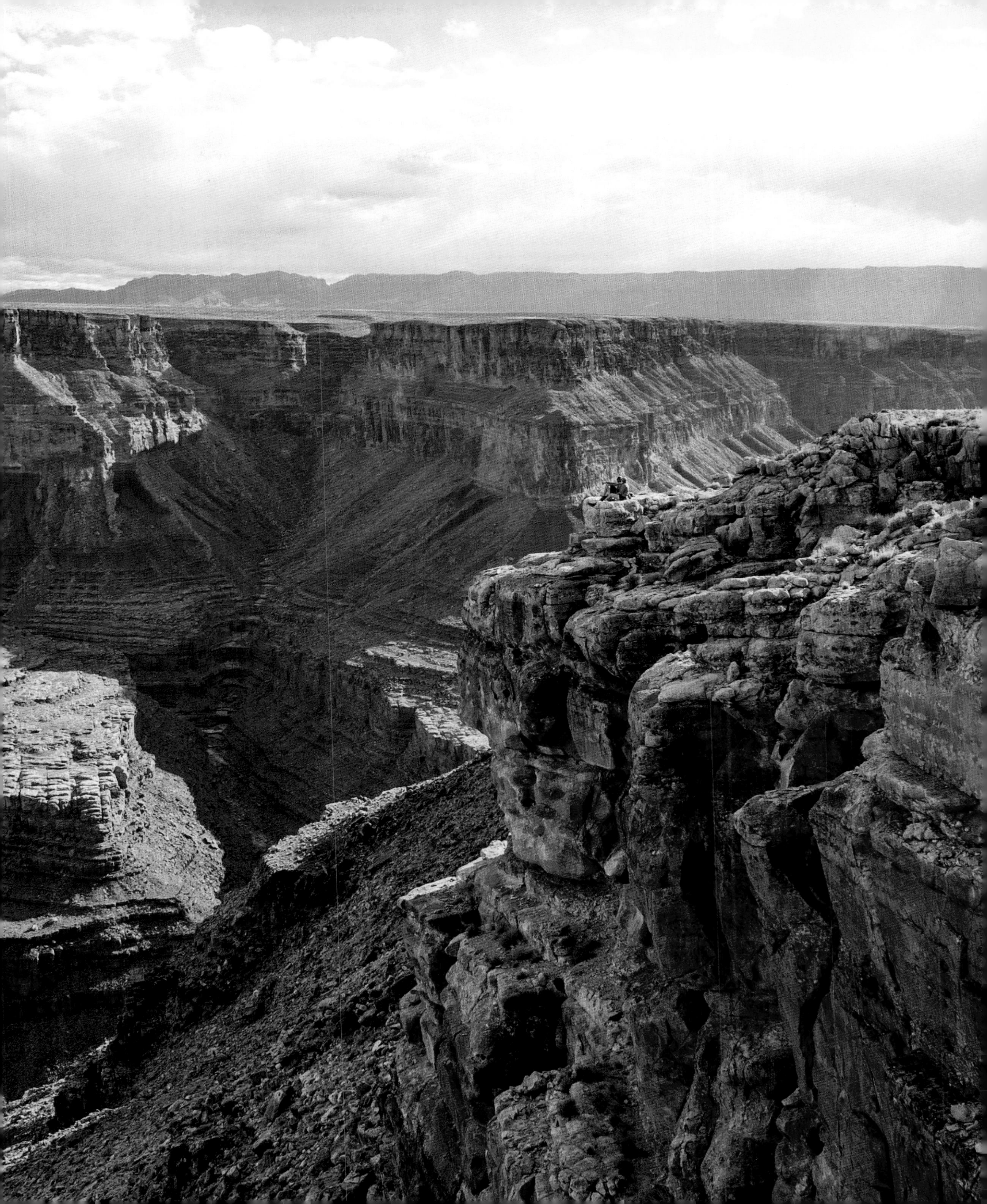

READY FOR AN ULTRA

Don't listen to anyone who is being negative. Most people think you must be ultra-fit, ultra-fast (and ultra-crazy!) to attempt an ultramarathon. And yet, "When you reach the point where you can run a marathon and then jog from the finish line back to your car, you're ready for an ultra," says ultrarunner and personal trainer Lloyd Clark, director of Ultramarathon. The reason? An ultra is any race that's longer than 42.2km. This means you can call yourself an ultrarunner by simply doing the Nottingham Ultra 50km or Gloucester 50km (both of which are just 8km longer than a marathon), and you can delay doing the 89km Comrades Marathon in South Africa, the 217km Badwater Ultramarathon in Death Valley or the 243km Marathon des Sables in Morocco, until you've got a shorter ultra under your belt.

The other good news about ultras is that they actually suit slower runners, and everyone, bar the elite athletes, will walk at some point during an ultra race, so it isn't just one long, relentless, breathless slog. However, what makes an ultra such a challenge is convincing your brain that it's actually possible to push your body past its limits; it's often said, "Ultras are 80 per cent in your mind."

That said, you still need to commit to a structured training plan and know that you have the time available to do it. And you need to make sure you have the full support of your loved ones. Running coach Richard Coates, from Full Potential, encourages anyone thinking of doing an ultra to speak to their family first and get them on board. "A lot of runners tell me they want to do ultras, and the first thing I say is, 'Great, but have you got agreement from your family?' Sometimes they laugh, and I say, 'Well, have you asked them? Seriously, you need to chat it through with them.' That's what I would do with my wife. Just say, 'Look, I'm training for this ultramarathon, is that OK?'

"If you work extremely long hours and you're going to go off and run for hours at the weekend, you need that level of support. People laugh when I say it, but your family and loved ones run the ultramarathon with you because they're there every single day listening to you about how this training run was terrible and you're never going to run again and how you got this niggle. So they're all there and cheering you on the sidelines and supporting you. Support is something special."

If you're already marathon-fit, how long should you allow to train for an ultra? Of course, it depends on the distance you're covering but, on average, shorter ultras will need at least 12 more weeks of training, while a major ultra such as Comrades Marathon (approximately 89km or 55.6 miles) will need at least 21 weeks of training. Other skills also come into play: you need a reasonable level of skill when it comes to navigation; you need to be able to change your running pace; and you'll need to have a lot of spare time on your hands, or at least be very organized with your time management.

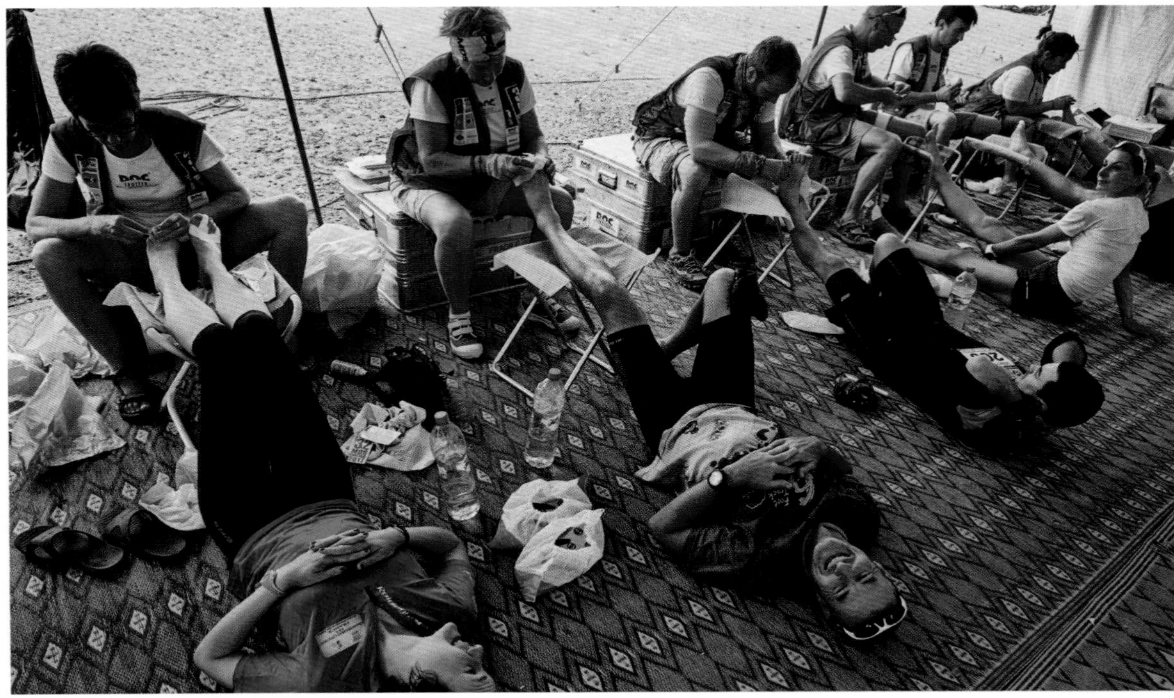

▶ Competitors receive much-needed treatment during a gruelling 250km ultra in Morocco.

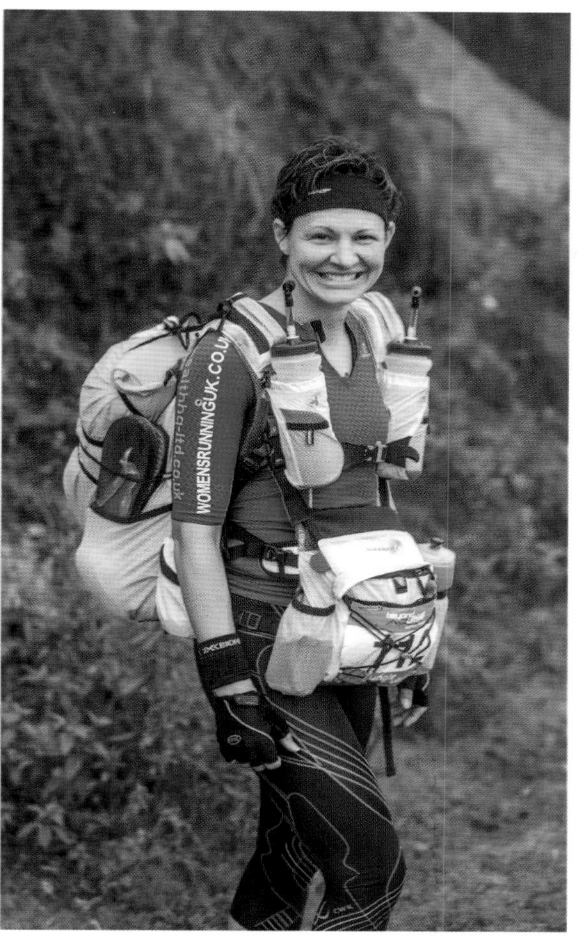

▲ Anne-Marie Lategan fully equipped for any situation.

▼ Not many marathons can claim to include a raft down a jungle river section.

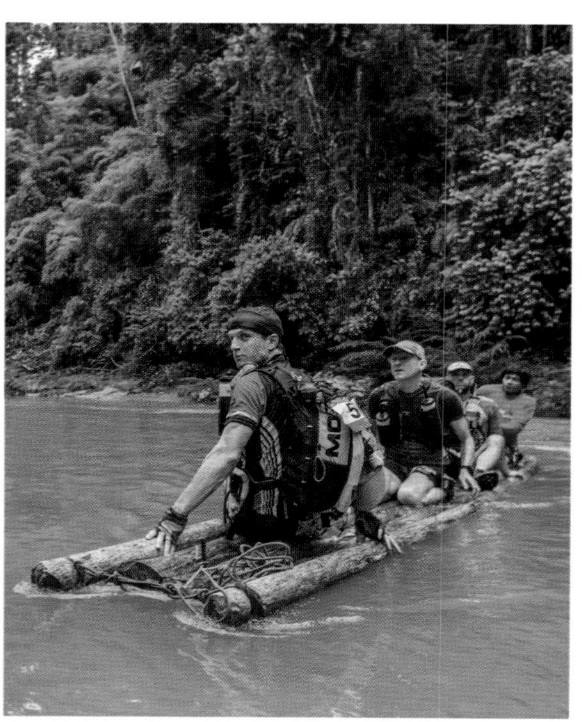

BEFORE YOU SIGN UP FOR AN ULTRA

- You'll need to commit a lot of time to training. You will be out for hours and hours. Longer runs at the weekend could be up to 65km.
- You'll need to slow your pace down. Many ultrarunners are quite open about the fact that they walk on the harder, more challenging parts of the course. Abandon your worries about pace, take the pressure off and park your ego when it comes to speed. Just concentrate on thinking about completing the course and don't worry about whether or not you feel as if you're running too slowly.
- Ultras exist in many different parts of the world. You don't have to settle for one in the UK – there are many scenic, exotic and beautiful locations where you can complete an ultra. So shop around, but bear in mind you'll want to pick an ultra in an environment that suits you. If you hate the cold, you don't want to be taking part in the Antarctic Ice Ultra, where temperatures plunge to subzero. Conversely, if you dislike the heat, the Marathon des Sables, where temperatures can soar to 120 Fahrenheit, may not be for you.
- You'll need to get used to eating on the go – *Women's Running*'s fitness editor and ultrarunner Anne-Marie Lategan has trained her body to get used to absorbing proper food while she is out training, such as malt loaf, sandwiches and wraps. Energy gels may be handy, but you'll need to get some proper food into your body over such a long distance.
- You'll probably have to carry your own gear – many ultras will require you to take essential items and transport them with you while you run, including a backpack with food, a change of clothes, water and overnight items if you're doing a race over a set number of days. It makes sense to do some training runs in advance where you carry a backpack and the items you'll be taking with you on race day, so that you get used to running with the weight on your back before the race. Check all of your kit before race day. Test it all out on long training runs to make sure it's comfortable and not chafing or causing you any discomfort. You certainly don't want a backpack that swings around excessively while you run.
- Find out if there's a cut-off time for your chosen race – many ultra-races have a cut-off time and checkpoints along the course that you need to reach in a certain timeframe. You'll be forced to pull out of the race if you don't reach a checkpoint within a timeframe specified. Choose an ultra that you know you have a realistic chance of completing.
- Check the terrain of the course and try to train on something similar. Some ultras will take place on rocky terrain, others on muddy trails, and some even involve wading through rivers. Know the course before you commit, and make sure it's suitable for you.
- Give yourself time to adjust to a new environment – if you're doing an ultra abroad in a faraway location that entails a long-haul flight, go out as early as you can before the race starts – ideally at least a week – so that you've got time to recover from jetlag and adjust to local temperatures.
- Check to see if there's high altitude. It's difficult to know how you'll respond to high altitude until you experience it, so if you think this may be a struggle then it's one to avoid.
- Check if navigation is needed. Ultras tend to take place off-road, on trails and in remote areas, so you normally need to have some skills when it comes to navigation to ensure you don't get lost.
- Some ultras require you to have a certain number of points before you can enter, such as UTMB. You may not be able to enter automatically.

COMRADES MARATHON

ENJOY 89KM OF "THE ULTIMATE HUMAN RACE"

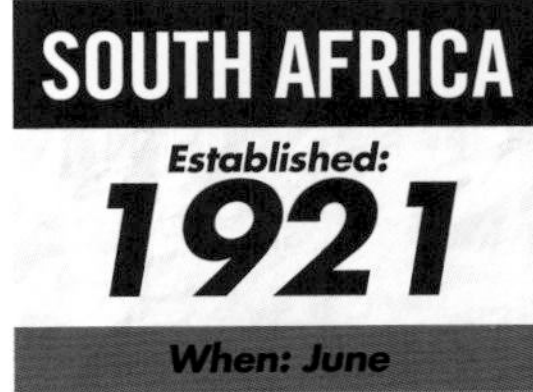

The Comrades race distance varies year on year depending on whether the course goes up or down, and the route changes slightly each year. In 2018, it was a downwards run that started at the City Hall in Pietermaritzburg and finished in Durban.

It's billed as "The Ultimate Human Race", a description that's particularly apt because what makes South Africa's Comrades Marathon so special isn't the spectacular Valley of a Thousand Hills scenery, or the fact that in 2010 it became the world's biggest ultramarathon with 14,343 finishers: it's the people who run it. The course covers approximately 89km in the KwaZulu-Natal Province of South Africa between Durban and Pietermaritzburg (the capital of the province of KwaZulu). The race has a limit of 20,000 runners so, by ultra standards, it's a biggie.

The very first Comrades Marathon took place in May 1921 and, apart from a break during World War II, it has taken place every year since. During the very first Comrades event, 34 runners took part and only 16 were able to complete the race. At the time of writing, more than 300,000 runners have completed this gruelling event.

The race has a cut-off time of 12 hours and you must reach various cut-off points around the course within a specific time. It has some unusual rules too: those who have run up to nine marathons must wear a yellow number; and, if you've completed ten marathon events, you wear a green number, which is allocated to you permanently for future races.

Those who complete the course in less than 12 hours receive a medal, while the first 10 men and women will receive a gold medal. South Africans entering the event must belong to a running club, while anyone entering from overseas must supply proof that they have completed a marathon in under five hours to be eligible to enter. Or you must have completed an 89km ultra in under 12 hours, or a 100km ultra in under 13 and a half hours. It is consequently not an easy race to enter, but it is worth it for the amazing experience.

The ultra has been attempted three times by *Women's Running* contributing editor Lisa Jackson, who completed it twice. Lisa has so far completed 106 marathons to date.

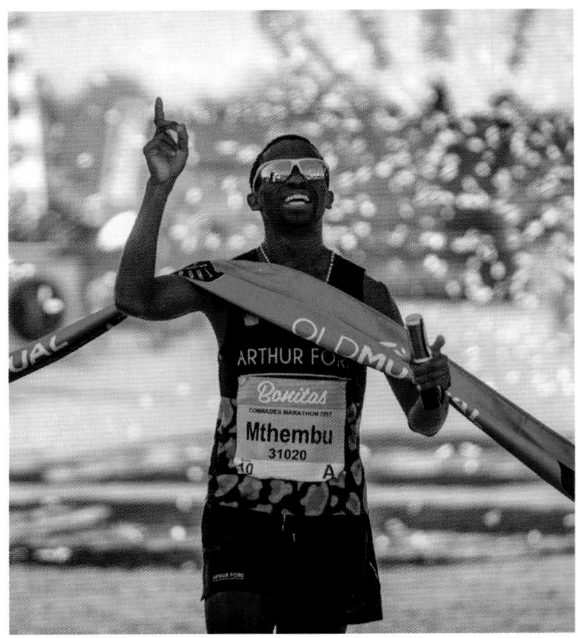

◀ The feeling of winning any ultramarathon can't be compared, let alone winning the world's biggest.

▶ Over 17,000 people competed in 2017's Comrades race.

LISA'S RACE EXPERIENCE

"I felt incredibly privileged to be able to take part in this race, which is famed for its camaraderie. For much of the race, I spoke to numerous fellow runners who, thanks to the inclusion of our names on the race numbers, were all on first-name terms. A highlight was spotting a lady called Nikki Campbell, founder of a super-inspiring website called www.alsorunners.info, which was aimed at helping slower runners complete Comrades. She told me she had suffered from depression for many years and running had helped lift her mood and improve her life. It's something you often hear when you talk to runners.

"When I reached the Wall of Honour, where runners who had completed Comrades before could have a plaque erected, I took out some tinfoil from my race belt and carefully sprinkled my late mother's ashes below the brick bearing my name (from a previous Comrades). I stood gazing at the names of all the people who had made this journey and marvelled at how this incredible race always gave me the chance to connect on a really meaningful level with total strangers. It was a totally unforgettable experience. There were crowds willing me along every step of the way and the comradeship among the runners was second to none. I sang, chanted and talked all the way, and crossing that finish line was one of the most exhilarating moments of my life. If you think you only have one ultra in you, make it this one, it will inspire, challenge and excite you like no other."

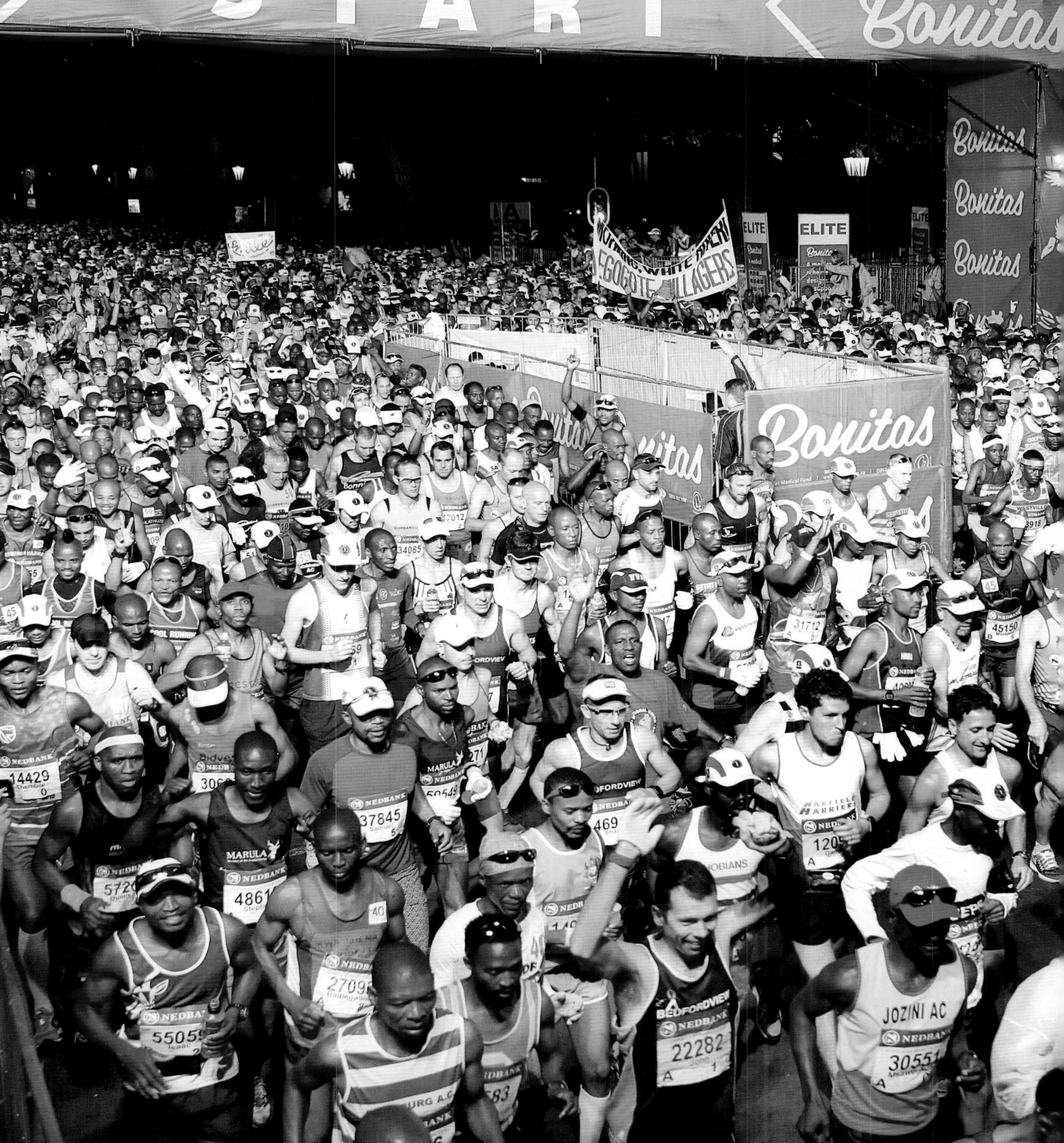

ULTIMATE HUMAN RACE
START
Bonitas
ELITE
NEDBANK
BEDFORDVIEW
JOZINI AC
MARULA

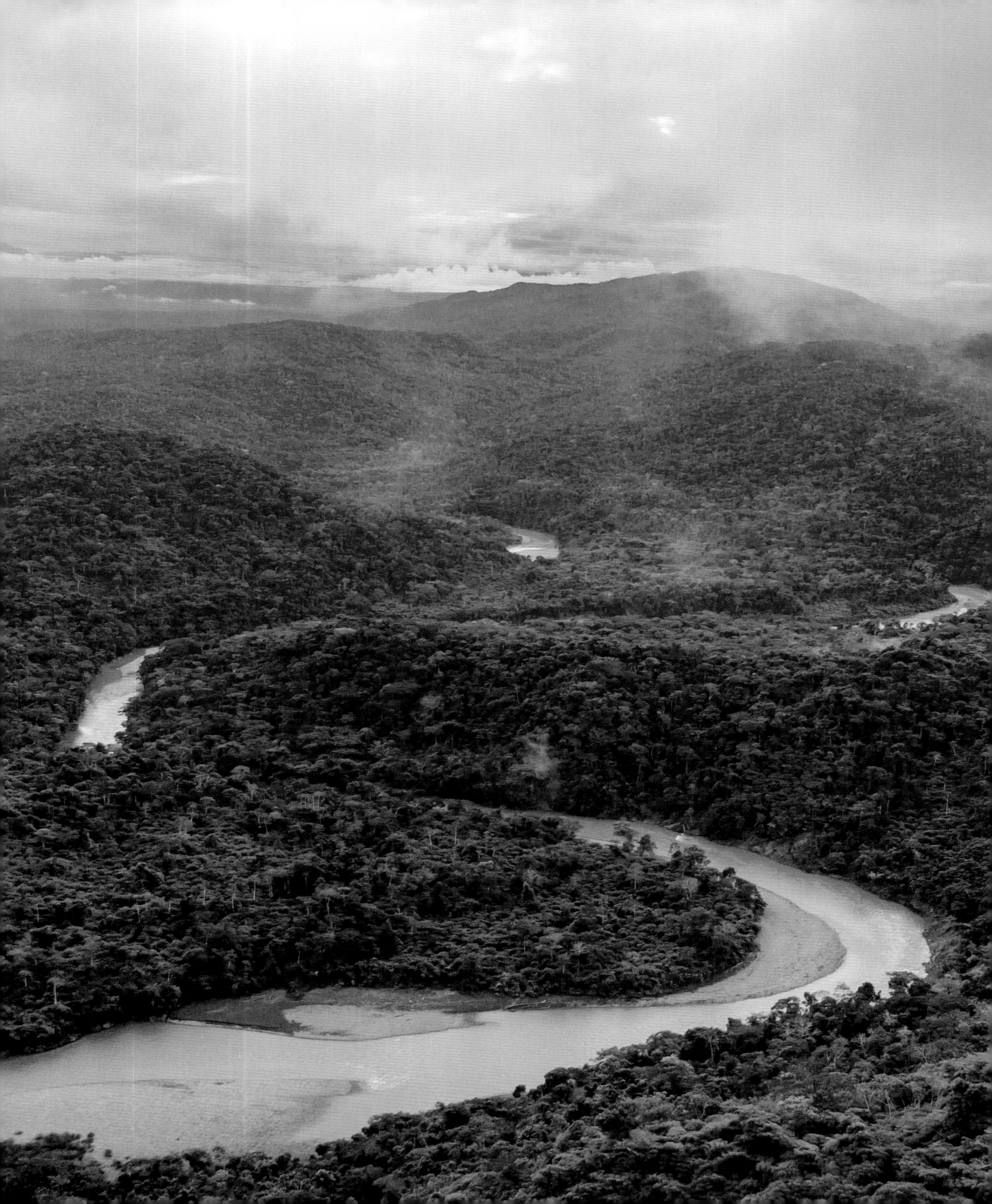

THE JUNGLE ULTRA

AN INTENSE 230KM RACE THROUGH THE AMAZON

This event takes place in the Manu National Park in the Amazon Rainforest, a humid jungle and cloud forest that goes from the Andes Mountains to the Madre de Dios River.

The race is split into five stages and you'll need to be able to cope with the humidity, as well as mud and rain. It's not for the faint-hearted, as you'll be expected to carry all of your kit, including food and safety equipment. You'll also need to carry water, which you'll need to fill up at various checkpoints during the race. Fortunately, you will have accommodation provided at research stations and lodges.

Sounds tough? You bet, but the reward is that you get to enjoy amazing scenery, see some incredible wildlife – and even stand above the clouds. The race runs through a UNESCO world heritage site, and wades across a river. Hot, humid, challenging – but a memorable experience that will stay with you for a lifetime.

Completed by Anne-Marie Lategan, *Women's Running*'s fitness editor and a regular ultrarunner.

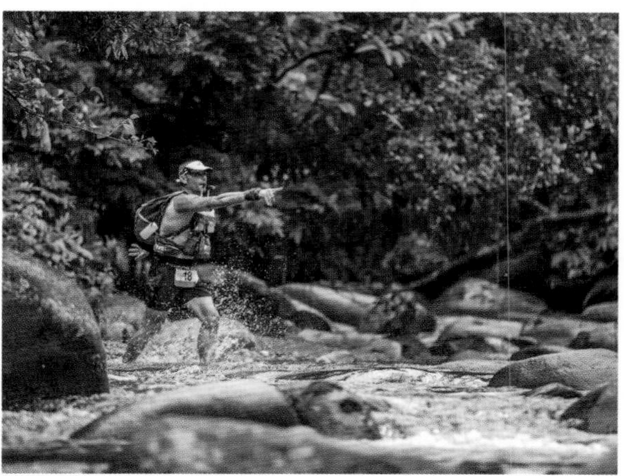

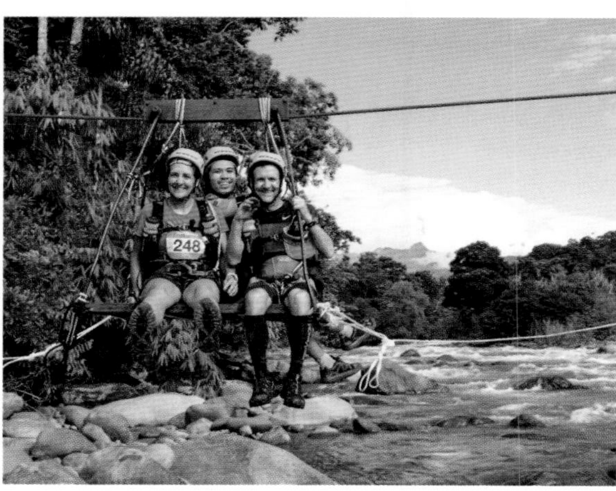

▲ You'll struggle to find a more unique marathon.

◀ Don't let the incredible beauty of this race fool you, it's one of the toughest.

▲▲ A splash through the river brings a welcome respite from the heat.

ANNE-MARIE'S RACE EXPERIENCE

"I grew up in South Africa, so the humidity during the race didn't bother me, but it could easily affect anyone not used to it. I had to carry my own sleeping bag and hammock. After each stage of the race, I had to put my hammock in the campsite and make sure I didn't get any ants or other creepy crawlies or mosquitoes in it with me. Every morning I had to pack everything into my backpack and get ready to move to the next campsite.

"During a stage race like this, the challenges are different every day. At the beginning of the race, you have normal pre-race nerves. Each stage has its own challenges. The combination of mental and physical challenges is probably the toughest element of this race. I found the second day the hardest. I had to stop early on to treat blisters from the first day, and then, when we ran through a village, local schoolchildren cheered us on, which was amazing, but it suddenly made me realize how much I missed my daughter. It was a privilege to run through parts of the rainforest which are now so protected that the public is not allowed in these areas without guides, as well as experiencing how powerful and unforgiving the rainforest can be. It's such a beautiful place but also very sad to see that parts of the forest have been destroyed.

"The longest stage of the race was the last day. The winners were supposed to finish towards the late evening and the rest of us were supposed to finish the next day at some point. But things didn't go to plan, which is what happens sometimes with ultras. We set off early in the morning and it was pouring with rain. This didn't bother us, as we were used to these conditions, but the river crossings were sometimes so deep that we had local men dragging us through the rivers, which were normally shallow but the water had risen to neck depth.

"On the last day, we almost got lost as it was hard to see the flags that marked where the route should have been. Crossing the finish line at the end was amazing and local villagers came out and cheered us on. The cheering was amazing."

MARATHON DES SABLES

JOURNEY ACROSS APPROXIMATELY 250KM OF GRUELLING DESERT

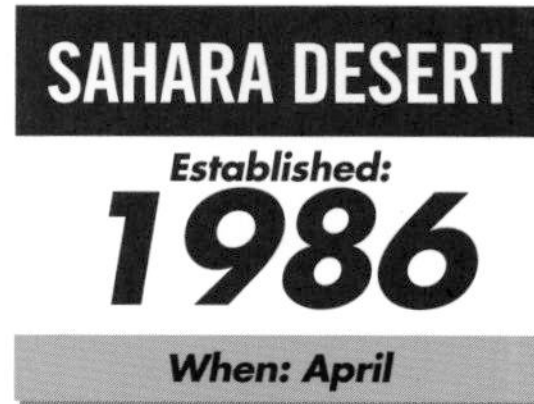

This gruelling event was dubbed the "Toughest Footrace on Earth" by the Discovery Channel, and is a multi-stage, six-day ultra through the Sahara Desert. This is not for the faint-hearted. Apart from coping with blistering heat (temperatures can rise to around 120 degrees Fahrenheit), you'll also need to deal with sleeping in tents and be self-sufficient during the race, which means being able to carry all of your own food and equipment on your back for the whole week. You'll sleep in tents pitched (and supplied) for you but you will be expected to carry them. Water is rationed (not what you want to hear in the desert) and exceeding your ration results in a time penalty.

The course consists of dunes, rocky jebels (mountains and hills) and hot salt plains with the sun on your back.

This event is the distance of approximately six marathons (although the course varies from one year to the next, which means the distance does, too), so you'll need to be super-fit as well as having to worry about the heat. The very first event took place in 1986, and 23 people took part in the first race. By 2009, the event had attracted more than 1,000 runners.

The most famous participant to date was Ranulph Fiennes, who became the oldest Briton to complete the event in 2015, raising over £1 million for Marie Curie at the age of 71. Fiennes completed the event after having a double-bypass 12 years before and lost 10lb during the race, despite staying hydrated and eating regularly. He described the event as "like walking on a treadmill in the heat".

Women's Running contributor and blogger Susie Chan ran the Marathon des Sables three times.

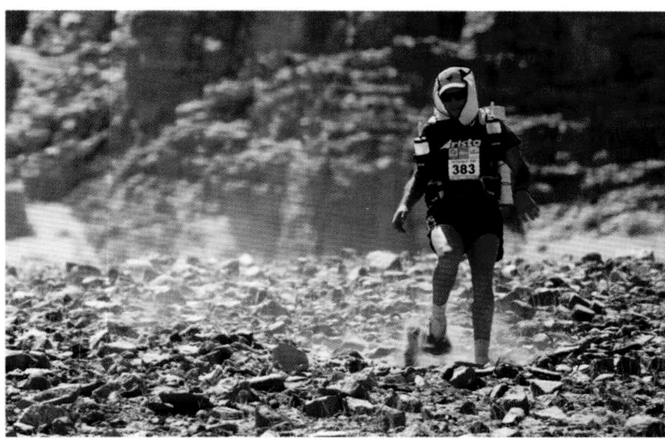

◣ Runners must be sure-footed for the variety of challenging desert terrain.

▶ The Sahara setting is tempting to many, but few are up to its challenges.

SUSIE'S RACE EXPERIENCE

"Some people who take part in the Marathon des Sables suffer from sleep deprivation. Fortunately, I have done this race three times and not had any issues with sleeping. When the sun went down at around 8 p.m., everyone went to sleep. I must admit that sleeping on a rocky ground did take its toll, but, as I felt more tired during the six days, the hard surface became easier to ignore.

"You can train your body to get used to the heat. It's hot for sure, and the heat can be dangerous if you're not ready for it. I got myself prepared for the heat by doing hot yoga (where temperatures in the class can be over 90 degrees Fahrenheit), and training in a heat chamber in the days leading up to the event. It's very important to do this in the weeks leading up to the event and to do it regularly (leaving it no longer than 48 hours between sessions). This will get your body gradually used to the heat, leaving you in best possible shape going into the Sahara.

"Thankfully, there is a huge team behind this race. The local Berbers are on hand, putting up and taking down the tents each day as the race moves across the desert. The tents are basically blankets on sticks and can be prone to letting in an awful lot of desert in a sandstorm! [...]

"I deliberately kept my bag as light as possible. I also did lots of strength training before the event to make sure my core was strong before the race. Having a comfortable, lightweight, backpack was key. [...]

"The course changes each year and so does the distance. Runners don't know how long the race is until they are off the plane in Morocco and on their way to the Sahara. On the three occasions I have done it, the distance has fluctuated by as much as 20km.

"I recommend this event. It's such an iconic race with so many runners. It really is unique. You are not allowed to use your phone, so communication is very limited, and it's like being in a bubble with other runners. You bond so well with your fellow runners and tent-mates. I have many happy memories from my time in the desert.

"Anyone thinking of doing it should be aware that feet and heat are the two things that can slow you down. You can prepare your feet for what they will take on. Toughen the skin on your feet and get heat training. That way you can focus on having a great time during the race."

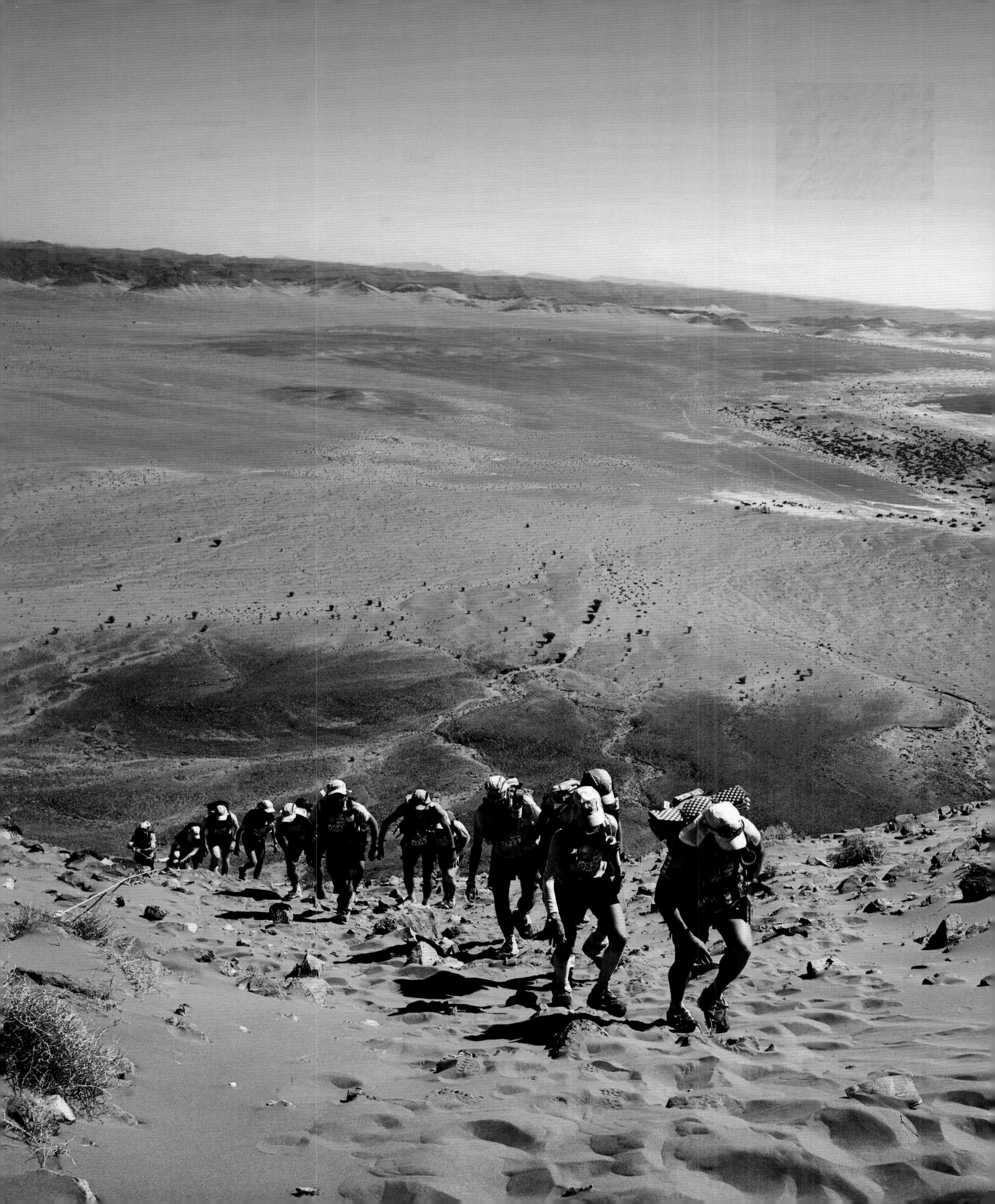

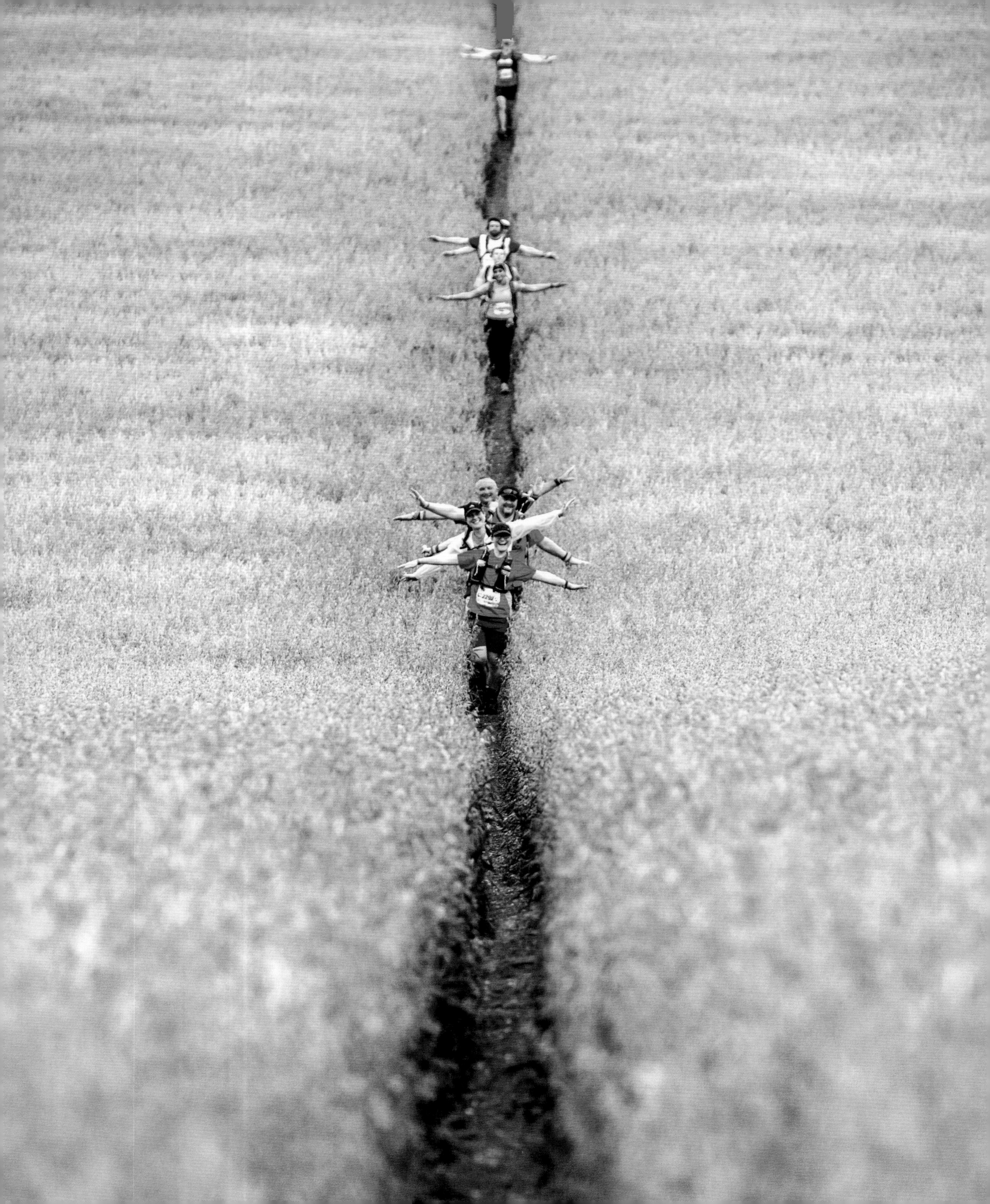

RACE TO THE STONES

50KM AND 100KM PAST THE FIELD OF DREAMS

CHILTERNS, UK
Established:
2013
When: July

A popular UK trail marathon, this event was voted the UK's Best Endurance Event at the Running Awards in 2016 and crosses one of the oldest trails in Britain, the Ridgeway, which crosses North Wessex Downs and the Chilterns. The course stretches from the Chilterns in Oxfordshire to the North Wessex Downs and follows high ground. Expect rolling hills, ancient woodlands and natural beauty.

The event offers you the flexibility either to complete the 100km distance in one day or to complete it over two days with an overnight stop where you'll camp for one night. Course highlights include the Field of Dreams – so named by participants because it is a crop field that has different colours – Grim's Ditch, Barbury Castle and Liddington Castle. There's also Avebury Stone Circle on the course – one of the largest stone circles in Europe. There's also a 50km distance for those new to ultrarunning, so you can choose the best option to suit you and your fitness levels.

Completed by Anne-Marie Lategan, *Women's Running*'s fitness editor.

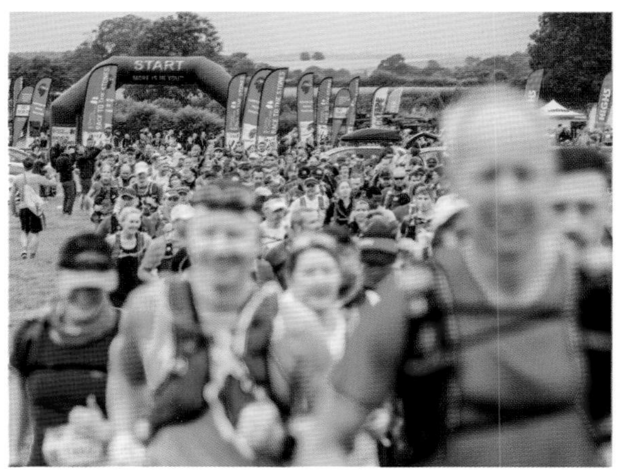

ANNE-MARIE'S RACE EXPERIENCE

"I ran this race as a single-stage event. I carried water, food and a head torch. My backpack weighed around 2 kilograms. There was a heatwave warning for the race and it was very hot. The amazing Ridgeway countryside was stunning and one of my favourite parts of the course. At one point, I ran past a jetty where there were boats on the river. I was so hot that I walked into the river and sat down. There was a family enjoying a picnic and I can just remember this little boy asking his mum why this woman had waded into the river. I turned around and said I was hot and wanted to cool down but they still thought I was mad.

"This is the only ultra I've done where I spent about 30 minutes at a checkpoint near the end to cool down. There wasn't a time limit on this race, so I decided to wait until it got dark before continuing. I teamed up with another runner and we completed the race together. I finished the race at 2 a.m. and then went back to my hotel for a bath at 3 a.m.

"The hardest part was the last few kilometres. When I got to the stones, where I thought the finish line was located, I was told the finish line was at the farm next to the stones and that I only had to run a few more kilometres. That broke my spirit and my ability to run. I wasn't happy, but I did it!"

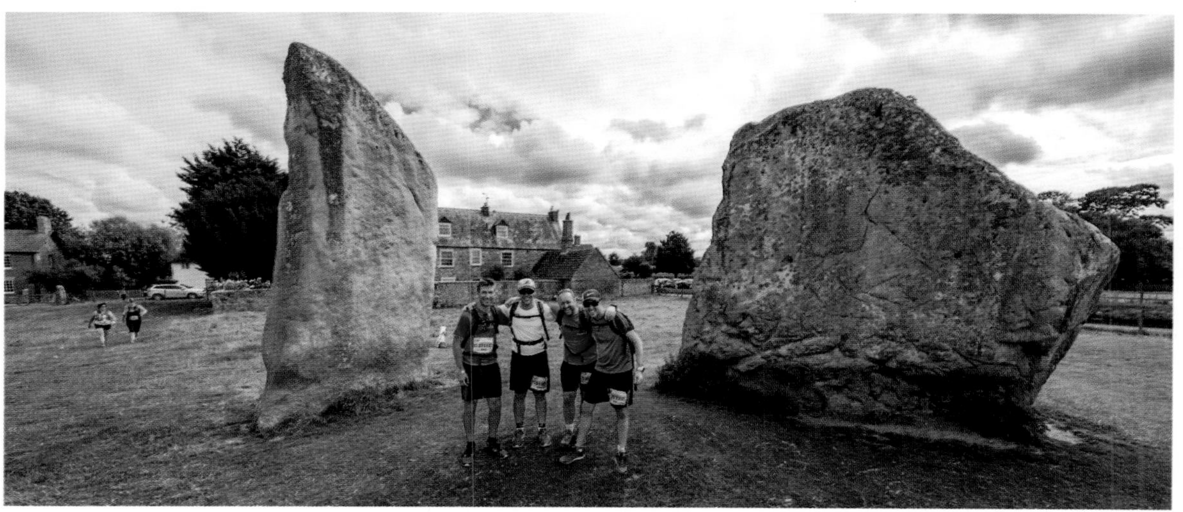

◤ A sea of colour spreads across the ancient route through the English countryside.

◀ Despite the marathon's title, the stones aren't quite the finish line.

◀◀ Not many marathons require competitors to go single-file, but it allows extra time to enjoy the views.

TRANSYLVANIAN BEAR RACE

A PAIR OF 50KM AND 80KM ULTRAMARATHONS IN MOUNTAINOUS ROMANIA

TRANSYLVANIA
Established: 2015
When: June

This beautiful but extremely challenging event takes you through Europe's last unspoiled wilderness. You'll follow a marked course through a scattering of ancient Saxon villages, including a ruined castle and open pastureland, soaking up the history as you go. You'll also run through rural village pathways.

There's a significant elevation of 950m and a cut-off time of 12 hours for the ultra. The course also has five stocked checkpoints and runners are required to make sure their race numbers are recorded as they go through each one – safety is understandably a priority here.

The ultra distance was completed by *Women's Running* contributing editor Lisa Jackson.

◢ The route takes runners along hills and mountains, rather than up them.

▼ Heading towards some of the verdant forest that makes up most of the route.

▶▶ Some people may be surprised enough to learn that Transylvania is real, let alone that it holds landscapes like this.

LISA'S RACE EXPERIENCE

"It was a race like no other. One where, over a single day, I transformed from a black-caped, blood-red-lipstick-wearing vamp into a dishevelled Drac, hauling myself wearily to the finish line in the birthplace of Vlad the Impaler, the inspiration for the world's most famous vampire. The Transylvanian Bear Race starts at Viscri's fortified Saxon church, a UNESCO World Heritage Site, and winds its way along forest tracks and village pathways before finishing at another UNESCO treasure, the hilltop town of Sighisoara.

"As usual, I was soon right at the back of the pack, splashing through the muddy puddles created by the heavy rains of the preceding week. Most of the route was through shady forest, where cuckoos called out encouragement from the branches overhead; but every so often we emerged to run across sunlit, flower-strewn meadows past shepherds and their dogs herding sheep, as they'd done for centuries. We'd been warned to make plenty of noise to frighten off any inquisitive bears – and told if we were to encounter one, we should frighten it off by singing. I, however, am a former soloist, and was concerned that, far from being deterred by my songs, the bears would gather round to listen more closely, so I chose to loudly crush my plastic water bottle instead. One runner, who'd decided to use honey-filled sachets instead of gels, had a 'honey explosion' at one point and spent the rest of the race looking over his shoulder for fear of turning into a bite-sized bear snack!

"Thankfully, my husband had come out along the course to lead me past Dracula's birthplace to the bottom of the Scholar's Stairs, where he cajoled me up every one of its 175 steps to the finish line. My time? 11 hours 15. The distance I covered? I have no idea. And it's still a mystery to me why I should have taken many hours longer than usual on a course that turned out to be surprisingly flat. But, then, as Carmen said, 'This is Transylvania – and things are very different here...'"

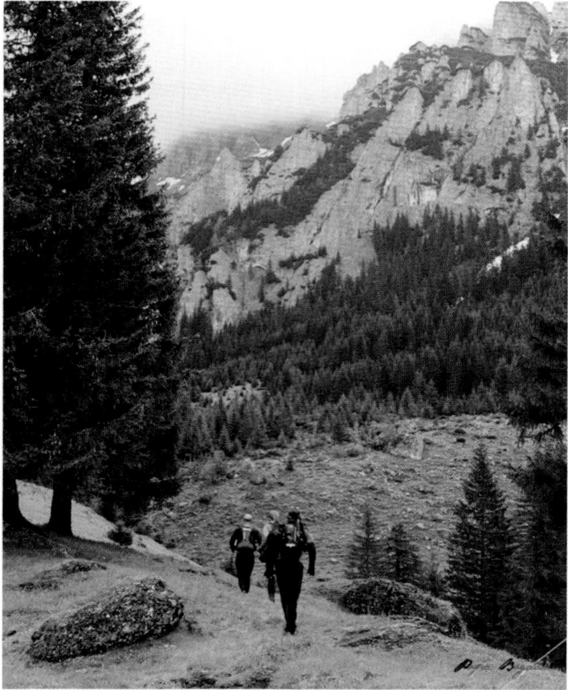

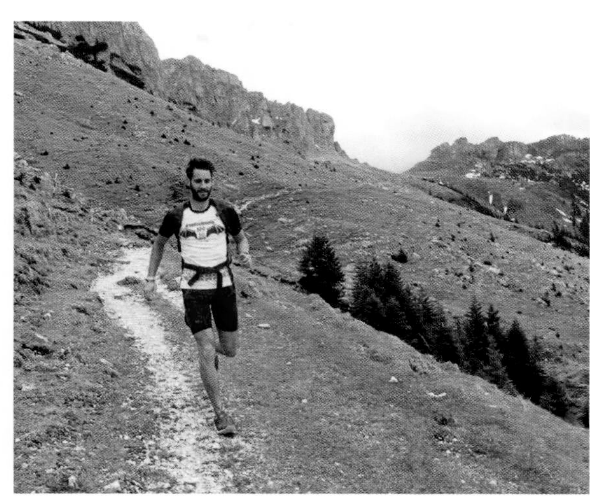

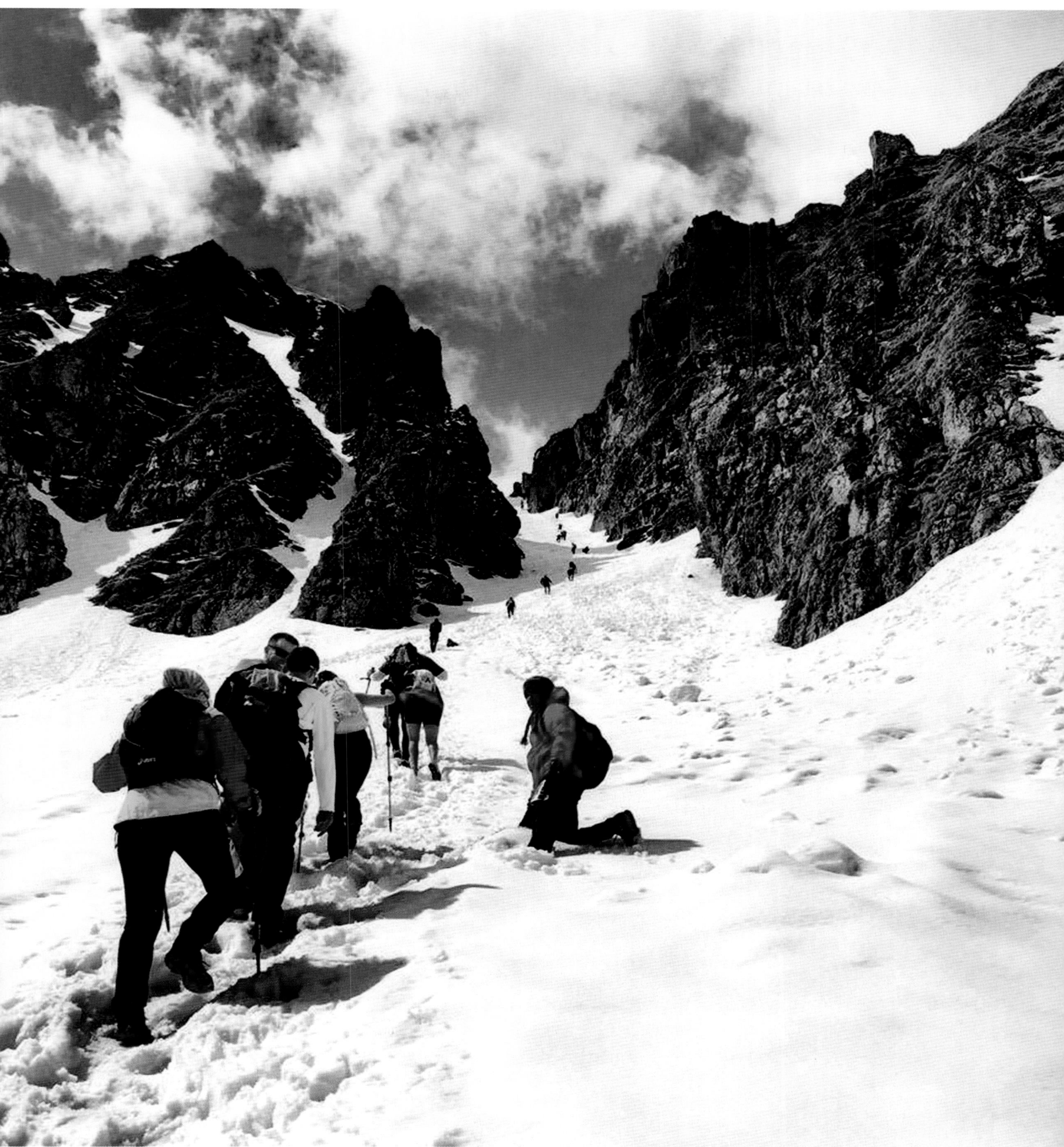

ULTRA-TRAIL DU MONT BLANC

A COOL 166KM REACHING ELEVATIONS OF 9,600M

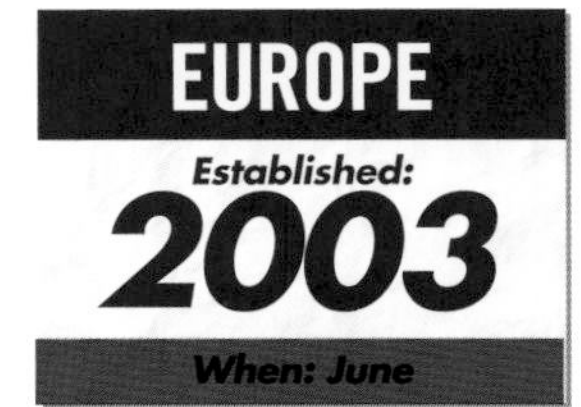

This single-stage mountain marathon takes place in high altitude of 2,500m and typically starts in the last weekend of August and runs into the first weekend of September. It has challenging weather conditions, including wind, cold temperatures and even the possibility of snow. The race starts in Chamonix and goes through France, Italy and Switzerland. It reaches a total elevation of around 9,600m. It takes place over a whole festival week and normally has around 2,000 starters.

Many people struggle to finish this race, usually due to the altitude, and it is described as one of the toughest races in the world. Fit runners would normally take around 20 hours to finish, while most runners take around 30 to 45 hours. The route varies slightly each year for safety reasons. The cut-off time is 46 hours 30 minutes.

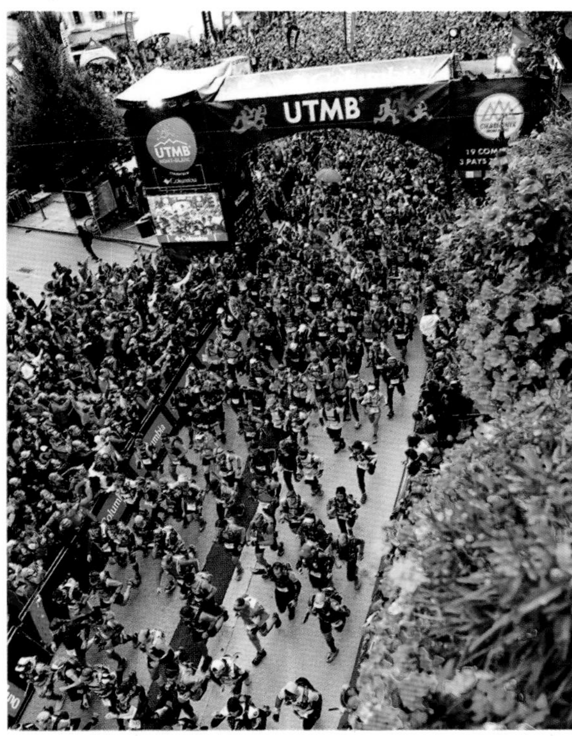

▲ A large portion of these eager starters won't make it to the finish line.

▶ The mountains create an imposing backdrop, and their altitude creates a tough race.

You need qualifying points to enter this race: the organizers look for you to have gained a minimum of 15 points from a maximum of three trail ultra-races, which must be on the UTMB's approved list.

The Ultra-Trail du Mont Blanc was completed by Anne-Marie Lategan, *Women's Running*'s fitness editor.

ANNE-MARIE'S RACE EXPERIENCE

"Two years of sweating, crying, victories and dreaming brought me to the goal I wanted to achieve the most: completing UTMB. I had trained for this event for so long and accumulated points from other ultras to qualify.

"This race is unpredictable and every participant had a difficult decision to make before they'd even crossed the start line. The challenge was knowing how to cope with the weather. Rain began to fall at the start. Runners had a decision to make. Should we put on rainproof jackets and stay dry, knowing that the high humidity would eventually make it too warm to run in? Or should we run without a jacket and then risk going into the night, ascending 2,500m with wet clothes, risking cold temperatures of the mountains? Of course, there was no right or wrong answer. During a race like this, all you can do is trust your instincts and do what feels right at the time. And you need to hope you've got your kit selection right.

"I knew this would be a race against the clock, and the tick-ticking sound of hiking poles and the noise of runners breathing heavily filled the cold mountain air. I was sold on the dream of breathtaking mountain views, but fog and darkness were the reality. Every runner was fighting their own battle, mentally and physically. At one point, I had to run on a ledge 2,500m high with a drop on both sides. It turned my legs to jelly! I realized that, despite all my night running, I just didn't have the skill to run or even brisk-walk over this terrain. I was scared of falling. I felt vulnerable. The risk was too great and I slowed down.

"I looked at my watch. I had 40 minutes left to reach the checkpoint but had no idea how far away it was. As the minutes ticked by, I realized I wouldn't make it. I wasn't brave enough to give it my all and sprint down a downhill slope at 4 a.m. after running for 10 hours. In the end, the rain and the darkness had got the better of me. Not finishing showed me that, despite my training, I needed to get more comfortable with the terrain and the challenging weather conditions. With UTMB, you need to be prepared for whatever Mother Nature may throw at you. It's not just about being fit enough: it's about being brave enough to cope with heights, bad weather and altitude."

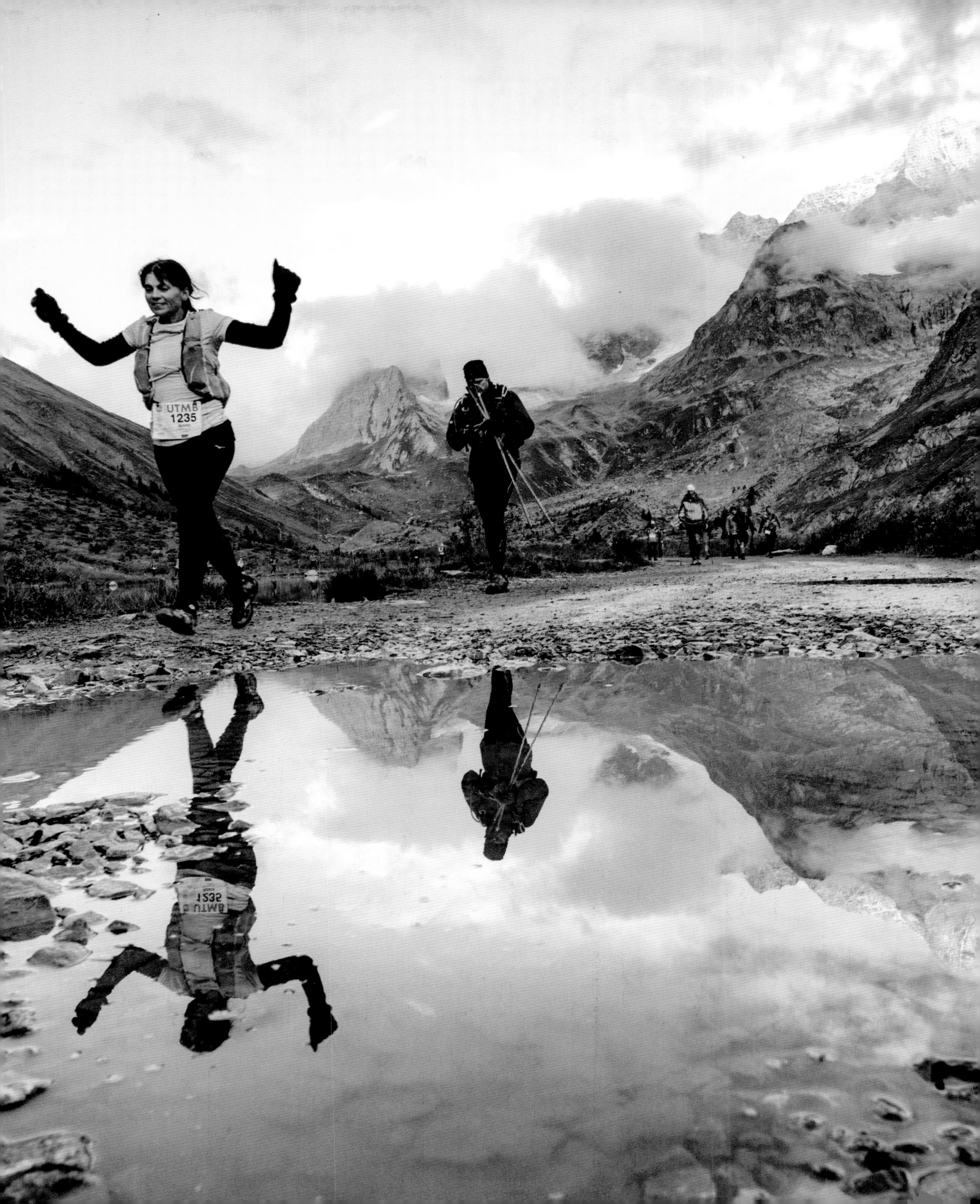
UTMB
1235

THE BEST OF THE REST

Like the sound of the challenge? If you still love the idea of completing an ultra, here are some of the most challenging, scenic, appealing and, in some cases, unusual marathons in the world . . .

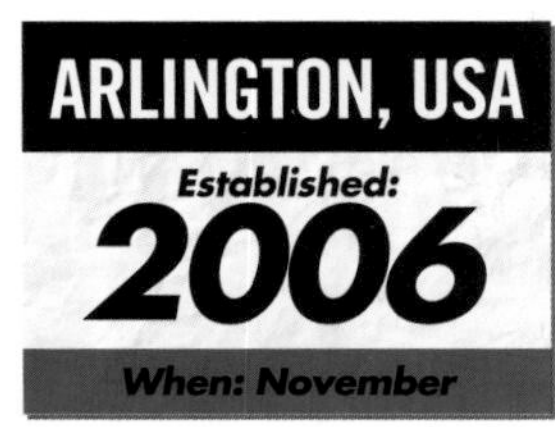

ANTARCTIC ULTRA RACE, 100KM

This is a single-stage event that attracts a fanatical group of around 25 runners and, trust us, it's not for the faint-hearted. The race takes place a few hundred miles from the South Pole and is described as "a run under the sun that never sets", offering hills, mountains and lots of ice.

Be prepared for snow and ice underfoot and an average wind-chill temperature of minus 20°C. The course has a typical elevation of around 3,000 feet. You have 24 hours to complete this race and participants are flown to the Union Glacier camp in Antarctica from Punta Arenas. Union Glacier is a full-service camp and competitors will stay in double-walled sleeping tents based on a proven design from William Shackleton's famous Endurance Expedition.

CALIFORNIA, USA
Established:
1987
When: July

BADWATER ULTRAMARATHON, 135 MILES

This famous race goes nonstop from Badwater Basin in Death Valley to Mt Whitney in California and is described as one of the most demanding races in the world. The start line is at the lowest elevation in North America, 85m below sea level, and the finish line is at Mt Whitney, after you've climbed 9,000 feet. The race can take on average approximately 60 hours.

The Badwater Ultramarathon was born in 1978, when around 100 runners took part. Not every participant reaches the finish line and some find the searing temperatures too much. Past temperatures have included 110 degrees Fahrenheit at the start, rising to over 130 further into the race.

This race was made famous by ultrarunner Pam Reed, who won the Badwater Ultramarathon twice – in 2002 and 2003. In 2002, Reed became the first woman to be the overall winner of this event, beating the male runner-up by 25 minutes in 28 hours and 26 minutes at the age of 42. She famously overtook the male lead after 111 miles. Reed is now race director of the Tucson Marathon.

▼ The crowds at this race may be small, but they're passionate enough to make up for it.

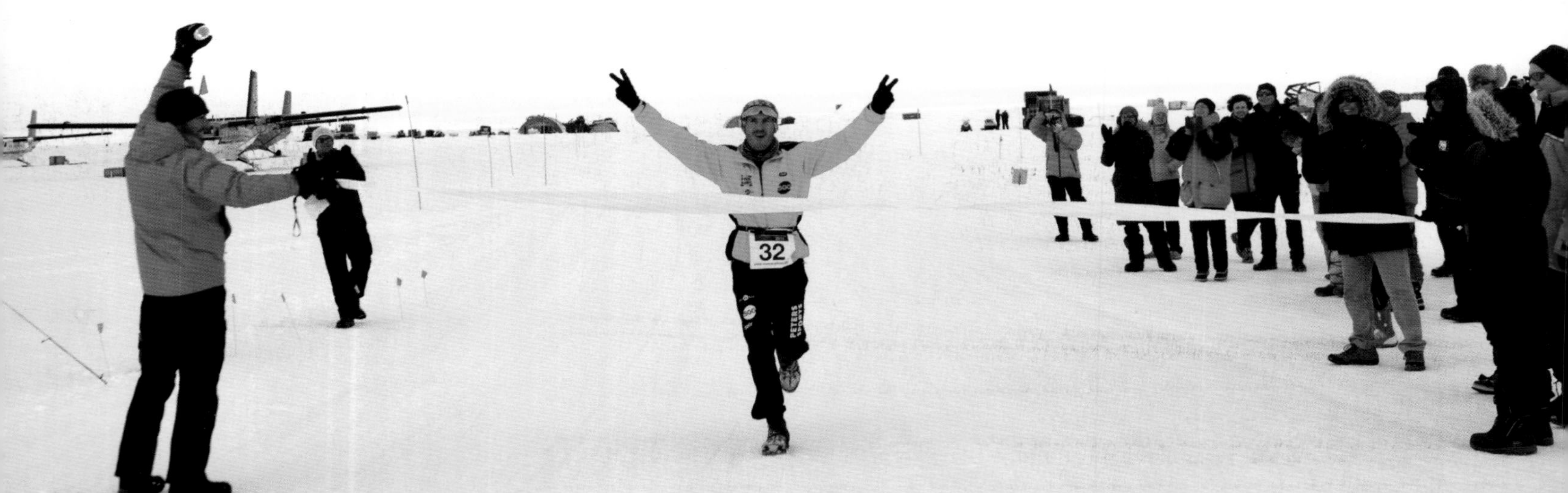

JORDAN
Established:
1995
When: April

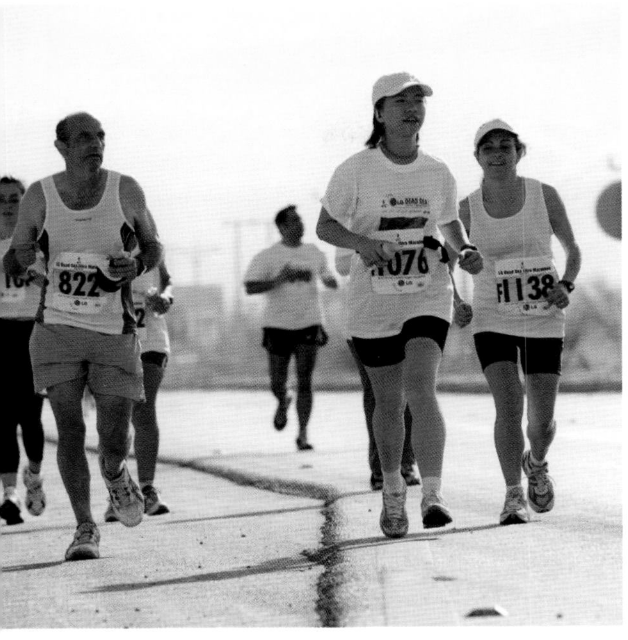

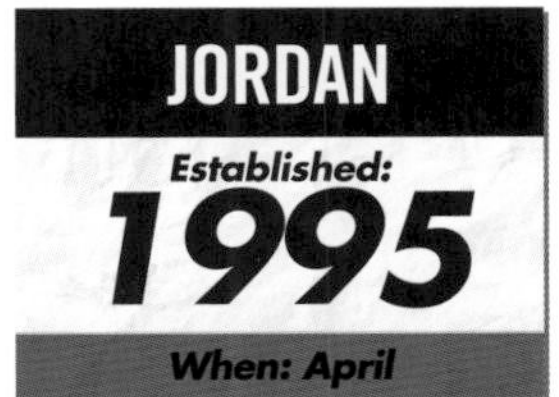

DEAD SEA ULTRAMARATHON, 50KM

This annual race held in Amman, Jordan, draws in thousands of runners from all over the world. The race starts from the peaks and highlands of Amman and runs down to the earth's lowest point on land, the Dead Sea. The race typically attracts runners from more than 50 countries, and is intended to promote athleticism among the young. The main event involves a 50km stretch, but there are also other, shorter, race options, including a half-marathon and a standard-distance marathon. The race finishes on the Amman Tourist Beach in Jordan. Terrain is described as "rolling", so expect it to be rugged, hilly and mountainous, with narrow sections. The race is marked at every kilometre and there are ambulances and first-aid crews available throughout the route all the way up to the finish line. There is a 12-hour cut-off time for the 50km distance.

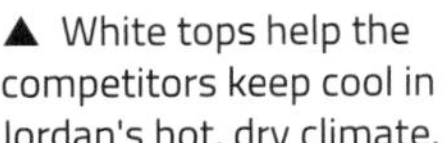

▲ White tops help the competitors keep cool in Jordan's hot, dry climate.

▼ Runners may begin 85m below sea level, but the finish is approximately 2,600m above it.

WALES
Established:
1992
When: May

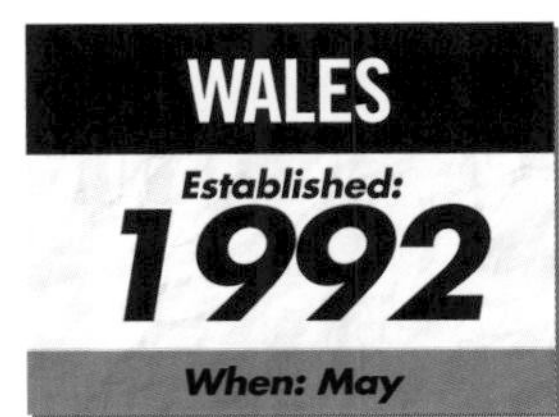

DRAGON'S BACK RACE, 315KM

This event follows the mountains of Wales from North to South and takes place over five days. During that time, you'll cover 315km and tackle 15,500 metres of ascent across uneven and unpredictable terrain. Tough and remote, this event began in 1992 and attracts mountain and fell runners from all over the world. The very first race was won by Helene Diamantides and her running partner Martin Stone, which firmly put female runners on the map and proved that women can and do run ultras very well. Reported to be the toughest five-day mountain race in the world, it's not for the faint-hearted.

PARK OFF PAVEMENT
ELEVATION
SEA LEVEL

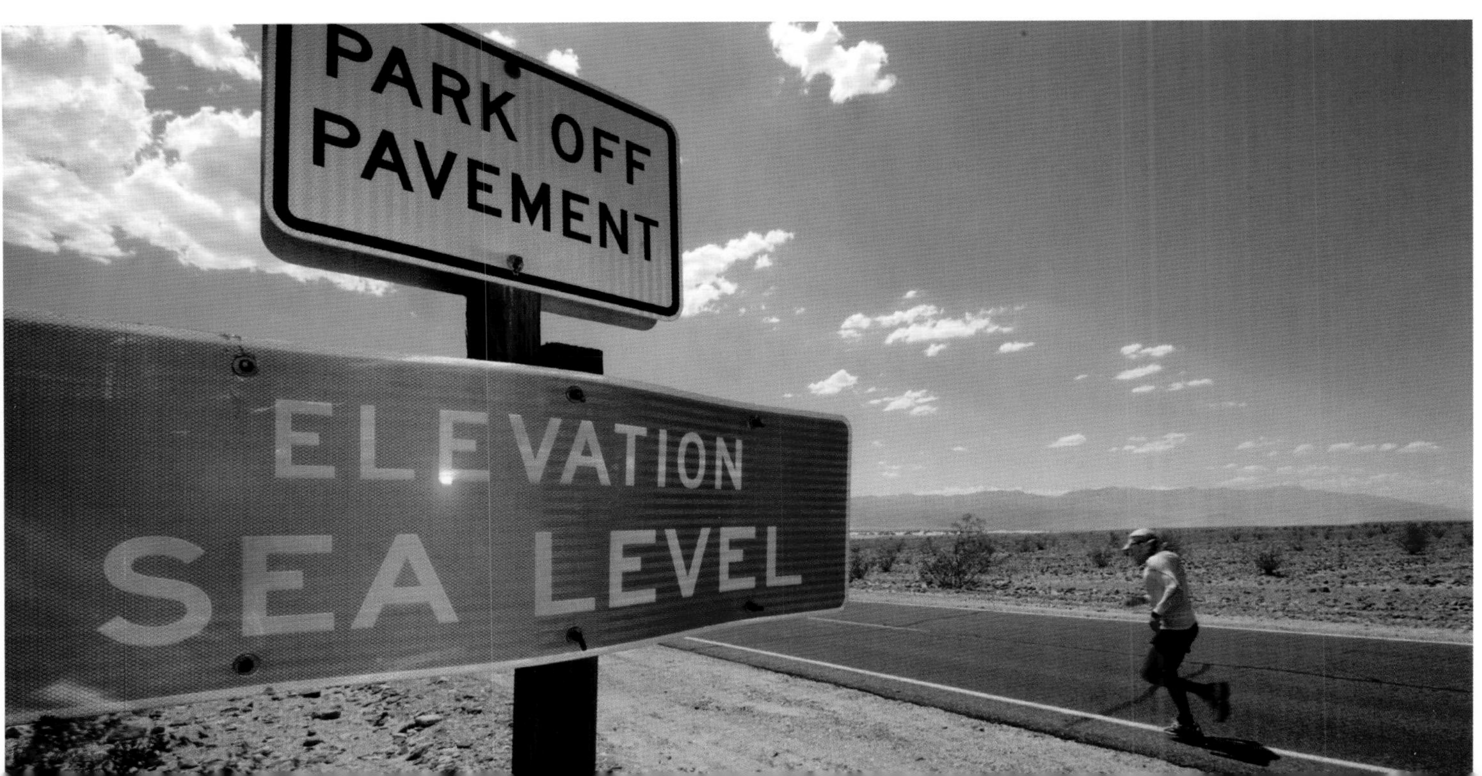

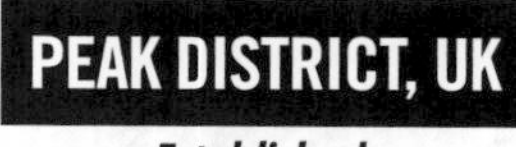

PEAK DISTRICT, UK

Established:

2012

When: October

DUSK TIL DAWN ULTRA, 50 MILES

One of the UK's most popular night races, this 50-mile ultramarathon starts at 5.45 p.m. in the village of Hope and you'll head from there to hills in the Peak District, where you'll have to make it back to Hope before sunrise. You'll cover Mam Tor (a hill in the High Peak of Derbyshire), Lose Hill in the Peak District and Shining Tor (another hill), to name a few, in this challenging route.

Sounds like enough of an adventure, but there's something else. Behind you runs the "Grim Sweeper". If you're too slow and it catches you, you'll be retired from the race. The event also includes marathon and half-marathon options.

SWITZERLAND

Established:

2013

When: July

THE EIGER TRAIL ULTRA, 101KM

This event takes place at the Eiger, a classic route in the Jungfrau used by climbers to access climbing routes on the north face of the Eiger. It's 3,970m above Grindelwald (a popular Swiss village) and offers amazing views. The route goes through Grosse Scheidegg (a mountain pass in the Bernese Alps), Faulhorn (another mountain), Wengen (a Swiss holiday resort) and Kleine Scheidegg (another mountain pass), before going along the base of the Eiger's north face itself. The race is challenging but the views are amazing, with runners having a chance to enjoy the panoramic views of the surrounding peaks towards Schynige Platte, a beautiful mountain ridge.

UTAH, USA

Established:

2012

When: September

GRAND TO GRAND ULTRA, 273KM

This challenging event goes through the Arizona desert in six stages over seven days. What's more, it's an entirely self-supported event and goes from one of the Seven Natural Wonders of the World (the north rim of Grand Canyon), to finish on the summit of Grand Staircase.

You'll go through sand dunes, canyons and hoodoos – it's not for the faint-hearted.

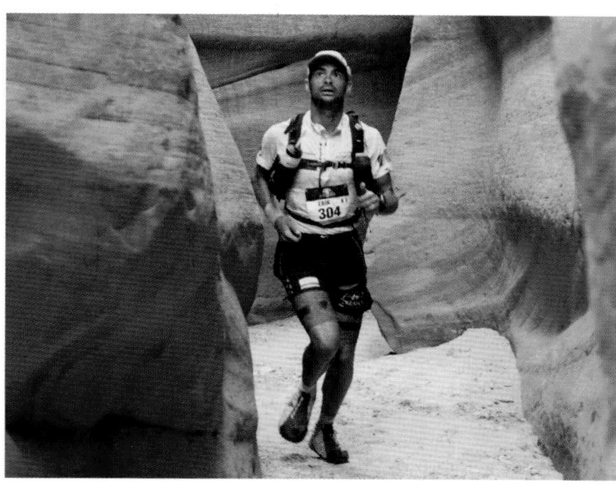

▶ Runners need to make sure to have plenty of water on them in the Arizona heat that radiates off the red rock.

▶▶ It's easy to forget that other runners are taking part when you find yourself alone in the vast canyons.

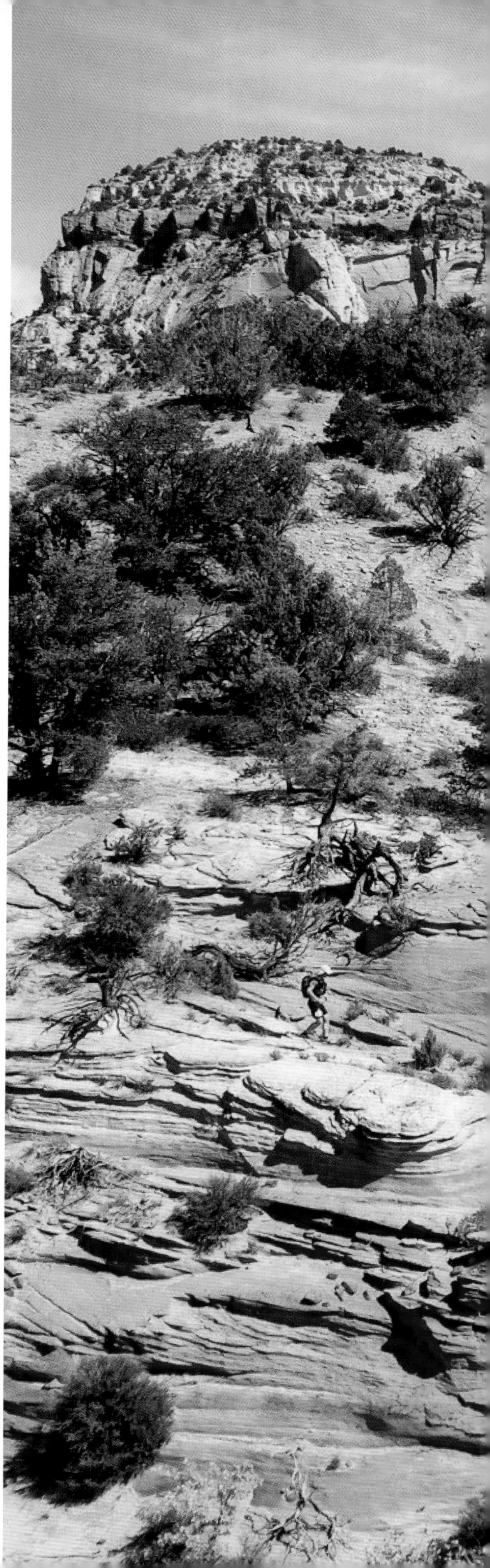

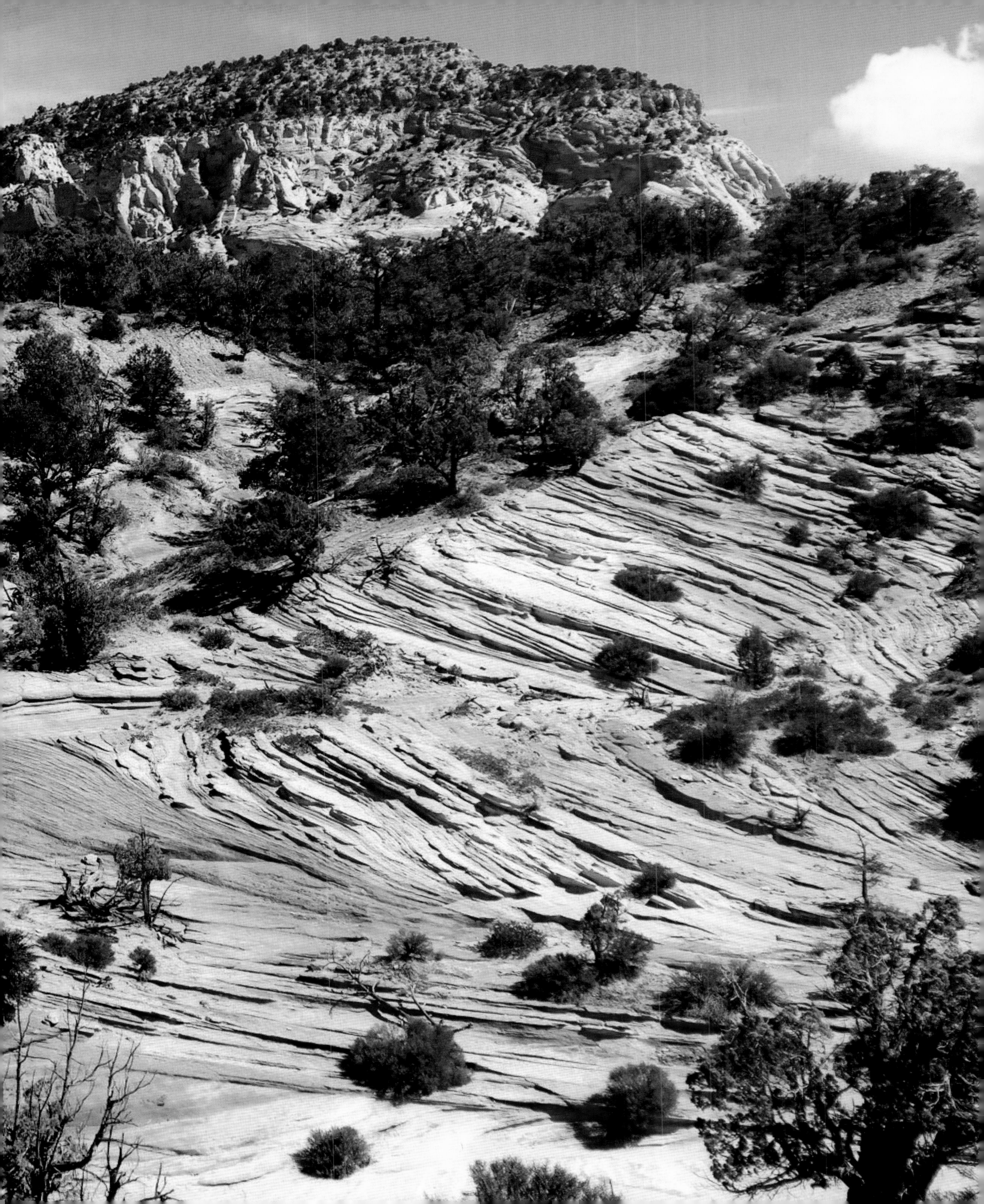

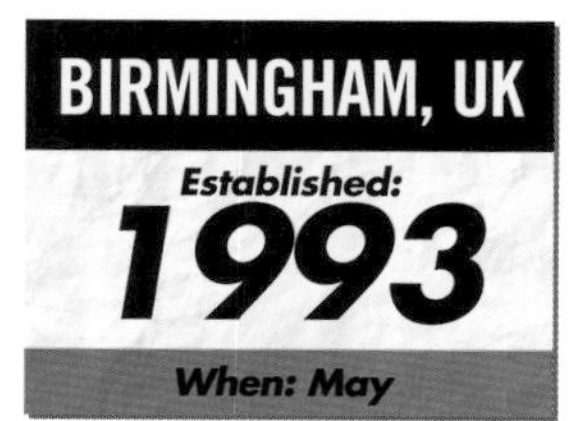

GRAND UNION CANAL RACE, 145 MILES

This race goes from Birmingham to London along towpaths. It starts at 6 a.m. and typically attracts around 100 runners. Previous participants have included famous ultrarunner Mimi Anderson, who has won the event, and Debs Martin-Consani, who won the race in 2012 despite falling into the canal. The course is narrow, so participants have been known to fall over, strike their heads on tree branches or go the wrong way, so it's one where you need to keep your wits about you, even when you start feeling tired. You must complete the event within the 45-hour time limit and many runners with time to spare make the most of this by stopping to enjoy some pub food along the way.

COLORADO, USA
Established:
1992
When: July

HARDROCK 100, 100 MILES

This is a 100-mile endurance race covering 66,100 feet of elevation change that is completed on dirt trails and across country in the San Juan Mountain Range of Southern Colorado. It goes through some of the most beautiful, rugged mountains in the world.

The race starts in Silverton, Colorado, and goes through a town of Telluridge, Ouray, travelling above 12,000 feet of elevation 13 times. The highest point of the course is the summit of Handies Peak, a high mountain. Instead of crossing a finish line at the end, participants must kiss a "hardrock" – a picture of a ram's head on a large block of stone-mining debris.

The race has a cut-off time of 48 hours and the average runner normally takes around 41 hours to finish. It has a 6 a.m. start, so you should see the sun set twice before you finish.

Weather conditions can be unpredictable – expect rain, hail or high winds as well as the possibility of severe thunder storms. It's worth carrying additional layers of clothing in your backpack so you've plenty of spare, dry kit if you need it. It's also advisable to carry your own food. The event has a limit of 140 participants and the entire course is clearly marked.

▼ The sun may occasionally peak out but runners in Colorado need to be prepared for all weather.

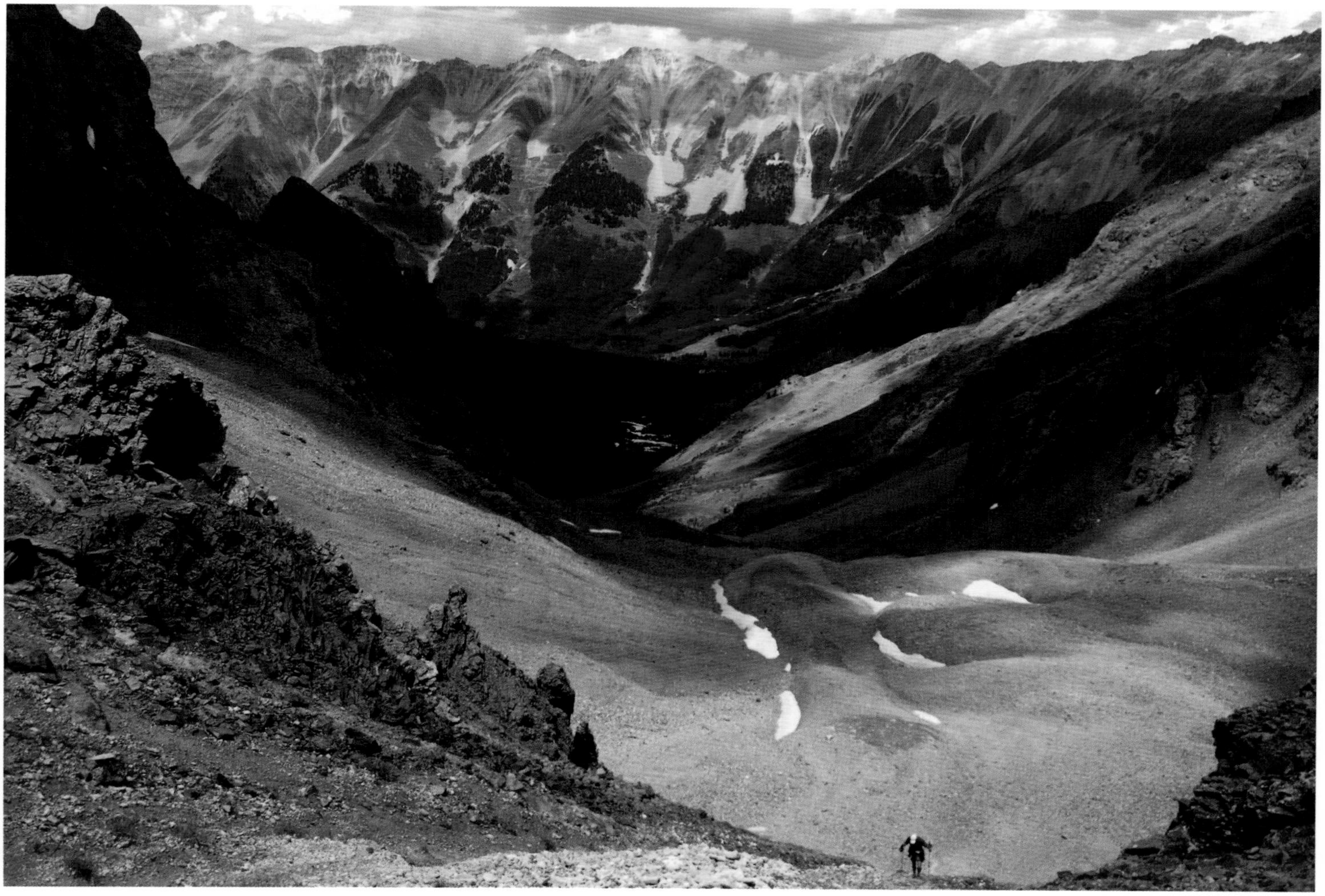

ALASKA, USA
Established:
1973
When: February

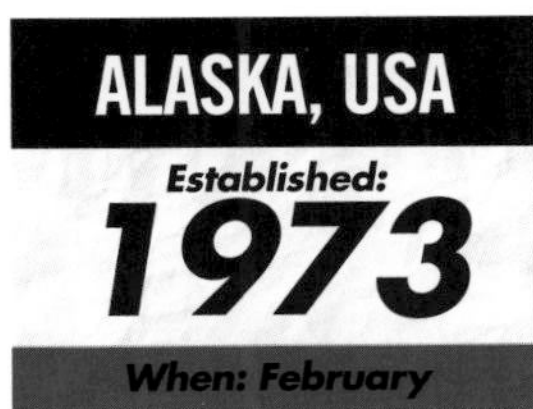

IDITAROD TRAIL INVITATIONAL, 130 MILES, 1,000 MILES

You've got to be able to cope with the cold as well as the distance, as this event, one of the most challenging ultras you can find, provides extreme physical and mental challenges. Participants will move along the Iditarod Trail on bike, foot or skis. What's more, you'll need to be self-sufficient (there are only three snow machines in front of the leaders) in this race, which goes from the Trail of Knik to the village of McGrath across the Yukon River and to Nome, a city in Alaska.

The famous sled-dog route has gone 1,000 miles through Alaska every winter since 1973. Participants must be able to take care of themselves but can choose any route they wish to follow, so long as they go past the checkpoints. You have a maximum time of 10 days, 23 hours, 59 minutes and 59 seconds to finish this race.

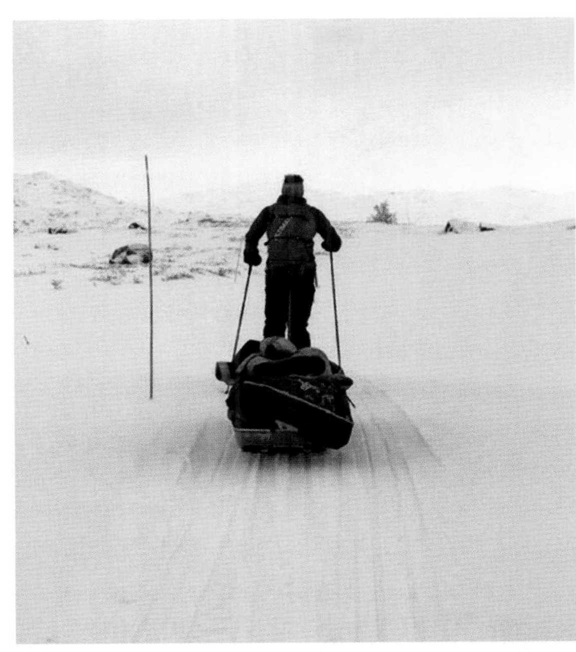

▶ Who needs sled-dogs when you can pull your own supplies behind you?

DORSET, UK
Established:
2005
When: July

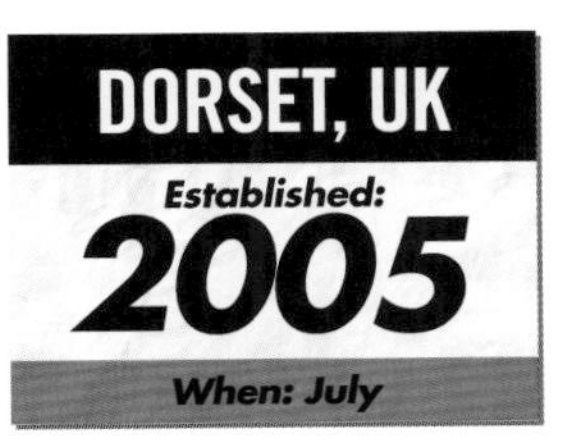

JURASSIC COAST CHALLENGE, 78 MILES

This event consists of three marathons in three days, starting from the Jurassic Coast Challenge Headquarters at Poole Harbour and running along the stunning Jurassic Coastal Path on a challenging route. The event is promoted as being suitable for walkers, joggers or runners – each of whom will start the route at a different time each day (and you can even take part as one of a team). The routes are marked on maps you'll be given and require little navigation as the footpath along the coast is well marked. Meals and massages are located at the HQ and shuttle buses are provided throughout the day to and from accommodation that is provided as part of the race entry.

On the first day, you'll go from Weymouth and Portland National Sailing Academy; on Day Two, you'll cover Portland Ferry Road and Lulworth Cove; and on the third day, you'll go from Lulworth Cove all the way to Shell Bay. The terrain on the route has challenging hills and the course will finish on the third day at the National Trust Shell Bay Car Park.

This well-organized event has everything for ultra-running fans – the organization is fantastic and you'll be transported to the start at the beginning of each day from the headquarters. At the end of the race on the third day, you'll be taken back to the event HQ. Everything will be taken care of, so you'll need to worry only about completing the distance.

INDIA
Established:
2012
When: September

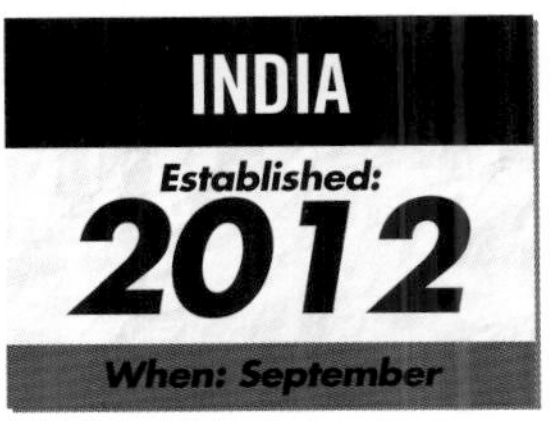

KHARDUNG LA CHALLENGE, 72KM

This event is reported to be the highest ultra-marathon in the world. The race has a limit of 150 runners and is tough and challenging, with the organizers emphasizing that it's suitable only for fit and experienced runners. The harsh conditions make it a tough race and you'll be running approximately 60km of the race at above 4,000m. The organizers recommend you arrive at least two weeks before the race if you are visiting from overseas, and give yourself time to prepare and get used to the high altitude.

The race begins at Khardung Village (3,975 metres) and involves a steady climb to the top of the Khardung La. Then you'll head downhill to Leh Town (a high city desert in the Himalayas) and get to enjoy spectacular mountain views. The race has a cut-off time of 14 hours. There's also a marathon and a half-marathon for those who prefer a shorter distance but still want to have the experience of running in this amazing location.

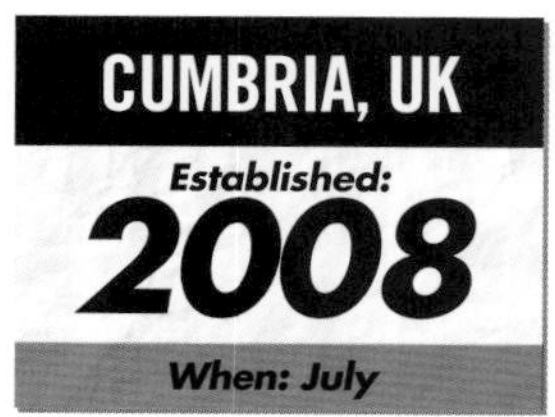
CUMBRIA, UK
Established:
2008
When: July

THE LAKELAND 50, LAKELAND 100, 50 MILES, 100 MILES

One of the greatest ultrarunning challenges in Europe, these events offer a 50-mile option and a 100-mile option, both of which take place in the Lake District. The 50-mile course starts from Ullswater (the second largest lake in the Lake District) and follows the eastern shoreline to Howtown. The route visits Long Sleddale, Kentmere, and Ambleside, to name a few locations, before finishing at Coniston.

The course offers six manned compulsory checkpoints on the course, with food and drink available at each one. The 50-mile option starts from Dalemain Estate and has a time limit of 24 hours.

The 100-mile route takes in all of the Lakeland fells and has around 6,300m of ascent. It starts in Coniston and ends in the Dunnerdale Fells.

There are cut-off times for checkpoints – you need to reach a lake cabin in four hours after the first 22km of the race – and the organizers encourage you to be realistic about your chances of being able to complete the event. Runners are sorted into four groups based on their estimated finish time, with faster runners starting at the front. There are breathtaking views with scenery at virtually every part of the course.

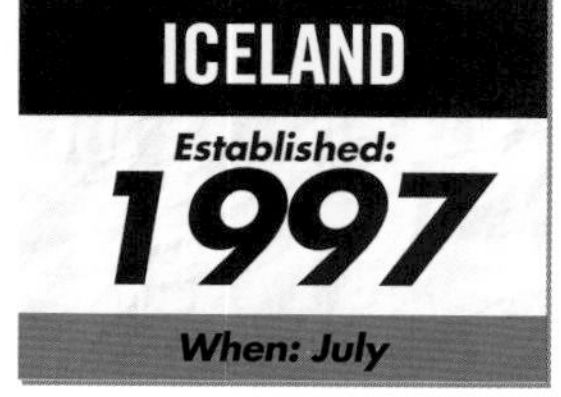
ICELAND
Established:
1997
When: July

LAUGAVEGUR ULTRAMARATHON, 55KM

This is a mountain race in the Southern Highlands of Iceland, which takes participants through the natural beauty of the area over four days. The course is multi-terrain and goes over sand, gravel, grass, snow, ice and rivers. You'll even cross a river with a rope stretched over it that's about 4km long.

The first part of the course runs from Landmannalaugar, located in the Highlands of Iceland, to Hrafntinnusker, a mountain, with an elevation of 5,000m. The second part of the course goes from Hrafntinnusker to the lake of Álftavatn and is a high part of the course consisting of snow and ice. The third section goes from Álftavatn to Emstrur and there's a drop in elevation, before you head to Emstrur, a desolate grazing area to Húsadalur, a valley with challenging hills. The organizers recommend you hold back in the earlier stages of the race in order to cope with the hills on this part of the course.

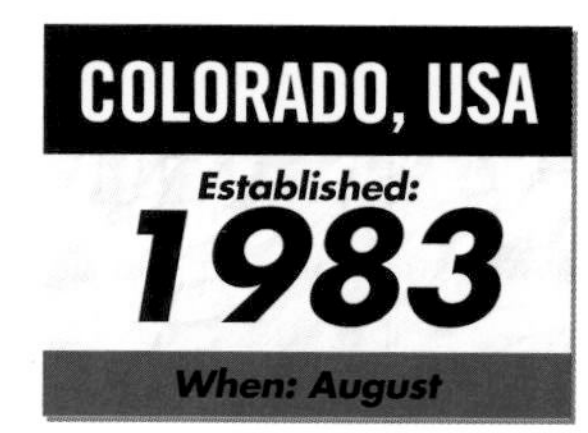
COLORADO, USA
Established:
1983
When: August

LEADVILLE TRAIL 100 RUN, 100 MILES

Known as the "Race Across the Sky", this event started in 1983 with just 45 runners. It offers participants 100 miles of extreme Colorado Rockies terrain and thousands of runners now take part. This out-and-back, up-and-down race and is the ultimate test of fitness and determination. Be prepared to cope with elevations of 9,200 to 12,600 feet. You'll need to love the trails, with much of the race taking place on forest trails with a few mountain roads.

The course has largely remained unchanged over the years, but there have been some alterations. In 2017 the organizers reverted to a course used in 2012. The route now entails starting at the Half Moon Road to Twin Lakes fire station, then using the Colorado Trail to Winfield. The race offers 11 well-stocked aid stations and there at cut-off times for each of them.

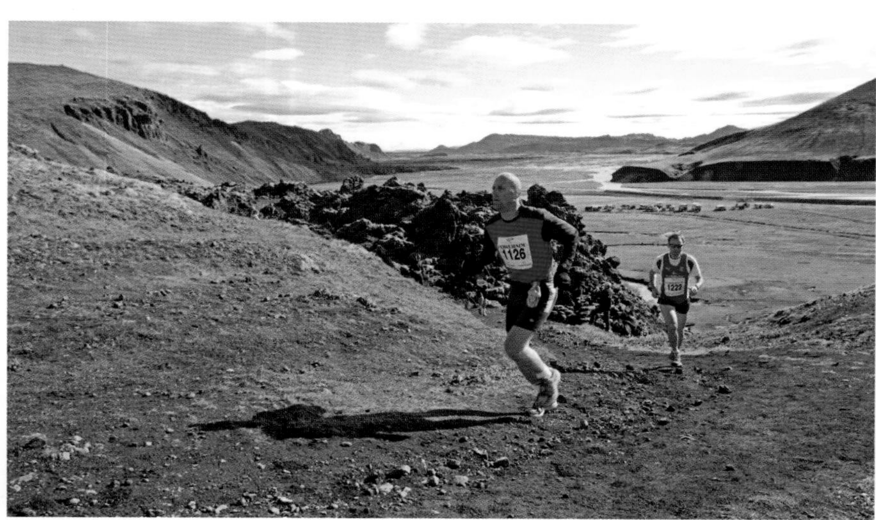

▼ Laugavegur contains many terrains, and ends in the beautiful natural reservation area of Thorsmork.

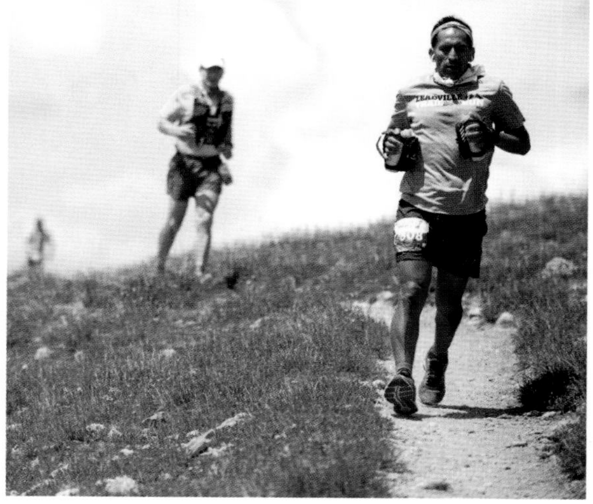

◢ Runners will be feeling on top of the world after the Leadville Trail 100 Run.

LONDON, UK
Established:
2002
When: May

LONDON 2 BRIGHTON CHALLENGE, 100KM

You have the option to walk, jog or run from London to Brighton. The course starts in Richmond and goes along the Thames, over the North and South Downs and through the Sussex countryside. You can do the full 100km distance, or cover half or a quarter of the course if you prefer. With around 2,500 participants, the 100km distance runs over two days, with a "daylight" option, and the course is fully supported. There are rest-stops with free food and drink and plenty of support.

HAWAII, USA
Established:
2017
When: May

MAUNA TO MAUNA ULTRA, 250KM

This race took place for the first time in May 2017 and is in six stages over seven days. It's self-supported, which means you're responsible for carrying your own supplies. Described by the organizers as the "remotest self-supported stage footrace in the world", it runs every two years, with the next event set to take place in May 2019. The race offers ascending volcanoes and lava flows, as well as a rainforest and open grasslines.

The course starts in the slopes of Mauna Loa, a large mountain, and passes around Mauna Kea, the tallest mountain on earth, which rises around 9,966m through the water and then a further 4,200m above sea level. There are also lots of beautiful beaches to take in, which means you're guaranteed some great views.

◥ Pyrotechnics signal the start of another race for a collection of keen runners.

▼ The elite group of runners who completed the first Mauna to Mauna Ultra in 2017.

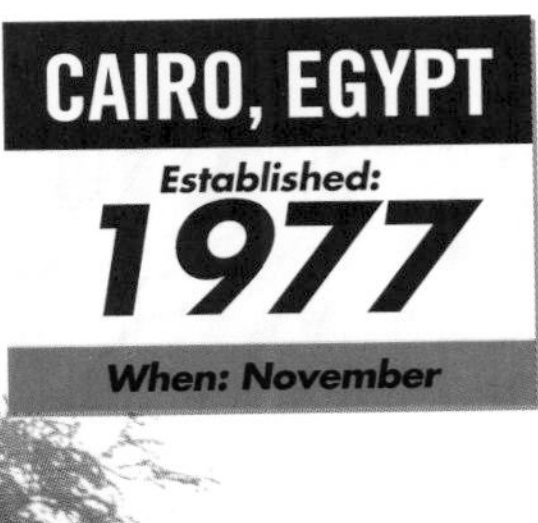

PHARAONIC RACE, 100KM

The idea for this race was born in 1977, when the Egyptian Egyptologist Ahmed Moussa discovered a piece of rock that revealed the story of the Pharaonic soldiers running a race of 100km way back in 690 BC during the reign of King Taharka (a Pharaoh of ancient Egypt). The king went to inspect an army camp and found the soldiers in perfect physical condition, so the race must have been doing them some good. This desert race takes place in one day and takes you through the glamorous sites of Sakkara (an ancient burial ground), Dashure, which is where you can view the red Pyramids of King Snefru, and then on to List and Meidum, an archaeological site where the first pyramid in Egypt was built. Stunning, historical and a perfect race adventure.

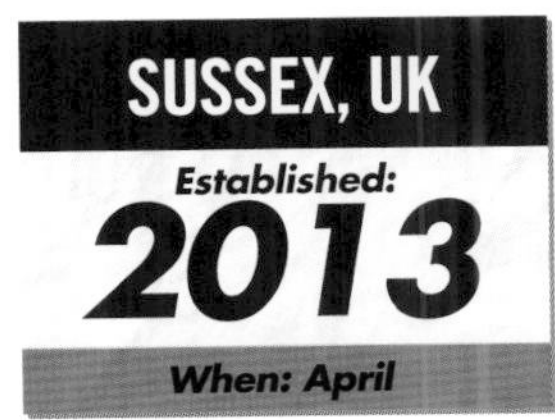

SOUTH DOWNS WAY 50, 50 MILES

This 50-mile race offers great scenery, as it goes along the South Downs Way National Trail, starting from Worthing in Sussex and finishing in Eastbourne. You'll start off by weaving your way around six miles of chalk footpaths and bridleways, then climb up to join the South Downs Way at Chanctonbury Ring, before finishing at Eastbourne Sports Club Athletics track, doing a lap of the track to finish. The race has a climb of 5,700 feet and the course is marked with red and white tape and Centurion Marker Arrows.

There are seven aid stations along the course and all of them are very well stocked with water, coke, chocolate, sweets, sandwiches, nuts, fruit, energy gels, wraps, sandwiches and savoury snacks. The organizers recommend that you check out the route before race day and carry a map and compass with you on the day, just in case. The race has a 13-hour cut-off time.

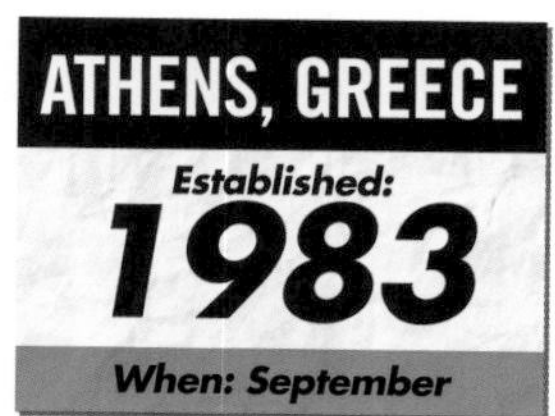

SPARTATHLON, 246KM

A British wing commander named John Foden was the inspiration behind this event, a historic, ultra-distance foot race described as one of the most difficult and satisfying ultra-distances in the world. It first took place in 1983 and traces the footsteps of Pheidippides, an ancient long-distance runner who is said to have run from Marathon to Athens, before falling dead, in 490 BC.

Spartathlon covers 152 miles in less than 36 hours. The course has around 72 numbered water stations roughly 4km apart and ranges from sea level to 1,200m along a mixture of roads, trails and footpaths. Around 390 participants take part.

SWITZERLAND
Established:
1986
When: July

SWISSALPINE IRONTRAIL, VARIOUS DISTANCES

This has breathtaking tracks with great scenery and a choice of 12 exciting races. There are the T127, which is 127km, starting at midnight with a full moon, and covering an altitude of 3,022m on the Alp Muntasch; the Piz Nair, a mountain; and the Chamanna, a charming mountain resort – to name a few. Finishers will receive six qualifying points for UTMB.

There's also an 88.1km distance, which is a trail run from the Rhaetian Railway and Davos to St Moritz. The breathtaking running trail is scenic and goes from the alpine village of Bergün via the Keschhütte (a mountain hut) and the Sertig Pass to the alpine town of Davos. The T88 can also be run as a team event – as a couple or as a team of four. There are also a 39.1km event and various other distances.

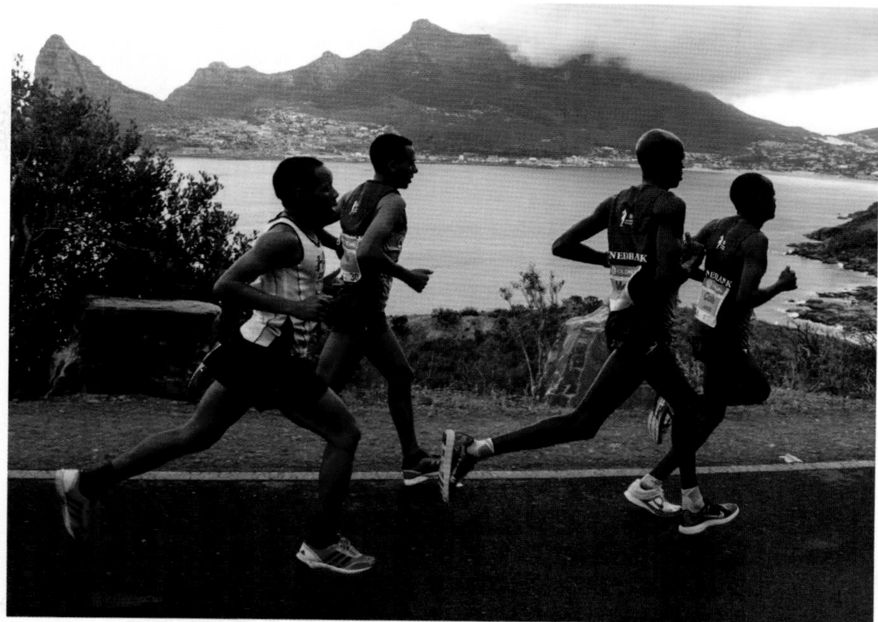

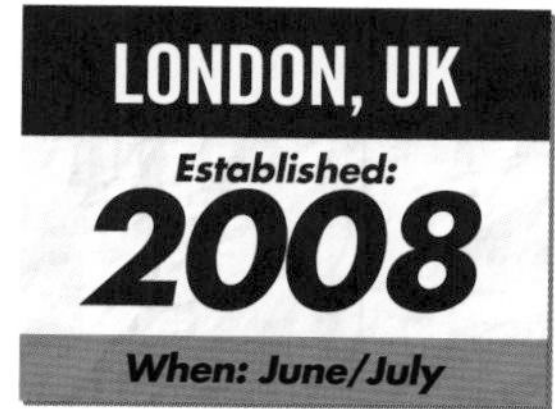

THE THAMES RING 250, 250 MILES

As the name suggests, this is a 250-mile trail race that starts in the village of Streatley-on-Thames and goes along a series of twisting and turning canal and river paths heading anticlockwise. It's a relatively flat course and runners have 100 hours to complete it.

You need to be a competent navigator, as you'll be using maps to find your way, and there will be checkpoints at around every 25 miles. A tough event, this race runs only every two years. Around 30 to 40 per cent of entrants are expected to complete the course.

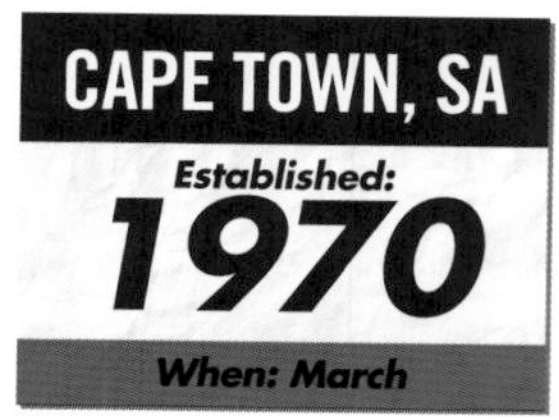

TWO OCEANS MARATHON, 56KM

This event is claimed to be the world's most beautiful marathon and takes place around the Cape Peninsula. The race begins at 6.30 a.m. on Easter Saturday and starts outside SA Breweries on Main Road, Newlands, and is run against a backdrop of amazing scenery through the Cape Peninsula. The event was launched in 1970 and is a popular race.

The route is almost circular and finishes at the University of Cape Town campus. There is also a half-marathon and a 5km fun run. Around 16,000 participants take part in total. The half-marathon goes along Edinburgh Drive, which is the main M3 highway, and turns into forest roads where half-marathon runners meet with the ultramarathon participants. The half-marathon is the biggest such race in South Africa.

◀ The biggest race in Africa is also one of the most scenic and spectacular.

MT FUJI, JAPAN
Established:
2012
When: May

▼ Brave runners from 32 countries have previously taken part in the Ultra-Trail Mt.Fuji.

◢ The conditions and terrain of the Western States Trail don't stay as sunny and flat as pictured here.

ULTRA-TRAIL MT.FUJI, 170KM

This event is an extreme long-distance race through mountains that circle Mount Fuji and is one of the toughest, most challenging ultras you could attempt. The event began in 2012 and is part of the Ultra-Trail World Series. It starts and ends at the Yagizaki Park in Fuji-Kawaguchi in Yamanshi Prefecture, and circles around Mt Fuji. There is a cut-off time of 46 hours and you'll need to have acquired a minimum of six points (in a maximum of three qualifying races) in races that are registered with the International Trail Run Association before you can enter this race.

This is described as one of the longest and most difficult long-distance endurance races, and it's reported that, from the 1,400 runners who enter, fewer than 50 per cent make it to the finish line. The fittest runners usually complete the race in around 20 hours. One of the biggest challenges, apart from the cumulative altitude gain of around 8,000m and the rocky, rough terrain, is the fact that you run through day and night. You also need to deal with changing weather conditions on your own, such as low temperatures, strong winds, rain and snow, along with any muscle aches or pains you may encounter during the event. Runners are asked to wear bells to scare off dangerous animals that may be lurking in the mountains. The race organizers stipulate that you must be responsible for your own safety and be able to navigate the trails. Sounds like the adventure of a lifetime, if you're brave enough!

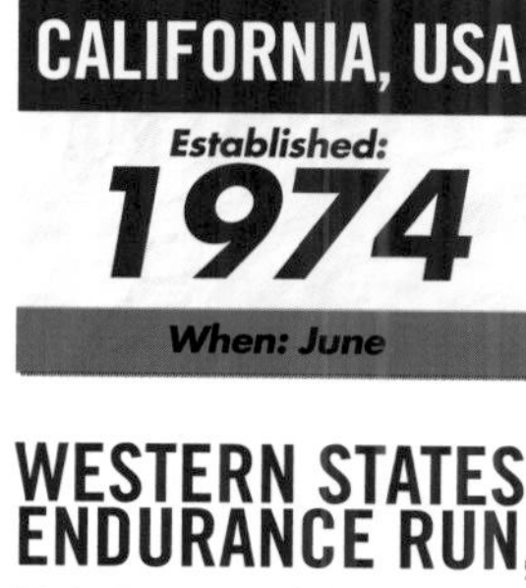

WESTERN STATES 100-MILE ENDURANCE RUN, 100 MILES

This is one of the world's oldest 100-mile trail events, and starts in Squaw Valley, California, near the location of the 1960 Winter Olympics. The course ends just over 100 miles later in Auburn, California. The race was first held in 1974 and follows the historic Western States Trail. Race participants are expected to climb over 18,000 feet and then descend 23,000 feet before they reach the finish line. There's a cut-off time of just under 11 hours and runners are encouraged to get used to trail running before they enter this event, as the race covers many trails, some of which you will need to complete in the dark. You're expected to carry two LED flashlights or wait for another runner if your lights fail.

It's worth doing your homework on this course first, as much of the race course is accessible only by foot, horse or helicopter. Good navigation is key and, if you do decide to visit the location and do a training run in advance, you're strongly advised to take someone with you or buddy up with a native guide.

Temperatures during this event are wide-ranging, going from 20 degrees to 110 degrees Fahrenheit, so you'll need to be used to running in extreme weather.

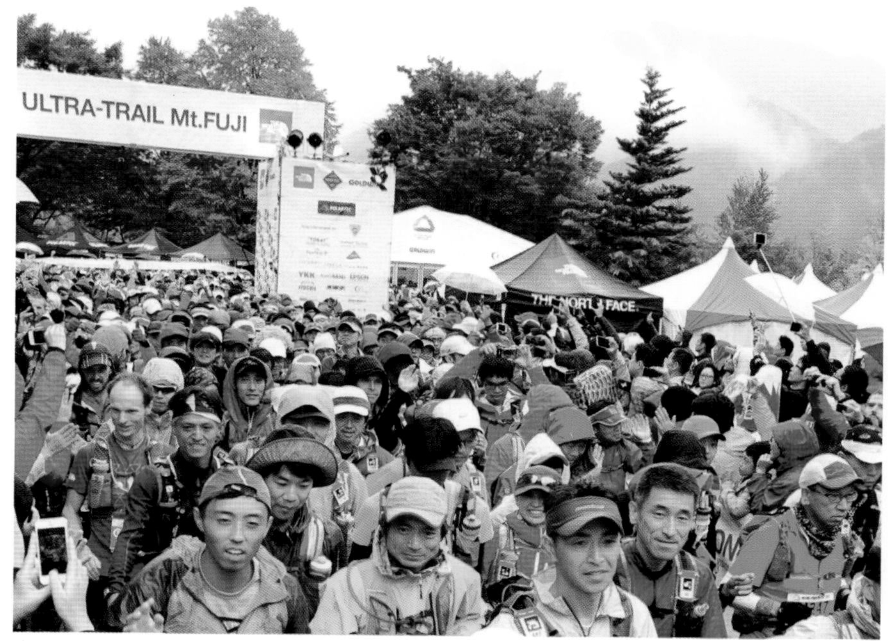

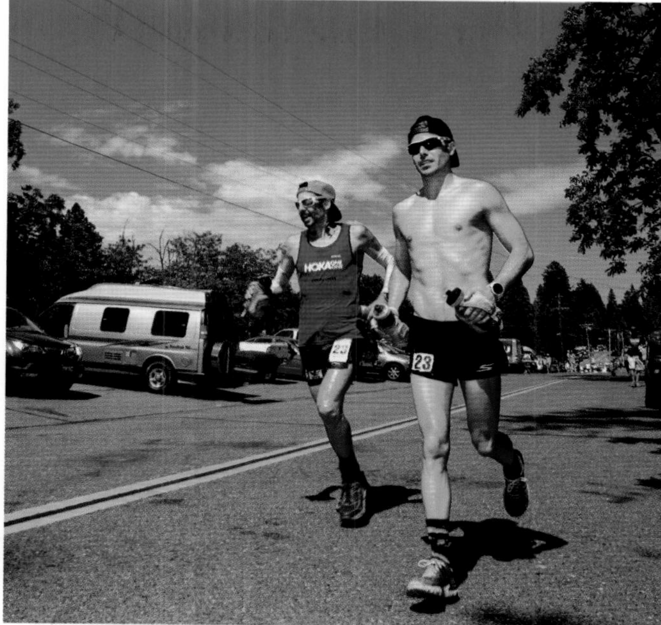

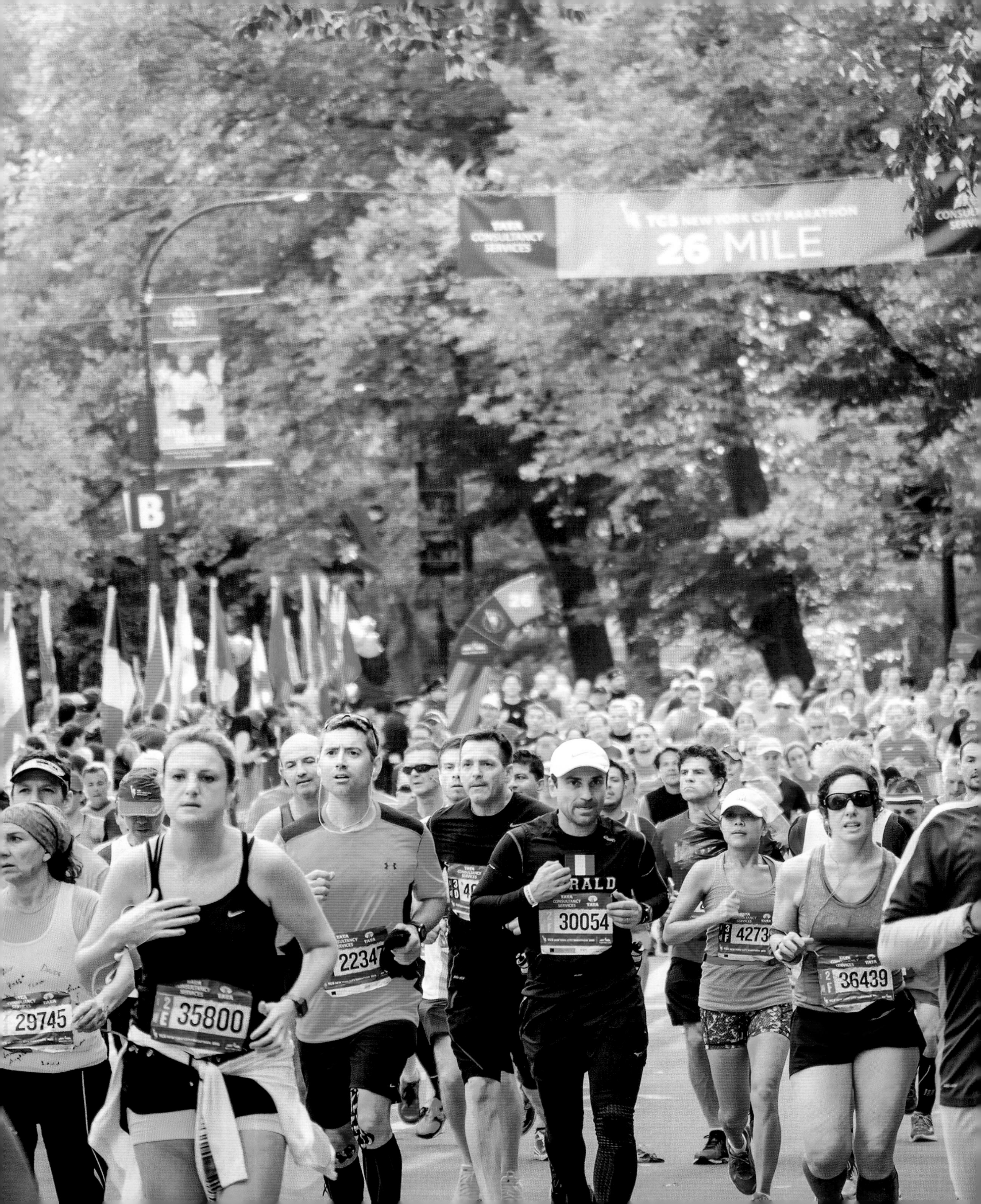
TATA CONSULTANCY SERVICES
TCS NEW YORK CITY MARATHON
26 MILE
B
29745
35800
30054
36439

PLANNING & PREPARATION

PLANNING & PREPARATION

The key to running a marathon successfully and having a positive race-day experience is to ensure you follow a structured training plan. You need to put the miles in, which will give you confidence in your running ability, but it's also important to not overdo it and not to train too hard. It's important to build up your mileage gradually and give your body time to recover in between long runs or harder sessions.

PREPARING FOR A RACE ABROAD

If you're flying out to Japan or any other distant territory to run a marathon, it's essential that you're well organized and well prepared in advance. Here are some tips about taking part in a race abroad where a long-haul flight is involved.

- Fly out at least a week before race day to give yourself plenty of time to get over jetlag and become acclimatised to the different environment. Don't leave it till the last minute to fly out, as you'll still be in a different time zone.
- Be prepared with your kit. Take all the usual running essentials, such as the clothing you've trained in that you know is comfortable and doesn't rub or chafe, and don't forget your trainers! Make sure you also take other useful items you may not find abroad, such as a small first-aid kit, plasters for nipples or toes, waist belt, water bottle, energy gels, safety pins and other essentials that you may not find abroad. While you may be able to buy some of these items, you may not be able to find the same brands.
- Bring a choice of running outfits – a warm one and a cooler one so that you're prepared for all temperatures, since you just can't predict the weather and it's best to be prepared for whatever conditions you face on race day.
- Know the course route well – make sure you know where the start and finish lines are located and how far the start line is from your hotel. Have a plan in place for how you're going to reach the start line and walk the route before race day, so that you're absolutely clear on how to get there before the event.
- Know the terrain well – are you going to be on a nice flat course or are you going to have to endure hills, uneven surfaces or unusual terrain, such as rocks? The Osaka Marathon is mostly on flat tarmac but other marathons may offer all sorts of unpredictable terrain. Do your homework.
- Be prepared for the likely temperature on race day. If it's going to be humid, cold or even foggy, you need to know that in advance and be prepared. Running a few half-marathons in hotter weather, for instance, can prepare you for heat. Do your research and know what you're letting yourself in for.

We have three training plans on the pages that follow (see pages 176 to 181), aimed at beginner, intermediate and advanced runners, along with some useful tips on how to avoid overtraining. Follow the advice in this chapter and you'll give yourself the best possible chance of completing a marathon and feeling great at the finish line.

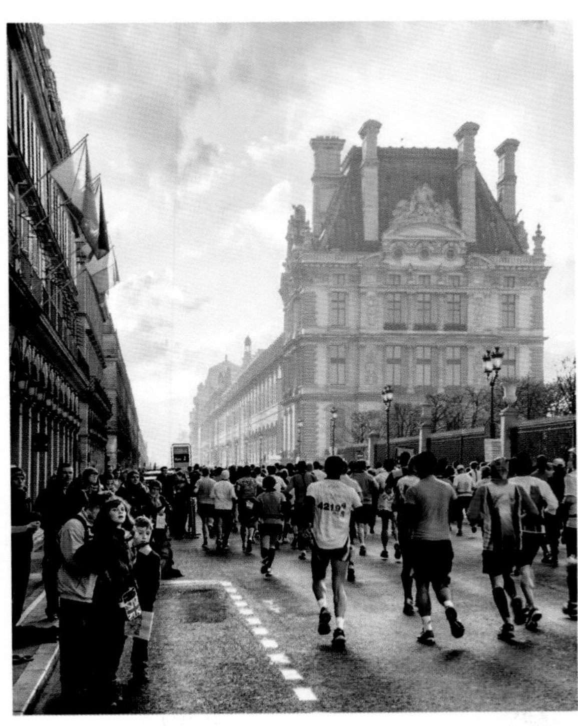

▲▶ With the right planning, running a marathon can become part of the trip of a lifetime.

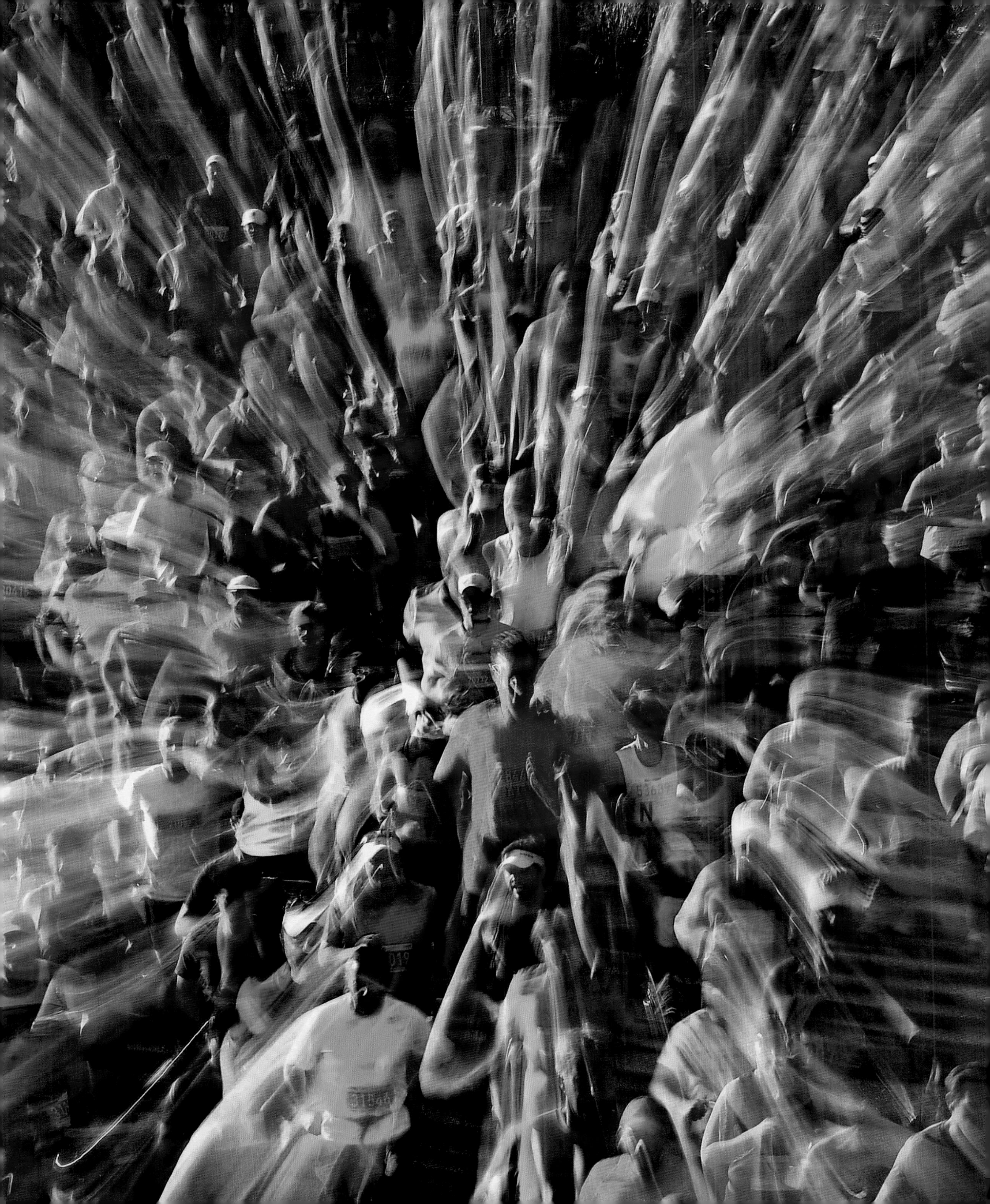

WHY BECOME A GLOBETROTTER?

Like the idea of running a marathon abroad? The excitement of running on streets you've only ever seen in TV travel shows or Sunday supplements, and eating exotic food you've never even heard of, tend to be some of the main reasons why many runners keep entering foreign races. There's also the opportunity to meet runners from across the globe – you could end up making friends in countries ranging from Italy to India as a direct result of your marathon globetrotting.

DON'T LEAVE HOME WITHOUT A FEW ESSENTIALS

- Your passport and printouts of your air or rail ticket, details of your hotel, proof of your race entry, race information including directions to the registration venue and start/finish.
- Your favourite gels, sports drink and racing snacks. With foreign races, it's far harder to train with the refreshments that are going to be provided, so it's best to take your own. When Lisa Jackson first ran the Rome Marathon several years ago, they dished out a super-sugary sports drink en route. "I'll never forget the sight of hundreds of runners being sick over the railings of the ruins of Trajan's Markets," she says. "I, on the other hand, was fine, as I'd carried powdered sports drink with me and had simply diluted it with water."
- Finally, a lesson learned is a lesson shared. Jackson recalls, "I learned the hard way once again while I was in Rome – don't leave it to chance that the country you're visiting will have the things you regard as absolutely vital for a pleasant race experience. When I ran the Rome Marathon in 2013, I mislaid the blister-preventing Vaseline I usually slather my feet in and so spent over an hour fruitlessly going from pharmacy to pharmacy trying to buy some. It was only when I discovered that it's called Vaselina and is sold in pricey tubes, not giant budget-sized tubs, that I finally found some. Without it, I may well have ended up with feet that looked like bubble wrap!"

▶ Running the Rome Marathon is one of the more inventive ways of touring the city and taking in its sights.

▶▶ If you're traveling to Australia to run, then remember to factor in jetlag recovery time.

◥ Even if you're traveling solo, you're sure to meet many like-minded folks who are passionate about running.

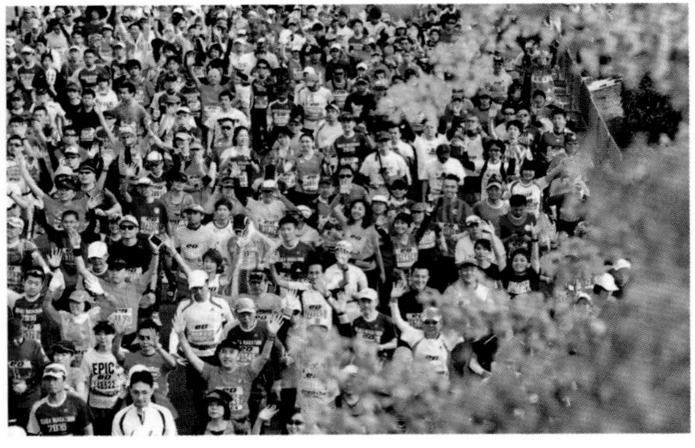

However, there are certain drawbacks to racing abroad. Race websites in foreign languages can prove an issue, and the language barrier can sometimes make obtaining essential information a struggle. Finding out where you have to collect your race number or even turn up to the start can be surprisingly tricky.

Certain countries, such as Italy and France, also ask that you provide a medical certificate attesting to the fact that you're fit enough to run, as we saw earlier. Some GPs charge for this service, meaning getting one can be costly in terms of time and money. Similarly, racing abroad means organising flights and accommodation in addition to race entry, but, if you combine an event with a holiday or city break, this could make for a more cost-effective trip – with the added bonus of a marathon included!

HOW TO HAVE A GREAT RACE EXPERIENCE ABROAD

- Engage with the locals. Let them know you've travelled all the way from the UK to experience their city and take part in the race. Tell them how excited you are to be experiencing the delights their city has to offer.
- Put your name on the front and back of your race T-shirt so that you get more crowd support and spectators can cheer for you by name.
- Remember to pack your blisters and first-aid kit. Don't leave it at home. Beware of chub-rub. Chafing will make race day memorable for all the wrong reasons. Try out plasters, Vaseline or an anti-chafing balm such as Glide, in training, to see what works best for you.
- Arrange a proper rendezvous with friends and loved ones at the end of the course or on the route if they have flown out to support you. Make sure you know enough of the city or the route so that you can find them at the end of the race. Support during the race is key, too. Seeing friends and family along the route will give you more energy than slugging a dozen gels, but in big marathons you need to make sure they can spot you. Arrange to meet up at specific mile markers and don't forget to stipulate which side of the road they should stand on.
- Snack sensibly. No matter how much research has gone in to a particular gel or energy snack, if you don't like the way it tastes, you're much less likely to consume it during a race, so experiment in training to find your favourite.
- Don't overdo the pre-race carbs. Yes, you are going to be burning a lot of calories during the marathon, but the Italians famously like their food and are well known for eating meals with many courses. Enjoy the pasta but don't overdo the tiramisu. There's always a chance to indulge after the race!
- Create race-day memories. Carrying your mobile phone with you means you can not only dial for assistance should you need it, but you can also capture special moments on camera. Fabulous scenery, a runner in a fabulous fancy-dress outfit, your face at every mile marker – give yourself something to inspire you for your next marathon!

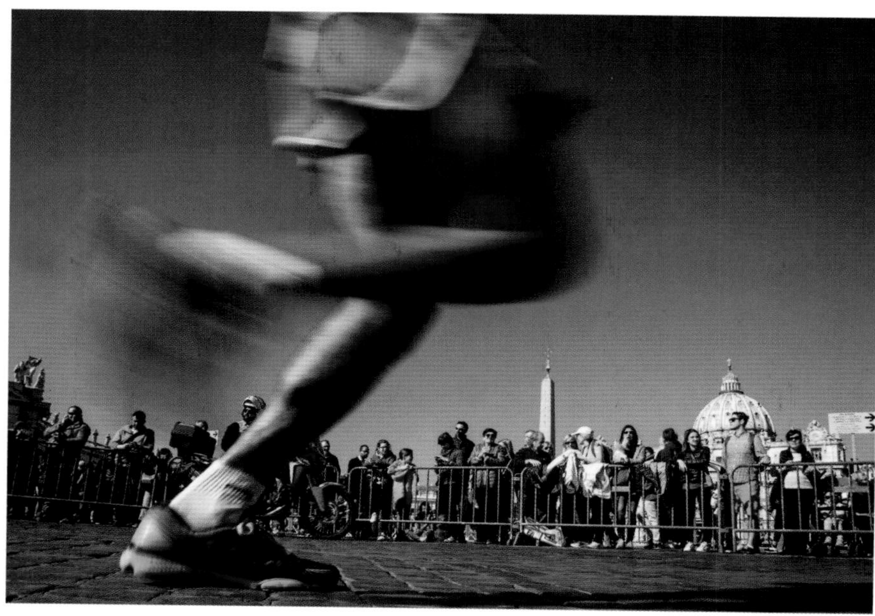

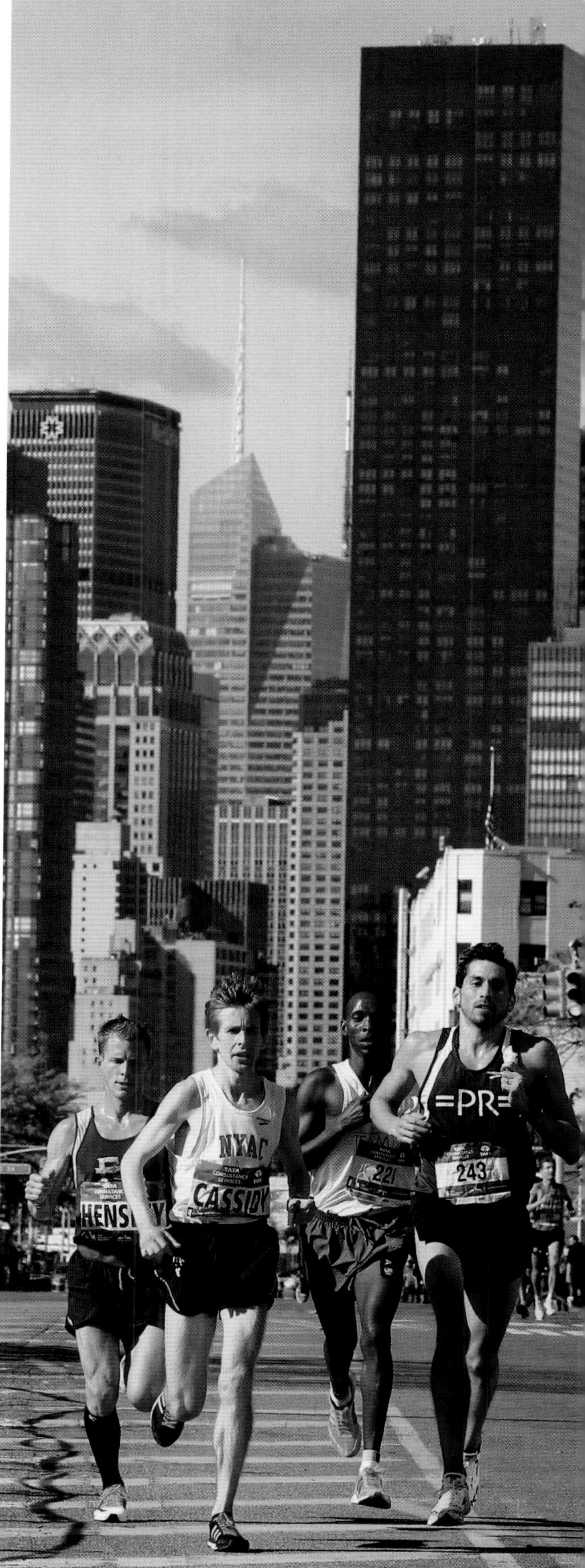

BEGINNER'S MARATHON TRAINING PLAN

NEW TO MARATHON TRAINING? THEN THIS IS THE PLAN FOR YOU . . .

WEEK	MONDAY	TUESDAY	WEDNESDAY	THURSDAY	FRIDAY	SATURDAY	SUNDAY
1	Rest or light swim or aerobic cross-train session for 30 mins. Stretch well afterwards	Threshold run for 3 x 4 mins with 3 mins jog recovery +15-min warm-up and 15-min cool-down jog	Pilates, yoga or core body conditioning	Continuous hills. 3 x 4 mins effort with 15-min warm-up and cool-down jog. 3-min rec between sets	Rest	Rest or 30-min relaxed cross-train/swim	Long run 45 mins, easy conversational pace
2	Rest or light swim or aerobic cross-train session for 30 mins. Stretch well afterwards	Threshold run for 4 x 4 mins with 3 mins jog recovery +15-min warm-up and 15-min cool-down jog	Pilates, yoga or core body conditioning.	Continuous hills. 3 x 5 mins effort with 15-min warm-up and cool-down jog. 3-min rec between sets	Rest	Rest or 30-min relaxed cross-train/swim	Long run 45–60 mins, easy conversational pace
3	Rest or light swim or aerobic cross-train session for 30 mins. Stretch well afterwards	Threshold run for 3 x 5 mins with 3 mins jog recovery +15-min warm-up and 15-min cool-down jog	Pilates, yoga or core body conditioning	Continuous hills. 3 x 5 mins effort with 15-min warm-up and cool-down jog. 3-min rec between sets	Rest	Rest or 30-min relaxed run or cross-train/swim	Long run 60 mins, easy conversational pace
4	Rest or light swim or aerobic cross-train session for 30 mins. Stretch well afterwards	Threshold run 4 x 5 mins effort with 3 mins recovery jog between	Pilates, yoga or core body conditioning	Continuous hills. 2 x 7.5 mins effort with 15-min warm-up and cool-down jog. 3-min rec between sets	Rest	Rest or 30-min relaxed run or cross-train/swim	Long run 75 mins, all easy conversational pace
5	Rest or light swim or cross-train session for 30 mins. Stretch well afterwards	Threshold run 5 x 5 mins effort with 3 mins recovery jog between	Pilates, yoga or core body conditioning	Continuous hills. 2 x 10 mins effort with 15 min warm-up and cool-down jog. 3 min rec between sets	Rest	Rest or 30-min relaxed run or cross-train/swim	90 mins, all easy conversation pace
6	Rest This is a recovery week	Recovery run 30 mins	Pilates, yoga or core body conditioning	30 mins run to include 5 mins easy/5 mins threshold ALL x 3	Rest	Rest	Long run 60 mins
7	Rest or light swim or cross-train session for 30 mins. Stretch well afterwards	Threshold run 4 x 6 mins effort with 2 mins recovery jog between	Pilates, yoga or core body conditioning	Continuous hills. 4 x 6 mins effort with 15-min warm-up and cool-down jog. 3-min rec between sets	Rest	Rest or 30-min relaxed run or cross-train/swim	Long run 90 mins with last 30 mins at target marathon pace
8	Rest or light swim or cross-train session for 30 mins. Stretch well afterwards	Progression run – 10 easy, 10 steady and 10 at threshold as a continuous 30 mins	Pilates, yoga or core body conditioning	Continuous hills. 5 x5 mins effort with 2 mins jog recovery between	Rest	Rest or 30-min relaxed run or cross-train/swim	Long run 105 mins, all conversational pace
9	Rest or light swim or aerobic cross-train session for 30 mins. Stretch well afterwards	Progression run – 15 easy, 15 steady and 15 at threshold as a continuous 45 mins	Pilates, yoga or core body conditioning	Continuous hills. 4 x 7 mins effort with 3 mins jog recovery between	Rest	Rest or 45-min relaxed run or cross-train/swim	Long run 120 mins, all conversational pace

WEEK	MONDAY	TUESDAY	WEDNESDAY	THURSDAY	FRIDAY	SATURDAY	SUNDAY
10	Rest This is a recovery week	Pilates or core conditioning + recovery run 30 mins and stretching	Intervals – 4 x 5 mins at threshold pace with 2–3 mins recovery jog	Rest or 45 min relaxed cross-train/ swim	Rest	Recovery run 15 mins + stretch	**HALF-MARATHON** at target marathon pace.
11	Rest or light swim or aerobic cross-train session for 30 mins. Stretch well afterwards	Pilates or core conditioning + recovery run 30 mins and stretching	45 mins cross-training and stretching	Threshold run 4 x 6 mins effort with 3 mins recovery jog between	Rest	Rest or 45-min relaxed run or cross-train/swim	Long run 140 mins with last 40 mins at target marathon pace
12	Rest or light swim or aerobic cross-train session for 30 mins. Stretch well afterwards	Pilates or core conditioning + recovery run 30 mins and stretching	45 mins cross-training and stretching	Medium long run, 80 mins with the middle 45 at 3 min threshold/3 min easy alternating	Rest	Rest or 45-min relaxed run or cross-train/swim	Long run 160 mins, 60 easy, 60 at target marathon pace and 40 easy
13	Rest or light swim or aerobic cross-train session for 30 mins. Stretch well afterwards	Pilates or core conditioning + Recovery Run 30 mins and stretching	45 mins cross-training and stretching	60 mins incl 3 x 10 mins at threshold off 3-min jog recovery	Rest	Rest or 30-min relaxed run or cross-train/swim	Long run 180 mins with first 2 hours very easy and last hour at target marathon pace
14	Rest or light swim or aerobic cross-train session for 30 mins. Stretch well afterwards	Pilates or core conditioning + recovery run 30 mins and stretching	45 mins cross-training and stretching	45 mins incl 4 x 5 mins at threshold off 2-min jog	Rest	Rest or 30-min relaxed run or cross-train/swim	90–105 mins all easy pace
15	Rest	Pilates or core conditioning + recovery run 30 mins and stretching	45 mins cross-training and stretching	5 x 5 mins at threshold off 90-sec recovery	Rest	Rest or 30-min relaxed run or cross-train/swim	Long run 60 mins all easy
16	Rest	30 mins recovery run	30 mins incl. 3 x 5 easy/5 at MP	15–20 easy jog or rest	Rest	15-min very easy jog	**MARATHON**

TRAINING NOTES

- Do a 15-minute warm-up and cool-down before threshold, continuous hills and interval sessions.
- If you're feeling OK, you may wish to consider a 20–30-minute recovery run in the morning before any of the quality sessions above.
- Always substitute cross-training for running if you are injured, very sore or it is not safe to run.
- Add Pilates or yoga classes once or twice a week if you have time.
- Try to stretch every day for at least 10 mins.
- Always eat within 20–30 mins of finishing a run.
- Always train at your target pace, don't compromise or run too hard. Tiredness always catches up.

IMPROVER'S MARATHON TRAINING PLAN

WANT TO IMPROVE ON A PREVIOUS MARATHON TIME? PUT IN SOME QUALITY SESSIONS WITH THIS PLAN. . .

WEEK	MONDAY	TUESDAY	WEDNESDAY	THURSDAY	FRIDAY	SATURDAY	SUNDAY
1	Core conditioning class, yoga or Pilates	Recovery run 30 mins	Threshold run 2 x 10 mins' effort with 2-min recovery jog between efforts	30-min cross-train or 30-min recovery run + core conditioning	Rest	4 x 5 mins continuous hill reps. 2-min jog recovery	Long run, 90 mins, relaxed pace
2	Core conditioning class, yoga or Pilates	Recovery run 45 mins	5 x 5 mins at threshold off 2-min recovery jog	45-min rec run or cross-training + core conditioning	Rest	2 x 10 mins continuous hill reps. 2-min jog recovery	Long run, 105 mins
3	Core conditioning class, yoga or Pilates	Recovery run 30 mins	45 mins incl. 15 easy/15 steady/15 at threshold	45-min rec run or cross-train + core conditioning	Rest	4 x 6 mins continuous hill reps. 2-min jog recovery	Long run, 120 mins, all easy pace
4	Core conditioning class, yoga or Pilates	Recovery run 40 mins	8 x 3 mins off 2 mins recovery. Odd nos at threshold and even at 10km pace	45-min rec run or cross-train + core conditioning	Rest	5 x 5 mins at threshold on a hilly route off 2-min jog recovery Include hills naturally	120–35 mins relaxed
5	Core conditioning class, yoga or Pilates	Recovery run 30 mins	Rest Easy week	30 mins incl. 5 mins easy/5 mins threshold all x 3	Rest	4 x 6 mins at continuous hills off 90-sec recovery	Easy long run 60–75 mins + core conditioning
6	Core conditioning class, yoga or Pilates	60 mins including 3 x 10 mins at threshold off 2–3-min jog recovery	30-min recovery run	Intervals – 5 x 5 mins at 10km pace off 90-sec recovery	Rest	30–45-min recovery run or cross-train	135 mins with last 45 at marathon pace
7	Core conditioning class, yoga or Pilates	4 x 6 mins at continuous hills off 90-sec recovery	30–45-min recovery run or cross-train	10-min threshold + 4 x 3 mins at 10km pace + 10 mins threshold (all off 2 mins rec)	Rest	45 mins with 15 easy/15 steady/15 at threshold + core conditioning	150-min long run, all easy pace

WHY OVERTRAINING CAN BE A PROBLEM

Without proper recovery, your body cannot grow stronger. Worse than that, if you're training on fatigued muscles, you can do more harm than good and you will be at an increased risk of injury. Signs of overtraining can include:

- Choosing additional exercise sessions rather than observing rest days;
- Training more than once a day;
- Stealing time from sleep at the beginning or end of the day to squeeze in some extra training;
- Skipping social engagements to exercise;
- Scheduling extra training sessions and then not enjoying them.

WEEK	MONDAY	TUESDAY	WEDNESDAY	THURSDAY	FRIDAY	SATURDAY	SUNDAY
8	Core conditioning class, yoga or Pilates	45 mins recovery run	Threshold run, 5 x 6 mins, effort with 90-sec jog recovery	Recovery run 30 mins + core conditioning	Rest	45-min recovery run	90–105 with last 45 at marathon pace
9	Core conditioning class, yoga or Pilates	45 mins recovery run	6 x 3 mins. Odd nos at threshold and even at 10km pace. All off 90-sec recovery	30–45-min recovery run + easy core conditioning session	Rest	25–30-min recovery run	**HALF-MARATHON** at PB pace. Run at MP if still building fitness. Add 30 mins slow warm-down
10	Core conditioning class, yoga or Pilates	45 mins recovery run	45-min rec run or cross-train	45 mins incl. 4 x 6 mins at threshold off 2-min jog	Rest	45-min recovery run + core conditioning	165-min long run, last 45 mins at MP
11	Core conditioning class, yoga or Pilates	45 mins recovery run	45-min rec run or cross-train	15 mins MP + 5 x 3 mins at 10km pace + 15 mins MP (all off 2-min rec)	Rest	45-min recovery run + core conditioning	Long Run 180 mins last 60 mins at MP
12	Core conditioning class or Pilates	30 mins recovery run	45-min rec run and no hard session	75 mins incl. 3 x 10 mins at threshold	Rest	45-min recovery run + core conditioning	Long run 120 mins, last hour includes 3 x 15 at MP
13	Core conditioning class, yoga or Pilates	30 mins recovery run	45-min recovery run or cross-train.	90 mins with middle 60 at 3 mins threshold/3 mins steady continuous	Rest	5 x 5 mins at threshold off 90-sec rec	Long run 60 mins, easy pace + core conditioning
14	Rest	30 mins recovery Run + core conditioning	40 mins with 5 mins easy/5 mins at MP x 4	25-min rec run or cross-train	Rest	15-min jog	**MARATHON**

HOW TO PREVENT OVERTRAINING

- Establish how many rest days you need each week. Ensure you have two days off exercise each week. The balance is different for everyone and, with experience, you'll work out what suits you.
- Review your training schedule regularly and honestly. Assess how your progress is going and whether you'd benefit more from extra training or more recovery. Keep notes on what each session consists of, how motivated you were to do it and how much you enjoyed it.
- Have a week of rest or at least an easier week of training. You won't lose fitness during this period but it will give you an opportunity to assess objectively how things are going. It will also provide an opportunity for your body to recover fully and for your mind to rediscover your enthusiasm for training. By the end of the period, you'll be itching to get going again.
- If you begin your training with a realistic schedule and take the time to review your progress regularly, you'll be able to make small adjustments to your plan where necessary. This regular review will also help you maintain sight of your objective, which is not to pack as much training into every day as possible, but to complete the marathon in good time, without injury and with maximum enjoyment.

EXPERIENCED MARATHON TRAINING PLAN

SERIOUS ABOUT THAT PB AND HAVE AN EXCELLENT FITNESS BASE TO WORK WITH? THEN TRY THIS PLAN…

WEEK	MONDAY	TUESDAY	WEDNESDAY	THURSDAY	FRIDAY	SATURDAY	SUNDAY
1	30–45-min recovery run and core conditioning session	a.m., 30-min recovery run; p.m., threshold session: 5 x 5 mins with 60-sec jog recovery	45-min relaxed running or cross-training	60-min run – 20 mins easy pace, 20 mins steady pace and 20 mins at threshold	Rest	a.m., Kenyan Hills, 4 x 6 mins with 90-sec jog recovery; p.m., 30-min recovery run or cross-training	Long run, 90 mins, relaxed pace
2	30–45-min recovery run and core conditioning session	a.m., 30-min recovery run; p.m., threshold session: 6 x 5 mins with 60-sec jog recovery	45-min relaxed running or cross-training	60-min run – 20 mins easy pace, 20 mins steady pace and 20 mins at threshold	Rest	a.m., Kenyan Hills, 4 x 8 mins with 90-sec jog recovery; p.m., 30-min recovery run or cross-training	Long run, 105 mins, relaxed pace
3	30–45-min recovery run and core conditioning session	a.m., 30-min recovery run; p.m., threshold session: 3 x 10 mins with 2-min jog recovery	45-min relaxed running or cross-training	45-min rec run or cross-train + core conditioning	Rest	a.m., Kenyan Hills, 3 x 10 mins with 90-sec jog recovery; p.m., 30-min recovery run or cross-training	Long run, 120 mins, easy pace
4	30–45-min recovery run and core conditioning session	a.m., 30-min recovery run; p.m., 45-min run with last 25 mins at threshold	45-min relaxed running or cross-training	10 mins at threshold + 4 x 3 mins at 10km pace + 10 mins at threshold – all off 90-sec jog recovery	Rest	a.m., Kenyan Hills, 3 x 10 mins with 90-sec jog recovery; p.m., 30-min recovery run or cross-training	Long run, 135 mins, relaxed pace
5 Easy Wk	Rest	30-min easy-pace recovery run + core conditioning session	75 mins with last 30 at MP	30-min rec run	Rest	30–45-min easy-pace recovery run	**HALF-MARATHON** race – run at marathon pace and add 30 mins easy-pace run afterwards
6	30–45-min recovery run and core conditioning session	60 mins including 3 x 10 mins at threshold off 2–3-min jog rec	a.m. 30 mins easy-pace recovery run; p.m. 30-min steady pace	10 mins at threshold + 5, 4, 3, 2, 1 mins off 90-sec jog recovery	Rest	a.m., Kenyan Hills, 6 x 5 mins with 90-sec jog recovery; p.m., 30-rec run or cross-training	Long run, 120-135 mins easy pace
7	30–45-min recovery run and core conditioning session	a.m., 30-min rec run; p.m., 45-min easy-pace recovery run	10 x 3 mins: run odd nos at threshold and even nos at 10km pace with 90-sec recovery	60–75-min easy-pace recovery run or cross-training	Rest	a.m., Kenyan Hills, 4 x 10 mins with 90-sec jog recovery; p.m., 30-rec run or cross-training	Long run, 150 mins, easy pace.

WEEK	MONDAY	TUESDAY	WEDNESDAY	THURSDAY	FRIDAY	SATURDAY	SUNDAY
8	30–45-min recovery run and core conditioning session	a.m., 45-min rec run; p.m., 45-rec run	15 mins at MP + 5 x 3 mins at 10km pace + 15 mins MP, all off 90-sec rec	60–75-min easy run or cross-training	Rest	45-min easy-pace recovery run	Long run, 90 mins, with last 30 mins at half-marathon pace/threshold
9 Easy wk	Rest	a.m., 30-min rec run; p.m., 8 x 3 mins or 1km – 1, 3, 5, 7 at threshold; 2, 4, 6, 8 at 10km pace, all with 75-sec recovery	45-min recovery run	30 mins with 10 easy/10 steady/10 at threshold if racing hard on Sunday OR run 75 today with last 30 at MP if not	Rest	15–25-min very easy-pace jog	**HALF-MARATHON** Go for a PB! If not fit, then run the race at marathon pace + add 30–45 mins easy-pace run afterwards
10	30–45-min recovery run and core conditioning	a.m., 30–45-min recovery run	60–80-min easy-pace run	a.m., 30 cross-training or rec run/ p.m., 45-min run with 15 easy/15 steady/15 at threshold	Rest	6 x 5 mins at 10km pace with 1-min jog recovery	Long run 165 mins easy pace
11	30–45-min recovery run and core conditioning session	a.m., 45-min rec run; p.m., 30-min recovery run or cross-training	20 mins MP + 5 x 3 mins at 10km pace, off 90 secs jog + 20 mins MP	60-min easy-pace recovery run	Rest	180-min long run incl last 60 mins at marathon pace	30 min rec run
12	30–45-min recovery run and core conditioning session	a.m., 30-min rec run; p.m., 10-min run at threshold + 6 x 3 mins at 5km pace with 2-min jog recovery	45-min rec run or cross-training	30 mins with 10 easy/10 steady/10 threshold OR run 60–80 mins with last 45 at MP if not racing the 10km this weekend	Rest	30-min easy-pace recovery run	**10Km** – run for a new PB time if fit, otherwise long run, 120 mins, with last 60 mins at marathon pace
13	30–45-min recovery run and core conditioning session	30 mins recovery run	45-min easy-pace recovery run or cross-train	90-min run with middle 60 mins incl 3 mins at MP and 3 mins at threshold, alternating continuously	Rest	5 x 5 mins with 2-min jog rec reps 1, 3, 5 at 10km pace; reps 2, 4 at threshold	Long run, 60–75 mins, easy pace.
14	Rest	40-min easy-pace recovery run	40 mins incl. 4 x 5 mins steady/5 mins at threshold pace	30-min easy-pace recovery run	Rest	15–20-min easy-pace jog	**MARATHON DAY** **GOOD LUCK!**

MARATHON DAY CHECKLIST

If you are racing abroad, you'll need to plan ahead and make sure you take some key items with you. Otherwise, you may get caught short. The more you've prepared and planned, the smoother race day will be for you. You should already have your race-day kit bag packed. The following often make up the seasoned runner's checklist:

- Race number, chip and safety pins ▪ Spare laces
- Spare race socks ▪ Vaseline for chafing
- Hat ▪ Gloves ▪ Waterproof top and bottoms
- Bin liner x 2 ▪ Toilet paper ▪ iPod (or similar)
- Mobile phone ▪ Spare change ▪ Energy gels
- Pre-race snacks and drinks.

▽ Never be afraid to ask for help – running communities are some of the most positive and helpful out there.

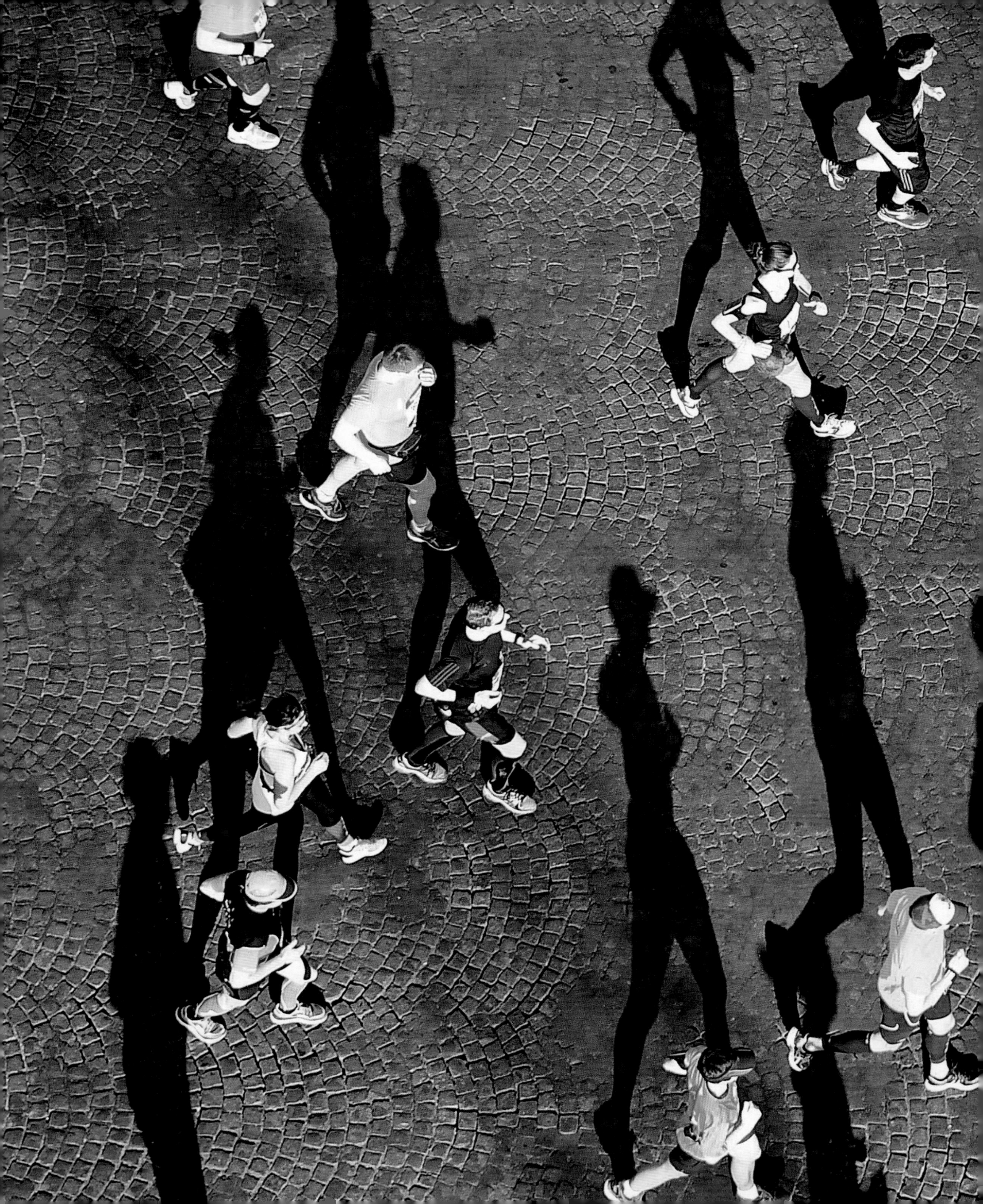

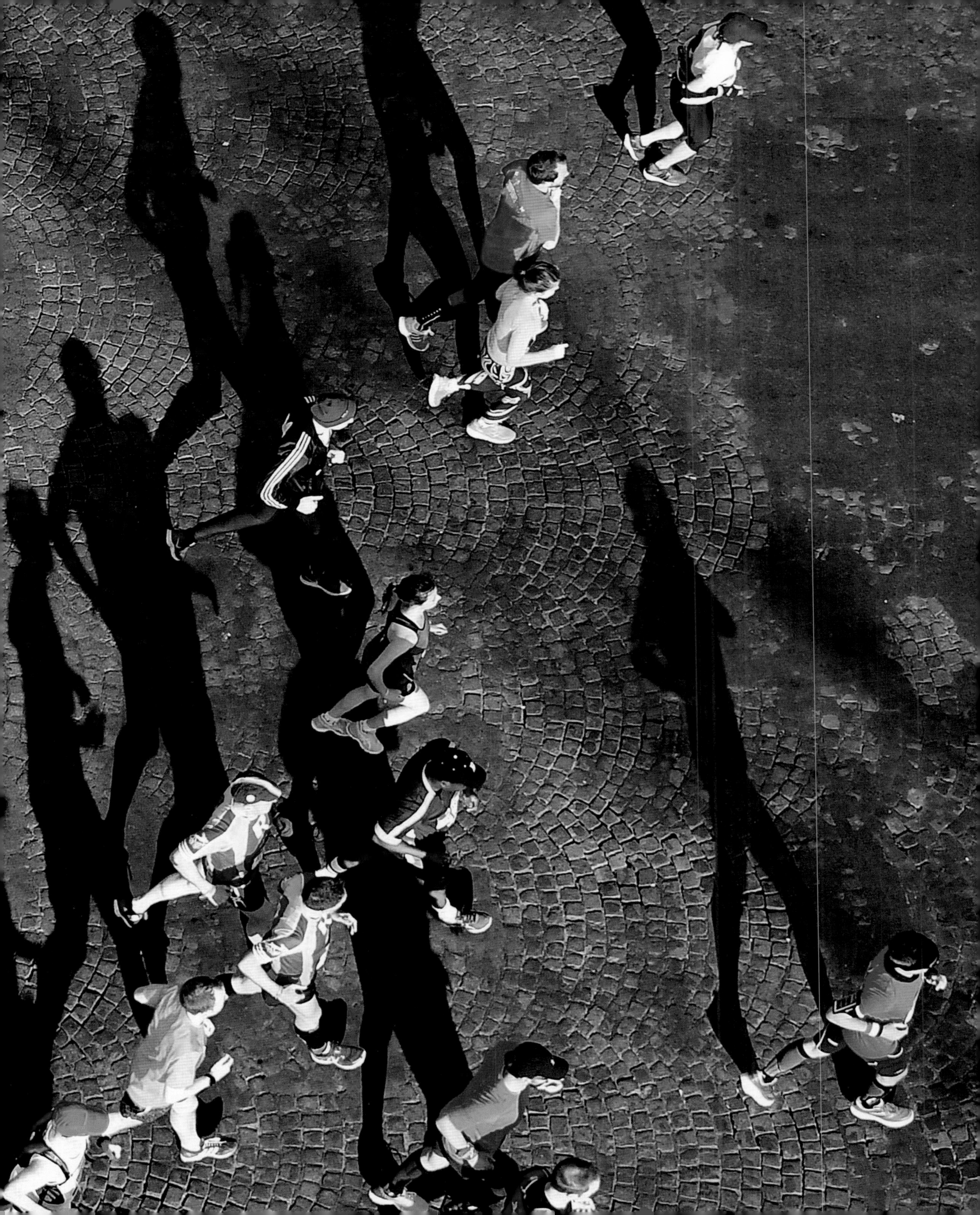

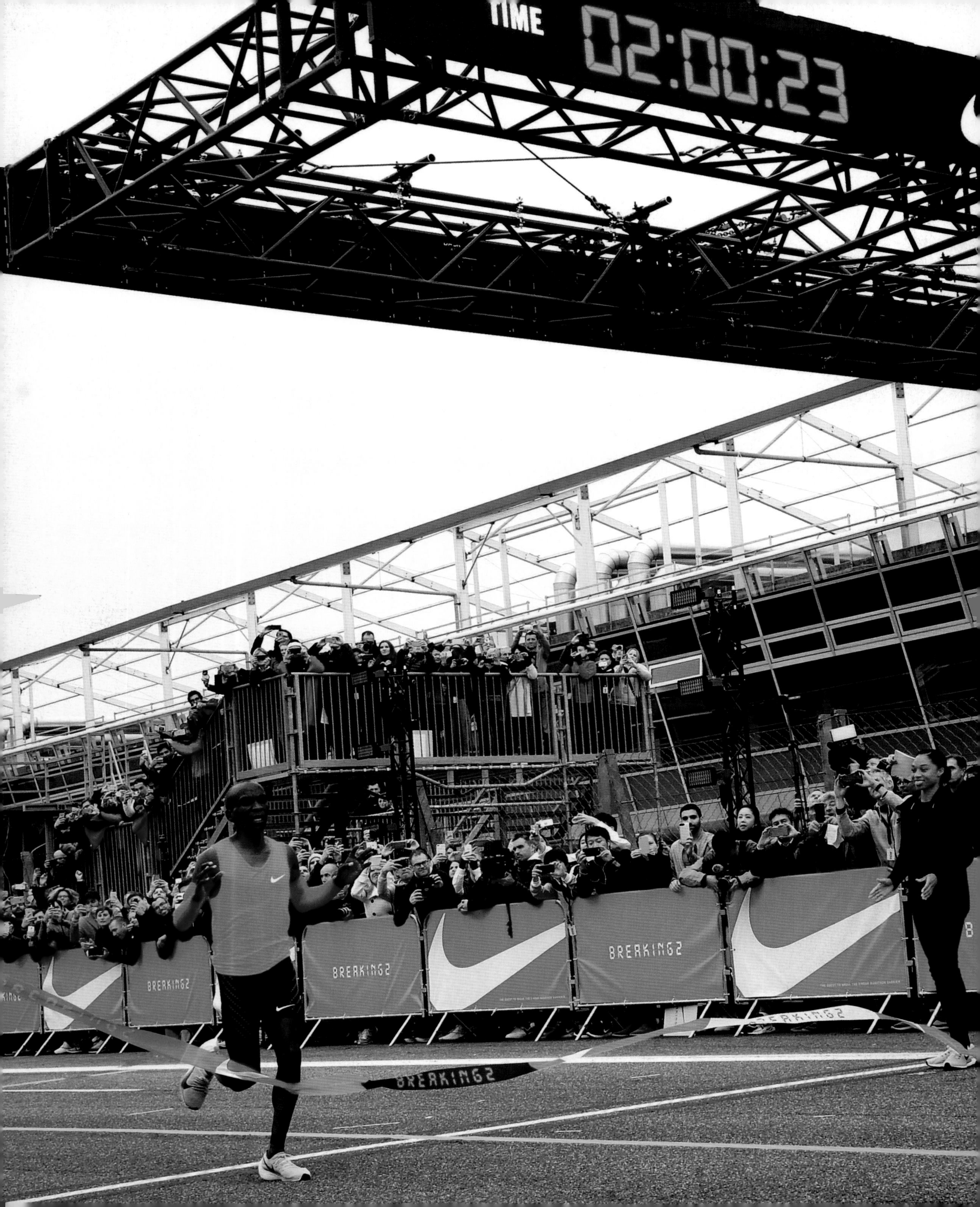
TIME
02:00:23
BREAKING2
BREAKING2
BREAKING2
BREAKING2

MARATHON RECORDS

PUSHING TO THE LIMIT

Amazing things can and do happen during marathons. It's not just the elite runners breaking world records: people of all ages, abilities and backgrounds have run marathons and, in the process, wowed spectators and accomplished extraordinary feats.

▶ Centurion Fauja Singh's marathon achievements are truly astounding.

▼ Paula Radcliffe's sensational world record has stood since 2003.

One of the best-known examples is Fauja Singh, who incredibly set a marathon personal best at the age of 92, or Steve Chalke, who has raised over £2.3 million for charity to date. And who could forget Paula Radcliffe, the British runner who broke her own world record in 2003 during the London Marathon?

Yes, running can help both ordinary people and elite athletes push themselves to the limits. Read on to discover some of the most amazing achievements in marathons and running . . .

FASTEST MARATHON:

PAULA RADCLIFFE, DENNIS KIPRUTO KIMETTO AND ELIUD KIPCHOGE

Paula Radcliffe completed the 2003 London Marathon in 2:15:25, beating her own record by almost two minutes in a race that included eight male pacemakers. Kenya's Dennis Kipruto Kimetto achieved the fastest male marathon time on 28 September 2014, when he ran the Berlin Marathon in 2:02:57. Interestingly, the Olympic champion Eliud Kipchoge has in fact run this distance more quickly on the Formula One racetrack in Monza, Italy, on 6 May 2017, but his time of 2:00:25 wasn't entered into the record books because he was helped by a team of 30 elite pacers who dipped in and out of the race, which is against the official rules of the International Association of Athletics Federations.

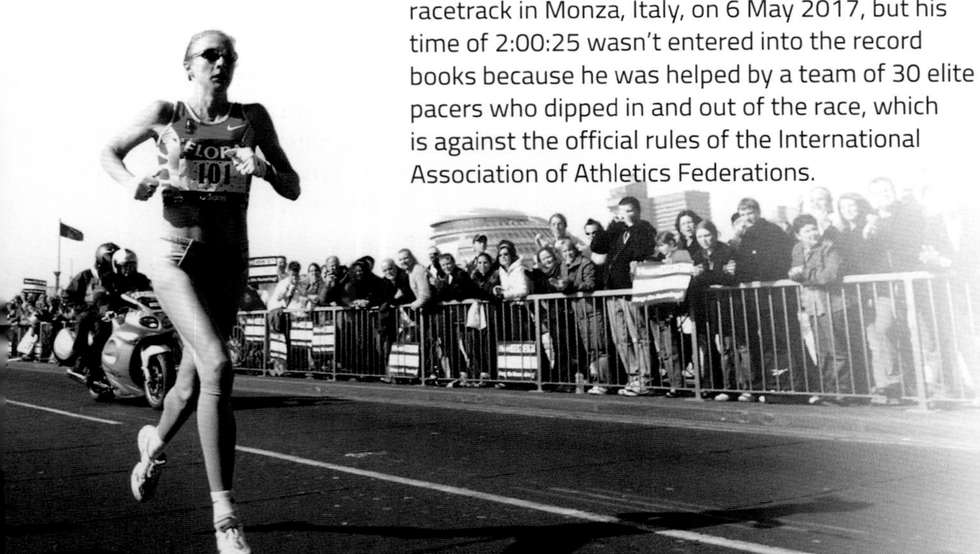

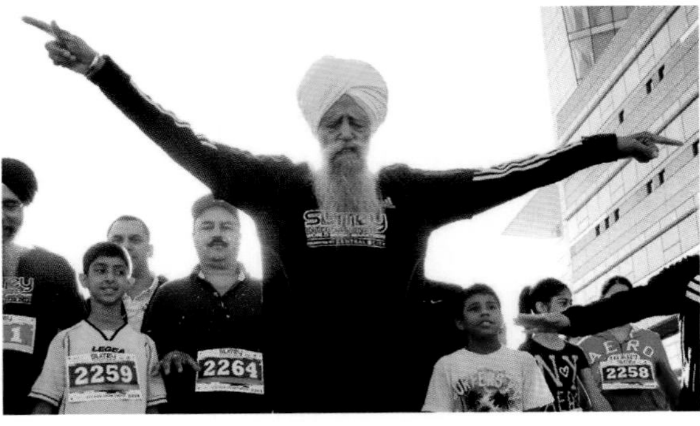

OLDEST MARATHON RUNNER:

FAUJA SINGH

Also known as the Turbaned Tornado, this Sikh runner is believed to be the world's oldest long-distance runner (his records remain unofficial because he's been unable to produce a birth certificate to prove his age). Punjab-born Fauja began marathon running at the ripe old age of 89, set a personal best of 5:40 at the age of 92, and became the face of Adidas in 2004. On 16 October 2011, he became the first 100-year-old to finish a marathon, completing the Toronto Waterfront Marathon in a gun time of 8:25:17.

FASTEST 1,000 MILES:

YIANNIS KOUROS AND SANDRA BARWICK

The legendary ultrarunner Yiannis Kouros (a.k.a. The Colossus of Roads) from Greece ran 1,000 miles (1,609km) in 10 days, 10 hours, 30 minutes, 36 seconds during the 1988 International Association of Ultrarunners (IAU) World Championship in New York City. Three years later, again in the Big Apple, New Zealand's Sandra Barwick ran the same distance (the equivalent of running from London to Seville) in 12 days, 14 hours, 38 minutes, 40 seconds during the Sri Chinmoy Ultimate Ultra.

MOST MONEY RAISED:

STEVE CHALKE

While many runners struggle to raise the required sponsorship minimum to get a guaranteed charity place in the London Marathon, Steve Chalke MBE seemed to have decided to "go large, or go home" in 2011. Through fundraising functions and events, press coverage and social media, this running reverend raised a staggering £2,330,159.38 for the Oasis Charitable Trust (a charity he founded with the original aim of opening a hostel for homeless young people), earning him an incredible third Guinness World Record for fundraising. His previous records? £1.25 million in 2005 and £1.85 million in 2007.

MOST MARATHONS RUN IN A YEAR:

RIK VERCOE

Despite having a day job as an operations director, dad-of-two Rik Vercoe, 47, from Walton-on-Thames, has made it his mission to pick up two Guinness World Records and a British record. In 2013, he ran 152 marathons and ultras, thereby setting the British record for the "Most marathons completed in 365 days". In doing so, he also set a world record for "The fastest aggregate time to complete 10 marathons in 10 days (male)", while running 16 marathons in Long Beach, California. Then, at the 2014 London Marathon, he set a new world record for the "Fastest marathon dressed as a cowboy" in a blistering time of 3:09:09, chopping a whopping 32 minutes off the previous record, a feat that left him, he admits, "walking like a cowboy for a week afterwards!"

▲ Rik Vercoe poses with just a few of the medals he's picked up over the years.

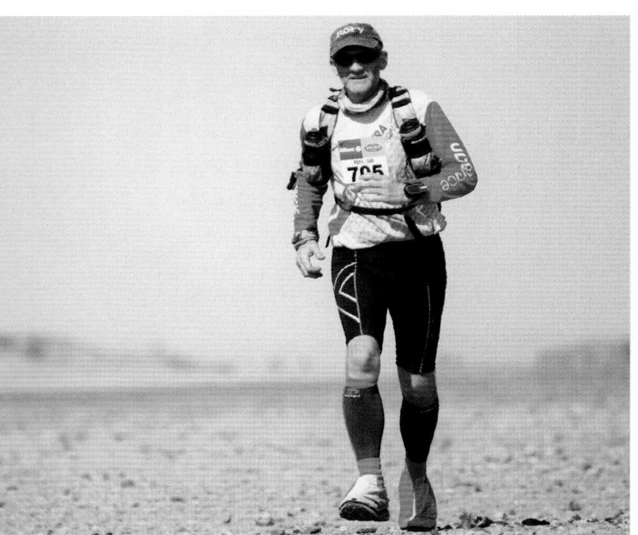

▼ Rory Coleman has completed the Marathon des Sables more than any Brit.

YOUNGEST PERSON TO COMPLETE 100 MARATHONS:

SOPHIE GOODWIN

Inspired by her marathon-mad mum, Carol, Sophie Goodwin, a 21-year-old masters student at the University of East Anglia in Norwich, became the youngest person to run 100 marathons, completed on 2 December 2017, aged 21 years and 152 days. "Achieving my record was an adventure in itself as I had to find so many marathons in such a short space of time – what turned out to be 31 months and eight days," says Sophie. "I did four marathons in four days at the Great Barrow Challenge, and then the next year did 10 marathons in 10 days in the same series."

NINE WORLD RECORDS:

RORY COLEMAN

Ultrarunner Rory Coleman has an astonishing nine Guinness World Records for running on treadmills (including doing 101.3 miles in 24 hours). Not only that, but he's completed the gruelling Marathon des Sables (dubbed "The World's Toughest Footrace") 14 times, more than any other British competitor. Despite being confined to a wheelchair in 2016 after being paralysed by Guillain-Barré Syndrome, Rory surpassed his 1,000 marathons goal in 2017. "On that very first run back in January 1994, my entire world changed," says Rory. "Being successful at something I love hasn't been hard, it's been incredibly liberating, enjoyable and a whole lot of fun."

RUNNING WHILE KNITTING OR CROCHETING:

SUSIE HEWER

After turning 50, Susie Hewer from East Sussex was determined not to act her age and stay at home with her knitting, as a friend had suggested. Instead, she decided to knit and run, and ended up setting a Guinness World Record at the 2007 London Marathon for "The longest scarf knitted while running a marathon". Not content with one record attempt, she began crocheting instead and, after setting a world record in 2010, went on to better that in 2014, when she crocheted a chain 139.42m long during the London Marathon.

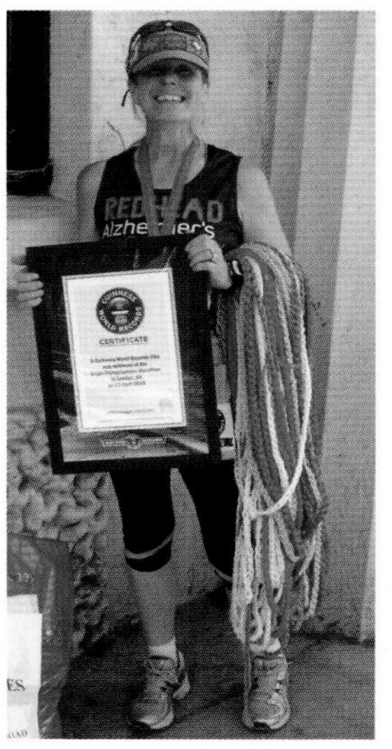

◀ Susie Hewer shows off her Guinness World Record – and her epic chain.

LONDON MARATHON RECORDS:
BIZARRE OUTFITS

The London Marathon not only attracts some of the world's most fleet-of-foot runners, it's also a magnet for the zaniest runners on the planet, many of whom are chasing rather bizarre Guinness World Records. Take British runner Susan Ridgeon, for example, who achieved a world record in 2017 in the "Fastest marathon dressed as a toilet roll (female)" category in a far-from-*loo*-dicrous time of 4:54.

Then there's John-Paul De Lacy, who, despite having to crawl through a couple of tunnels in a 7.04m-high giraffe costume made from papier-mâché and plastic tubing, bagged a world record in 2010 for "Tallest costume worn while running a marathon".

Another wacky record was set by the 22-person-strong Huddersfield University Marching Band in 2011, when they performed and marched round the marathon course in 7:55:00, thereby setting a world record for the "Fastest marathon by a marching band". Three years later, they did it again, smashing their record by almost an hour.

FASTEST MARATHON RUNNING BACKWARDS:
XU ZHENJUN

Many people regard running a marathon as a bucket-list challenge, aware that covering 26.2 miles on foot is no easy task. But, for one runner from China, this iconic distance was evidently not challenging enough, so Xu Zhenjun decided to run the 2004 Beijing Marathon backwards. His world-record-breaking time? An almost unbelievable 3:43:39!

FASTEST MILE:
HICHAM EL GUERROUJ AND SVETLANA MASTERKOVA

Completing a mile in under four minutes means running at a speed of over 15 m.p.h. and, in 1954, Sir Roger Bannister famously did just that at Oxford's Iffley Road track with his time of 3 minutes and 59.4 seconds. Although his record has been broken numerous times since, the male record of 3 minutes and 43.13 seconds, set by Morocco's Hicham El Guerrouj in Rome, has remained unbroken since 1999. The female record of 4 minutes and 12.56 seconds, achieved by Russia's Svetlana Masterkova, also dates from the 1990s, having been set in Zurich, Switzerland, on 14 August 1996.

BAREFOOT RUNNING:
ABEBE BIKILA AND EDDIE VEGA

Having trained barefoot in his native Ethiopia, Abebe Bikila famously shunned footwear to win gold at the 1960 Rome Olympic Games in a time of 2:15:16. Several decades later, thanks to Christopher McDougall's seminal book *Born to Run*, going barefoot took the running world by storm. One runner who took this trend to the max was Eddie "The Barefoot Bandito" Vega, from Raleigh in North Carolina. To maximize the amount of money he raised to provide shoes for underprivileged children, Eddie broke two Guinness World Records in 2014: "Most consecutive days to run an official marathon barefoot (male)" (he ran 10) and "Most barefoot marathons run in one year" (he ran 101). He's also done a marathon on all seven continents, six of them barefoot.

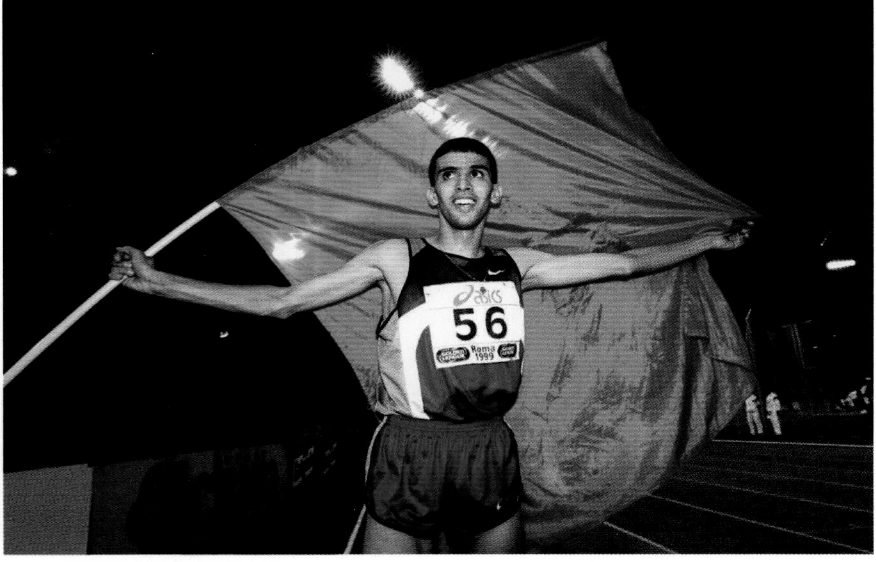

◀ Nobody has bettered Hicham El Guerrouj's sensational time for running a mile.

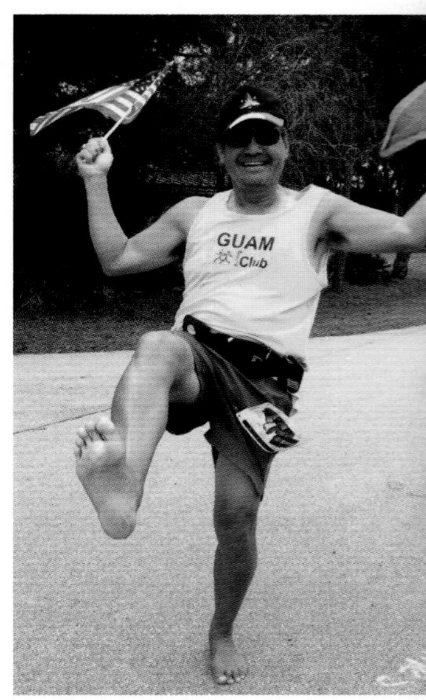

▶ Eddie Vega proudly shows off his trademark bare feet.

PARALYMPIC RECORDS:

RICHARD WHITEHEAD

British athlete Richard Whitehead set a world record in the T42 200m at the 2012 Summer Paralympics (and won gold again in Rio four years later, along with silver in the 100m). But his achievements don't end there: in 2013, he not only came 23rd in the London Marathon with a time of 3:15:53 but ran from John O'Groats to Land's End for charity.

THE FIRST WOMAN TO COME FIRST OVERALL IN THE BADWATER ULTRAMARATHON:

PAM REED

Not content with being the first woman to become the overall winner of the notorious Badwater Ultramarathon in 2002 (and in so doing set the women's course record), Pam went on to repeat this feat the following year and in total has completed this race 10 times, the only woman to do so. Also known as Satan's Fun Run, this 135-mile race in Death Valley, California, is run through one of the hottest deserts in the world in searing temperatures that can reach 55°C.

THE UK'S BIGGEST FUNDRAISER:

CANCER RESEARCH UK'S RACE FOR LIFE

Not only has Race for Life been instrumental in getting tens of thousands of nervous newbies to enter their first organized running event, but it's also notched up an incredibly impressive fundraising achievement of over £800 million. What's more, this race series has been the most successful mass-participation fundraising event in the UK for four years running.

NINE-TIMES COMRADES WINNER AND OVER-50-MILE RECORD HOLDER:

BRUCE FORDYCE

South African ultrarunner Bruce Fordyce is best known for having won the 89km Comrades Marathon in South Africa a record nine times, eight of which were consecutive. He also won the London 2 Brighton ultramarathon three years in a row: in the 1983 edition, he broke the world record for over 50 miles, a record that still stands. Now the CEO of Parkrun South Africa, he says, "I love Parkrun as much as I love Comrades, and that's saying something."

FASTEST MARATHON IN ORBIT (MALE):

TIM PEAKE

British astronaut Tim Peake had an out-of-this-world experience when setting his Guinness World Record: in the 3:35:21 it took him to finish the 2016 London Marathon, he'd also travelled more than twice around the earth. Although he wasn't the first man to run a marathon in orbit, the first person to do so was NASA astronaut Sunita Williams, who completed the 2007 Boston Marathon in 4:24 while aboard the International Space Station (ISS).

4-HOUR RUN WORLD RECORDS:

PATRYCJA BEREZNOWSKA AND YIANNIS KOUROS

Running as far as they could without stopping for a full 24 hours bagged Poland's Patrycja Bereznowska and Greece's Yiannis Kouros their world records of 258.339km (160.524 miles) and 303.506km (188.590 miles), respectively.

THE WORLD'S LONGEST CERTIFIED FOOTRACE:

THE SELF-TRANSCENDENCE 3,100 MILE RACES

Founded in 1996 by the Indian spiritual leader Sri Chinmoy, it has participants running around a single block in Queens, New York City, from 6 a.m. till midnight, when the course closes for the night. In order to complete the full 3,100 miles (4,989km) in the 52-day time limit, runners must average 59.6 miles per day. No wonder it's called the Mount Everest of Ultrarunning!

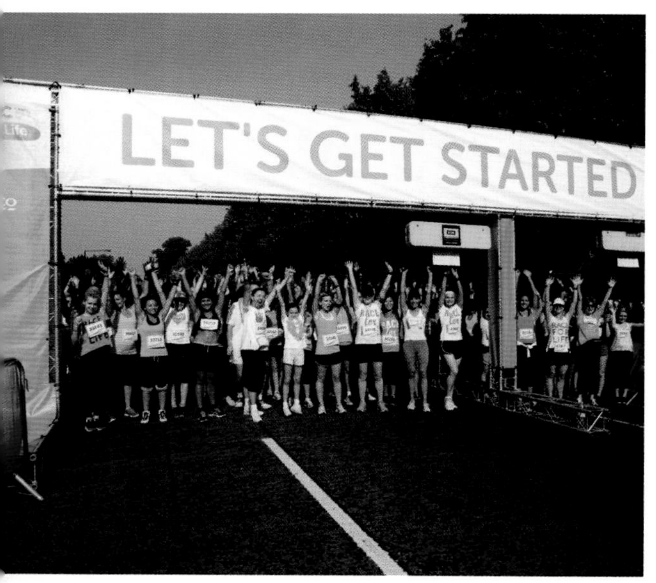

◀ Race for Life continues to raise millions for Cancer Research every year.

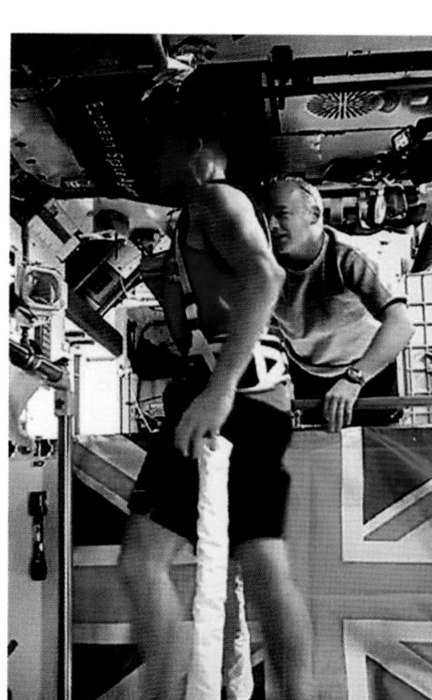

▶ Astronaut Tim Peake posted an excellent marathon time while orbiting the Earth.

INDEX

PICTURE CREDITS

The publishers would like to thank the following sources for their kind permission to reproduce the pictures in this book. T=top; B=bottom; L=left; R=right; C=centre; BK=background.

AMCM: /Yves Mainguy/De Tienda: 4(13), 125. **Action Challenge UK Ltd:** 167TR. **Alamy:** /James Boardman: 7; /CTK: 24TR; / Ashley Cooper: 141; /Mark Eite/Aflo Co. Ltd: 4(11), 78-79; / Philip Game: 36; /Sylvie Jarrossay: 69BR; /Nathan King: 68-69; /Craig Lovell/Eagle Visions Photography: 21TR; /Sandy Macys: 27BR; /PCN Photography: 73BR; /Marcin Rogozinski: 111; / Ingo Schulz/imageBROKER: 37L; /BJ Warnick/Newscom: 81, 107, 169BL. **Albatros Travel:** 23TR, 108, 110, 112, 113, 128. **The Authentic Athens Marathon:** 4(4); /Ioanna Fisilani: 20R; / Kris Tsatala: 20L. **Badwater.com:** /Ron Jones: 161B. **Bank of America Chicago Marathon:** 4(18), 46-47, 50T, 51TL, 53TL, 53BL. **Ryan Bethke:** 133, 134. **Beyond The Ultimate:** /Mikkel Beisner: 147BL, 151TL; /Ryan Lovejoy: 150; /Will Roberts: 151BL. **M. Bradford Photography:** 115BL, 115BR. **Susie Chan:** 4(10). **Dixons Carphone Race To The Stones:** 4(2), 144, 154, 155L, 155B. **Dublin Marathon:** /Ramsey Cardy/Sportsfile: 4(9) **Everest Marathon:** 116. **Fineman PR:** 26TR. **GSi Events Ltd:** / Paul J Roberts/Roberts Sports Photo: 4(12).
Getty Images: /Todd Anderson/Disney Parks: 138; /Drew Angerer: 72-73; /The Asahi Shimbun: 174; /Austrian Archives/ Imagno: 40; /Erbil Basay/Anadolu Agency: 37TL; Bettmann: 14T, 16T; /Bildquelle/ullstein bild: 30-31; /Andrew Burton: 77TL; / Jean-Pierre Clatot/AFP: 158; /Thomas Coex/AFP: 118; /Paul J Connell/The Boston Globe: 16B, 43TL; /Charlie Crowhurst: 67B; /Stephane de Sakutin/AFP: 135; /Matej Divizna: 18; /ESA/ NASA: 189BR; /Harry Engels: 62-63; /FPG: 49; /Eric Faferberg/ AFP: 90-91; /Baptiste Fernandez/Icon Sport: 84-85; /Franck Fife/AFP: 86, 182-183; /Stu Forster: 188BL; /Volkan Furuncu/ Anadolu Agency: 175R; /Ivo Gonzalez: 25L; /Henry Guttmann: 12-13; /Mark Hannaford: 166BL; /Ashraf Hendricks/Anadolu Agency: 168; /Hulton Archive: 8, 11; /Rajesh Jantilal/AFP: 148, 149; /Fred Kaplan/Sports Illustrated: 43TR; /Michael Kappeler/ AFP: 34; /Joe Kennedy/Los Angeles Times: 17; /Jean-Philippe Ksiazek/AFP: 2-3BK, 142, 146, 152, 153; /Matthew J Lee/ The Boston Globe: 45TR; /John MacDougall/AFP: 28; /Preston Mack/Disney Parks: 139BR; /Bob Martin: 33; /Adrian Murrell: 66TL; /Kazuhiro Nogi/AFP: 102, 104TL; /Jason O'Brien: 22; / Jeff Pachoud/AFP: 159; /Aydin Palabiyikoglu/Anadolu Agency: 26R; /Tom Pennington: 54-55, 58, 61L; /Günter Peters/ullstein bild: 32; /Daniel Petty/The Denver Post: 166BR; /Alberto Pizzoli/AFP: 92-93; /Popperfoto: 64; /Chris J Ratcliffe/AFP: 65; /Michael Reaves: 70-71; /Jessica Rinaldi/The Boston Globe: 42B; /Quinn Rooney: 173; /Andreas Solaro/AFP: 97; /Michael Steele: 186BL; /Boris Streubel/Bongarts: 35; /Pier Marco Tacca: 184; /Bob Thomas: 66TR; /John Tlumacki/The Boston Globe: 45TL; /Alex Trautwig: 41; /Yoshikazu Tsuno/AFP: 106; / Universal Images Group: 10; /Craig F Walker/The Boston Globe: 42TR; /Jared Wickerham: 38-39, 44; /Stuart C Wilson: 68BL; / John Zich/AFP: 51TR. **Golazo:** /Luka de Kruijf: 25R; /Pim Ras: 4(5). **Courtesy of Grand To Grand Ultra:** 145, 162BL, 163. **Green Events:** 123; /James Carnegie Photography/Whole Earth: 4(1). **The Grounded Events Company Ltd:** 4(6), 21B. **Guinness World Records:** 187L. **Hardrock Hundred:** 164. **Mike Hewer:** 187B. **Honolulu Marathon:** 4(17), 56, 59, 61BR; /Gregory Yamamoto Photography LLC: 60; /Ronen Zilberman: 58BR. **Iditarod Trail Invitational:** 165. **Junglemoon Images:** /Mark Gillett: 187BL. **James Kirby:** 4(8), 122, 140. **Loch Ness Marathon:** /Tim Winterburn: 4(14), 23BR. **Eddie MacDonald:** 6. **Marine Corps Marathon:** /Lance Cpl. Cristian L. Ricardo: 24B. **Courtesy of Mauna To Mauna Ultra:** 167B. **Midnight Sun Marathon:** /Tone Mette Yttergaard: 126. **Donald Miralle:** 132. **Cheryl Murdock:** 188BR. **Martin Paldan:** 147TL. **Pikes Peak Marathon Inc:** 129. **Public Domain:** 14B, 15. **Anna Rachel Photography:** 4(3). **Reggae Marathon:** /Karen Fuchs: 131. **Runcomm Global Ltd:** 26BL. **Saxons, Vikings and Normans:** 114BL; /Phil Batchelor: 4(15), 114BR. **Shutterstock:** /Aflo/REX: 103; /Alex Brandon/ AP/REX: 75; /J Henning Buchholz: 105; /Marianne Campolongo: 76; /Canadian Press/REX: 186R; /Angelo Carconi/Ansa/ REX: 175BL; /Stephen J Carrera/AP/REX: 52TL; /Ky Cho: 83; / Dennis Diatel: 119; /EPA/REX: 117; /EvrenKalinbacak: 23R; / f11photo: 170; /GSPhotography: 139TR; /Guillaume Louyot Onickz Artworks: 88, 89; /Max Herman: 48; /Kametaro: 100-101; /A Katz: 77BR; /Mike King/REX: 160; /Warren King: 67TL; /London News Pictures/REX: 127; /Tannen Maury/EPA/REX; /Andrew Medichini/AP/REX: 94; /Anna Muklinova: 3TR; / Fernanda Paradizo: 50R; /Thomas Persson: 95; /Philip Pilosian: 121; /James Pintar: 169BR; /Polifoto: 98-99; /REX: 74; /Franck Robichon/EPA/REX: 104BL; /RossHelen: 3TL; /Marco Rubino: 2TC; /Sergieiev: 172; /Geoffrey Swaine/REX: 130; /Tony4urban: 124; /Tupungato: 3TC; /ymgerman: 82; /Mohamed Zaid/REX: 161TL. **The Space Coast Marathon and Half Marathon:** 4(20), 136BL, 136BR, 137. **Matthew Stear:** 4(16). **Rebekah Taylor:** 189BL. **Transylvania Marathon:** 156R, 156BR, 157. **Unsplash:** /Henry Be: 2TR; /Liam Burnett Blue: 2TL. **Warsaw Marathon:** / Sportografica: 4(7), 27R. **Courtesy of Wild Frontiers (Pty) Ltd:** / Rachel Ambrose: 4(19), 120.

Every effort has been made to acknowledge correctly and contact the source and/or copyright holder of each picture and Carlton Books Limited apologises for any unintentional errors or omissions that will be corrected in future editions of this book.